"It all began with an improbable wager: ask 35 scholars to each write something intelligible about every single paragraph in one of the texts included in Jacques Lacan's *magnum opus*, *Écrits*, so as to generate a commentary on the entire 800-page volume. And yet, after years of preparation, the wager has paid off: we have here useful and at times brilliant examples of textual explication! Cryptic formulations are lucidly unpacked, and mysterious references are provided, giving the serious reader myriad keys to fascinating texts."

– **Bruce Fink**, translator of *Écrits: The First Complete Edition in English*

"Let's face it: Lacan's *Écrits*, one of the classical texts of modern thought are unreadable – they remain impenetrable if we just pick the thick volume up and start to read it. Vanheule, Hook and Neill provide what we were all waiting for: a detailed commentary which does not aim to replace reading *Écrits* but to render it possible. The three volumes do wonder, their effect is no less than magic: when, after getting stuck at a particularly dense page of *Écrits*, we turn to the corresponding pages in the commentary and then return to the page of *Écrits* which pushed us to madness, the same lines appear in all the clarity of their line of thought. It is thus a safe prediction that Vanheule, Hook and Neill's commentary will become a kind of permanent companion of the English translation of *Écrits*, indispensable for everyone who wants to find her or his way in its complex texture."

– **Slavoj Žižek**

"Lacan's teaching is notoriously hard to access and comprehend. But this is done on purpose: understanding the psyche, the subject and its interaction with socio-political reality cannot be a piecemeal operation. One needs to take into account the paradoxical and often counterintuitive effects of unconscious mechanisms, and of the extimate operation of the real within and beyond the symbolic and the imaginary. Coupling exegesis with multi-level interpretations, the numerous texts in this volume advance a commentary, both informative and suggestive, that will immensely help readers navigate the archipelago of the Lacanian *Écrits*, without reducing in the least their complexity and inspirational value, without sacrificing their ability to surprise, provoke and jolt us out of our complacency."

– **Yannis Stavrakakis**, Aristotle University of Thessaloniki

"These essays will be an invaluable resource not only for those approaching the *Écrits* for the first time but also for seasoned readers. Broad in scope yet following the detail of the text, they help guide us through Lacan's difficult prose, elucidating, contextualising and clarifying, and reminding us time and time again of the precision, power and originality of his rethinking of psychoanalysis."

– **Darian Leader**

READING LACAN'S ÉCRITS: FROM 'SIGNIFICATION OF THE PHALLUS' TO 'METAPHOR OF THE SUBJECT'

The *Écrits* was Jacques Lacan's single most important text, a landmark in psychoanalysis which epitomized his aim of returning to Freud via structural linguistics, philosophy and literature. *Reading Lacan's Écrits* is the first extensive set of commentaries on the complete edition of Lacan's *Écrits* to be published in English.

An invaluable document in the history of psychoanalysis, and one of the most challenging intellectual works of the twentieth century, Lacan's *Écrits* still today begs the interpretative engagement of clinicians, scholars, philosophers and cultural theorists. The three volumes of *Reading Lacan's Écrits* offer just this: a series of systematic paragraph-by-paragraph commentaries – by some of the world's most renowned Lacanian analysts and scholars – on the complete edition of the *Écrits*, inclusive of lesser known articles such as 'Kant with Sade', 'The Youth of Gide', 'Science and Truth', 'Presentation on Transference' and 'Beyond the "Reality Principle"'.

The originality and importance of Lacan's *Écrits* to psychoanalysis and intellectual history is matched only by the text's notorious inaccessibility. *Reading Lacan's Écrits* is an indispensable companion piece and reference-text for clinicians and scholars exploring Lacan's *magnum opus*. Not only does it contextualize, explain and interrogate Lacan's arguments, it provides multiple interpretative routes through this most labyrinthine of texts.

Reading Lacan's Écrits provides an incisive and accessible companion for psychoanalysts and psychoanalytic psychotherapists in training and in practice, as well as philosophers, cultural theorists and literary, social science and humanities researchers who wish to draw upon Lacan's pivotal work.

Stijn Vanheule is a psychoanalyst and Professor of Psychoanalysis and Clinical Psychology at Ghent University, Belgium. He is also a privately practicing psychoanalyst and a member of the New Lacanian School for

Psychoanalysis. He is the author of *The Subject of Psychosis: A Lacanian Perspective* and *Psychiatric Diagnosis Revisited – From DSM to Clinical Case Formulation.*

Derek Hook is Associate Professor of Psychology at Duquesne University in Pittsburgh and Professor of Psychology at the University of Pretoria. A former lecturer at the London School of Economics and at Birkbeck College, he is a psychoanalytic practitioner, and the author of *Six Moments in Lacan.*

Calum Neill is Associate Professor of Psychoanalysis and Cultural Theory at Edinburgh Napier University. He is the author of *Without Ground: Lacanian Ethics and the Assumption of Subjectivity*, *Ethics and Psychology: Beyond Codes of Practice* and *Jacques Lacan: The Basics*.

READING LACAN'S ÉCRITS: FROM 'SIGNIFICATION OF THE PHALLUS' TO 'METAPHOR OF THE SUBJECT'

Edited by Stijn Vanheule, Derek Hook and Calum Neill

Routledge
Taylor & Francis Group
LONDON AND NEW YORK

First published 2019
by Routledge
2 Park Square, Milton Park, Abingdon, Oxon OX14 4RN

and by Routledge
711 Third Avenue, New York, NY 10017

Routledge is an imprint of the Taylor & Francis Group, an informa business

British Library Cataloguing in Publication Data
A catalogue record for this book is available from the British Library

Library of Congress Cataloging in Publication Data
Names: Vanheule, Stijn, 1974– editor. | Hook, Derek, editor. | Neill, Calum, 1968– editor.
Title: Reading Lacan's Ecrits: from "Signification of the phallus" to "Metaphor of the subject"/ edited by Stijn Vanheule, Derek Hook and Calum Neill.
Description: Abingdon, Oxon; New York, NY: Routledge, 2019. |
Includes bibliographical references and index.
Identifiers: LCCN 2018014841 (print) | LCCN 2018018178 (ebook) |
ISBN 9780429459221 (Master) | ISBN 9780429860072 (Web PDF) |
ISBN 9780429860065 (ePub) | ISBN 9780429860058 (Mobipocket/Kindle) |
ISBN 9780415708012 (hardback: alk. paper) | ISBN 9780415708029 (pbk.: alk. paper)
Subjects: LCSH: Lacan, Jacques, 1901–1981. Ecrits. | Psychoanalysis.
Classification: LCC BF173.L1423 (ebook) |
LCC BF173.L1423 R43 2019 (print) | DDC 150.19/5–dc23
LC record available at https://lccn.loc.gov/2018014841

ISBN: 978-0-415-70801-2 (hbk)
ISBN: 978-0-415-70802-9 (pbk)
ISBN: 978-0-429-45922-1 (ebk)

Typeset in Times New Roman
by Out of House Publishing

FOR ATTICUS, DYLAN AND ELLIOTT.

CONTENTS

FIGURES

CONTRIBUTORS

Filip Geerardyn is Professor of Applied Psychoanalysis at Ghent University and Psychoanalyst. He is the author of several papers and books on psychoanalysis and applied psychoanalysis, and the Editor in Chief of the journal *Psychoanalytische Perspectieven.*

Yael Goldman Baldwin is Professor of Psychology and Chair of the Social Sciences at Mars Hill University in North Carolina, USA. She is the author of *Let's Keep Talking: Lacanian Tales of Love, Sex, and Other Catastrophes* and co-editor of *Lacan and Addictions: An Anthology*, in addition to various chapters and articles on Lacan.

Todd McGowan teaches theory and film at the University of Vermont. He is the author of *Only a Joke Can Save Us: A Theory of Comedy*, *Capitalism and Desire: The Psychic Cost of Free Markets*, *Enjoying What We Don't Have*, and other works.

Dany Nobus is Professor of Psychoanalytic Psychology at Brunel University London, and the Chair of the Freud Museum London. He is the author, most recently, of *The Law of Desire: On Lacan's 'Kant with Sade'*, and he has published numerous books and papers on the history, theory and practice of psychoanalysis.

Ed Pluth is Professor and Chair of the Philosophy Department at California State University, Chico. He is the author of *Signifiers and Acts*, *Alain Badiou*, and co-editor, with Jan De Vos, of *Neuroscience and Critique*.

Alain Pringels is a psychotherapist and creative therapist with a special interest in art and sublimation. He has published on psychoanalysis and art. He is the Director and founder of a Belgian theatre company: Compagnie couRage, and wrote, translated and adapted several plays (Shakespeare, Brecht, Tsjechow, Pasolini, Euripides, Boelgakov, Kafka).

Jean-Michel Rabaté is Professor of English and Comparative Literature at the University of Pennsylvania, co-founder and curator of Slought

Foundation, co-editor of the *Journal of Modern Literature*, a Fellow of the American Academy of Arts and Sciences, and has authored or edited forty books; they include *The Pathos of Distance*, *Think, Pig!*, *Les Guerres de Jacques Derrida*, *Rust* and *Kafka L.O.L.*

Theo Reeves-Evison is Senior Lecturer in Theoretical and Contextual Studies at Birmingham School of Art. He is the editor, together with Jon K. Shaw of *Fiction as Method*, and has published recent articles on art and cultural theory in journals such as *Paragrana*, *Parallax* and *Third Text*. His monograph *In The Shadow of Transgression* is to be published in 2018.

Stephanie Swales is Assistant Professor of Psychology at the University of Dallas and has a private psychoanalytic practice in Dallas, Texas. Her forthcoming book, co-authored with Carol Owens, on a Lacanian approach to ambivalence in the clinic and in contemporary times, will be published in early 2019. She has also written the book *Perversion: A Lacanian Psychoanalytic Approach to the Subject* and numerous shorter works in the area of Lacanian psychoanalysis.

Paul Verhaeghe is Senior Professor of Psychoanalysis at Ghent University. He has published nine books (seven are translated in English) and more than two hundred papers. His most recent books bring a critique on contemporary psychotherapy and on the link between contemporary society and the new disorders. Personal website with downloads: www.paulverhaeghe.com/index.html

Fabio Vighi is Professor of Critical Theory at Cardiff University, UK. His recent publications include *Crisi di valore: Marx, Lacan e il crepuscolo della società del lavoro* and *Critical Theory and the Crisis of Contemporary Capitalism*. His current research tackles capitalist crisis from a psychoanalytic perspective, focusing on Jacques Lacan's notion of discourse. He is also interested in Hegelian dialectics as a mode of thinking crisis; film as a prominent form of dialectical thinking; and ideology critique as a way to address unconscious attachments.

Eve Watson has a psychoanalytic practice in Dublin, Ireland, where she also lectures on university programs in psychoanalysis and teacher education. Her recent book is *Clinical Encounters in Sexuality: Psychoanalytic Practice and Queer Theory*, co-edited with Noreen Giffney. She is the editor of *Lacunae*, the *APPI International Journal for Lacanian Psychoanalysis*, and is a registered practitioner member of the Association for Psychoanalysis and Psychotherapy in Ireland (APPI).

ACKNOWLEDGEMENTS

Editing three volumes on the *Écrits* was a challenge, which above all made clear that by translating Lacan's single most important and intimidating text, Bruce Fink had already made a tremendous first effort. His translation of the *Écrits* and generous support of our project were most helpful. This is one of three volumes of commentary on Jacques Lacan's *Écrits*. The other two volumes are titled *Reading Lacan's Écrits: From 'Overture' to 'Variations on the Standard Treatment'* (edited by Calum Neill, Stijn Vanheule & Derek Hook) and *Reading Lacan's Écrits: From 'On a Purpose' to 'Remarks on Daniel Lagache's Presentation'* (edited by Derek Hook, Calum Neill & Stijn Vanheule).

We are also grateful that the publisher W. W. Norton & Company gave their permission to reprint the original figures from the *Écrits*, and thank the Department of Psychoanalysis and Clinical Consulting at Ghent University for the financial support and acquiring this permission. We are likewise grateful to the various institutions that have supported our work on this project over the last five years, including the Department of Psychology at Duquesne University in Pittsburgh, the Department of Psychosocial Studies at Birkbeck College, London, and Edinburgh-Napier University.

Last, but not least we want to thank all authors and reviewers. Without our authors' dedication these Volumes simply could not have been realized. Each chapter implied hard study and a continuous search for clear expression, which was achieved. Each chapter has been reviewed by at least two peers. Many thanks to those who engaged in this meticulous task.

JACQUES LACAN'S SEMINARS

Throughout this book the following abbreviations are used when referring to Lacan's seminars:

S1: Seminar 1 (1953–1954): Lacan, J. (1975/1988) *The Seminar. Book I: Freud's Papers on Technique*, trans. J. Forrester, ed. J.-A. Miller, Cambridge: Cambridge University Press.

S2: Seminar 2 (1954–1955): Lacan, J. (1978/1988) *The Seminar. Book II: The Ego in Freud's Theory and in the Technique of Psychoanalysis*, trans. S. Tomaselli, ed. J.-A. Miller, Cambridge: Cambridge University Press.

S3: Seminar 3 (1955–1956): Lacan, J. (1981/1993) *The Seminar. Book III: The Psychoses*, trans. R. Grigg, ed. J.-A. Miller, New York: W. W. Norton & Company.

S4: Seminar 4 (1956–1957): Lacan, J. (1994) *Le Séminaire. Livre IV: La relation d'objet*, texte établi par J.-A. Miller, Paris: Éditions du Seuil.

S5: Seminar 5 (1957–1958): Lacan, J. (1998) *Le Séminaire. Livre V: Les formations de l'inconscient*, texte établi par J.-A. Miller, Paris: Éditions du Seuil.

S6: Seminar 6 (1958–1959): Lacan J. (2013) *Le Séminaire. Livre VI. Le désir et son interprétation*, texte établi par J.-A. Miller, Paris: Éditions de la Martinière.

S7: Seminar 7 (1959–1960): Lacan, J. (1986/1992) *The Seminar. Book VII: The Ethics of Psychoanalysis*, trans. D. Porter, ed. J.-A. Miller, New York/London: W. W. Norton & Company.

S8: Seminar 8 (1960–1961): Lacan, J. (2001/2015) *The Seminar. Book VIII: Transference*, trans. B. Fink, ed. J.-A. Miller, Cambridge: Polity.

S9: Seminar 9 (1961–1962): *Le Séminaire IX, L'Identification*, unpublished.

S10: Seminar 10 (1962–1963): Lacan, J. (2004/2014) *The Seminar. Book X: Anxiety*, trans. A. R. Price, ed. J.-A. Miller, Cambridge: Polity.

S11: Seminar 11 (1964): Lacan, J. (1973/1994) *The Seminar. Book XI: The Four Fundamental Concepts of Psycho-Analysis*, trans. A. Sheridan, ed. J.-A. Miller, New York/London: W. W. Norton & Company.

S12: Seminar 12 (1964–1965): *Le Séminaire XII, Problèmes cruciaux pour la psychanalyse*, unpublished.

S13: Seminar 13 (1965–1966): *Le Séminaire XIII, L'objet de la psychanalyse*, unpublished.

S14: Seminar 14 (1966–1967): *Le Séminaire XIV, La logique du fantasme*, unpublished.

S15: Seminar 15 (1967–1968): *Le Séminaire XV, l'acte psychanalytique*, unpublished.

S16: Seminar 16 (1968–1969): Lacan, J. (2006) *Le séminaire de Jacques Lacan, Livre XVI: D'un Autre à l'autre*, texte établi par J.-A. Miller, Paris: Éditions du Seuil.

S17: Seminar 17 (1969–1970): Lacan, J. (1991/2007) *The Seminar. Book XVII: The Other Side of Psychoanalysis*, trans. R. Grigg, ed. J.-A. Miller, New York/London: W. W. Norton & Company.

S18: Seminar 18 (1970–1971): Lacan J. (2006) *Le Séminaire. Livre XVIII. D'un discours qui ne serait pas du semblant*, Paris: Éditions du Seuil.

S19: Seminar 19 (1971–1972): Lacan, J. (2011) *Le Séminaire. Livre XIX: … ou pire*, texte établi par J.-A. Miller, Paris: Éditions du Seuil.

S20: Seminar 20 (1972–1973): Lacan, J. (1998) *The Seminar, Book XX, Encore: On Feminine Sexuality, the Limits of Love and Knowledge*, trans. B. Fink, ed. J.-A. Miller, New York/London: W. W. Norton & Company.

S21: Seminar 21 (1973–1974): *Le Séminaire XXI, Les non-dupes errent*, unpublished.

S22: Seminar 22 (1974–1975): *Le Séminaire XXII, R.S.I.*, unpublished.

S23: Seminar 23 (1975–1976): Lacan, J. (2005/2016) *The Seminar. Book XXIII: The Sinthome*, trans. A. R. Price, ed. J.-A. Miller, Cambridge: Polity.

S24: Seminar 24 (1976–1977): *Le Séminaire XXIV, L'insu que sait de l'une-bévue s'aile à mourre*, unpublished.

S25: Seminar 25 (1977–1978): *Le Séminaire XXV, Le moment de conclure*, unpublished.

S26: Seminar 26 (1978–1979): *Le Séminaire XXVI, La topologie et le temps*, unpublished.

INTRODUCTION TO 'READING THE ÉCRITS': *LA TRAHISON DE L'ÉCRITURE*

Derek Hook, Calum Neill and Stijn Vanheule

What kind of book is Lacan's *Écrits*? This is a more pressing question than it may appear. Knowing what type of book the *Écrits* is would provide us with a strategy for how one might go about reading – if 'reading' is even the most appropriate imperative in this context – this baroque, intimidating, ever-elusive text.

An unwieldy, conglomerate 'urtext', the *Écrits* might appear to have no clear precedent. There is, so it would seem, no collection of writings quite like it. For Élisabeth Roudinesco (2014), however, certain other equivalents can be cited:

> *Écrits* is a summa that resembles both Saussure's *Course in General Linguistics* and Hegel's *Phenomenology of Spirit*…it functions as the founding Book of an intellectual system, which, depending on the era can be read, criticized, glossed or interpreted in many ways.
>
> (p. 99)

While there is certainly truth to this characterization, there are nonetheless a series of qualifications that should be made here in respect of Lacan's relation both to his own *Écrits* and to writing more generally.

In comparison to Freud's oeuvre that of course exists in the collected form of the *Standard Edition*, Lacan's written work exists in a far more scattered and diffuse state. Formally, this work occupies a place in the interstices between the performative and the textual, between an oral teaching and the written word. Lacan's oeuvre, we might say, resists collection, encapsulation, just as it appears to resist writing itself.

One initial response to the above question would simply be to say that *Écrits* is not a 'book' at all, at least not in the sense of being something an author produces with the express wish of being published, understood, or even read. If we are to follow Roudinesco's (2014) account, it appears that François Wahl – former analysand of Lacan's and editor at Éditions du Seuil – played a more important role in motivating and conceiving the text than Lacan did himself. Prior to the eventual 15 November 1966 publication date of the *Écrits*, Lacan's writings were in a fragmentary state, appearing in select psychoanalytic journals that few could access. And as Roudinesco intimates, Lacan preferred it that way: "Lacan feared plagiarism … he allowed the written trace of his spoken word to appear solely so as to have it circulate in the restricted milieu of Freudian institutions and journals" (p. 94). Staggered across various periods of his teaching and juxtaposed against the oral performance of his weekly seminar, the *Écrits* thus represented the slow and apparently unwilling accretion of Lacan's writings. As Bruce Fink (2004) speculates:

> Lacan may have only reluctantly agreed to publish his *Écrits* after Paul Ricoeur published his thick volume *De L' interpretation* translated as *Freud and Philosophy: An Essay on Interpretation* … Lacan certainly did not want Ricoeur to take credit for the return to Freud that Lacan himself had been championing. Lacan claims [in *Seminar XVIII*] that the texts in his *Écrits* had to be pried away from him.
>
> (p. 178)

Écrits then was reluctant text – or such is the myth that has grown around it – a much delayed 'book', published, largely, it would seem, at the urging of others, late in Lacan's life (he was 65). The factor of circumvention and delay seems telling. This consideration of deferred arrival – which contrasts so strongly to Lacan's frequent stress on anticipatory/pre-emptive modes of temporality in the *Écrits* – is in retrospect, indicative less of Lacan's reticence than – perhaps – of his *desire*.

Lacan had a famously low opinion of published writing as a means of disseminating psychoanalytic knowledge – hence his dismissive reference to '*poubellication*' (a contraction combining both garbage can and publication). In *Seminar XX*, during a session entitled 'The function of the written', Lacan offers a pronouncement on the *Écrits*:

> There is an anecdote to be related here, namely, that one day, on the cover of a collection I brought out – *poubellication*, as I called it – I found nothing better to write than the word *Écrits*.
>
> It is rather well known that those *Écrits* cannot be read easily. I can make a little autobiographical admission – that is exactly what I thought. I thought, perhaps it goes that far, I thought they were not meant be read. That's a good start.
>
> (1988, p. 26)

Commenting on this passage, Fink (2004) notes that Lacan never characterizes his seminars as *poubellication*, adding furthermore that while Lacan claimed to find no major errors in the published version of the seminars, such errors were to be found in the *Écrits*. Not only, then, is *Écrits* (as *poubellication*) apparently fit for the dustbin, it is also, effectively untitled: '*Écrits*' ('writings') is, one might argue, more a *description* than name, more the avoidance of a title than a title. Lacan's gesture here calls to mind Magritte's (1929) famous *La trahison des images*, proclaiming instead: *This is Not a Book*.

The medium of the spoken word, with all its lyricism, enunciative ambiguity and prospective revelation, was, for Lacan, a far more suitable medium than the published word for the transmission of psychoanalysis. In the opening of *The Instance of the Letter* Lacan professes concern that what he presents "might stray too far from speech, whose different measures are essential to the training I seek to effect (412, 1). He goes on to announce that what we are about to read will be "situated between writing and speech … halfway between the two" (412, 1). So whereas speech is associated with what is generative and valuable, writing, by contrast "allows for … [a] kind of tightening up" which "leave[s] the reader no way out than the way in, which I prefer to be difficult" (412, 2).

Elsewhere, Lacan similarly refers to the written text as something that "can only be woven by forming knots" (*Seminar XIX*, May 10, 1972). Writing here is presented not merely as challenging – puzzling, enigmatic – but also as willfully obstructive. These comments connote as much a celebration of the spoken word as an aversion to what is written, a suspicious relation thus – to paraphrase Magritte – to *La trahison de l'écriture*. One is left with an image of the text as an intricately and deceptively designed labyrinth. This may in fact be one particularly apt way of describing "writing in my [Lacan's] sense of the term" (412, 2), that is, as precisely *labyrinthine*. The *Écrits* then, following this thinking, is more maze than book.

In this context Jacques-Alain Miller (2010) states that Lacan's *Écrits* actually have a provocative function in relation to his seminar. The texts within *Écrits* don't provide us some synthesis of his oral teaching, but contain 'the waste' of his teaching: elements that he didn't discuss in public because of time restraints; and, more importantly, sensitive points to which his audience would have reacted with reluctance. Significant elements Lacan's audience could not easily accept, and which would be treated as the waste of his discourse, were condensed, and sent back to them in a written form. Thus considered, the *Écrits* constitute the symptom of the seminars.

This yields an interesting strategy for reading the *Écrits*. The *Écrits*, we might argue is pivotal to Lacan's oeuvre, but provides us with a non-'Standard Edition' of his ideas. Through Lacan's kaleidoscopic text ideas get compressed, distorted, disguised, subjected to the multiple dreamwork operations that separate latent from manifest contents of Lacan's theoretical desire. Whereas the Freudian text is a prime instance of the secondary process – contradictions are avoided wherever possible, rational clarity is attained throughout – the Lacan text is more akin to the primary process, 'structured like a language', making use of all and every rhetorical or linguistic device possible.

Lacan's description of his own style as "between writing and speech" provides us with a suggestion regards how we might go about commenting on his texts. Rather than attempting to fix the significations put in play by his style of 'spoken writing' we might seek to stress the multiple significations apparent therein, to invoke multiple voices speaking in – or through – what is presented on the page. Rather than the Rosetta Stone that enables the unlocking of other obscure writings, Lacan's *Écrits* is far more akin to a literary Babel. A text "not meant to be read" could, after all, mean a text that *should be made to speak*, and speak in multiple voices.

Alternatively, a text "not made to be read" might simply mean: not to be understood. Following this logic, the *Écrits* surely works less within the pragmatic goals of comprehension or rational intelligibility than as a means of inducing in us the perplexity and the suspension of knowledge that the analysand experiences in respect of the analyst and the analytic process itself. We might conclude that Lacan's assemblage of lectures-turned-writing is possibly less book than psychoanalytic tool – a desire- or transference-engendering device. "[W]hen all is said and done", opined Anthony Wilden,

> even if the curious mixture of penetration, poetry, and willful obscurity in the *Écrits* seems designed to force the reader into a perpetual struggle of his own ... perhaps there is a method [in this] madness. Lacan has always told his readers that they must, "*y mettre du sien*".
>
> (1968, p. 311)

The *Écrits*, in this further sense, is *not* a book: it is a type of infinite text; it does not end, it cannot be finished; it continues to escape the 'imaginarization' of our attempts at assimilation. We might then agree – at least in part – with Roudinesco's idea that

> the *Écrits* should be viewed less as a book than as the collection of a whole lifetime devoted to oral teaching. Hence the title Écrits, to signify trace, archive, something that does not come undone, does not vanish, cannot be stolen: a letter arriving at its destination.
>
> (2014, p. 96)

If it is not a book, then what is the *Écrits?* How does one view this dense, obscure, assemblage of signifiers? As a doctrinal text, perhaps, the 'Talmud' of Lacan's return to Freud? A manual of Freudian-Lacanian clinical practice? As the constitution (or more likely in Lacan's case a 'de-constitution') of his own emerging Freudian school of psychoanalysis? A hystericizing object of desire and interpretative scrutiny? An extended manifesto against the ossified norms of the ego psychologists and the International Psychoanalytic Association, indeed, a diatribe against a degraded form of psychoanalysis? Lacan's *magnum opus*? Perhaps a (love) letter to psychoanalysis and those allegiant to Freud's own inaugural psychoanalytic desire? The Lacanian answer to this extended line of questioning must surely be: Yes.

References

Fink, B. (2004). *Lacan to the Letter: Reading* Écrits *Closely.* Minneapolis, MN/ London: University of Minnesota Press.

Lacan, J. (1998). *The Seminar of Jacques Lacan, Book XX, Encore: On Feminine Sexuality, the Limits of Love and Knowledge, 1972–1973* (edited by Jacques-Alain Miller, translated by Bruce Fink). New York/London: W. W. Norton & Company.

Lacan, J. (2011). *Le Séminaire. Livre XIX: … ou pire* (1971–1972), texte établi par J.-A. Miller, Paris: Éditions du Seuil.

Miller, J.-A. (2010). *L'orientation Lacanienne – La vie de Lacan.* Unpublished Seminar. https://viedelacan.wordpress.com/2012/11/19/iv-lacan-contre-tous-et-contre-lacan/.

Ricoeur, P. (1965). *De l' interpretation.* Paris: Éditions du Seuil. (Translated as *Freud and Philosophy: An Essay on Interpretation*, trans. D. Savage. New Haven, CT: Yale University Press, 1970).

Roudinesco, É. (2014). *Lacan: In Spite of Everything.* London: Verso.

Wilden, A. (1968). *Speech and Language in Psychoanalysis: Jacques Lacan.* Baltimore, MD/London: The Johns Hopkins University.

1

THE SIGNIFICATION OF THE PHALLUS

Todd McGowan

Context

'*The Signification of the Phallus*' is the only one of Jacques Lacan's *Écrits* originally written in German. For his collected writings, Lacan produced his own unaltered translation of the talk that he gave on May 9, 1958, to the Max Planck Society in Munich. The essay contains the original German title '*Die Bedeutung des Phallus*' just under the French title at the top of the essay. It was given during the time of Lacan's fifth seminar entitled *Formations of the Unconscious* and presents ideas developed in this seminar and in the three preceding ones. It continues Lacan's preoccupation with signification and the symbolic order, as well as his polemics against those psychoanalysts who fail to take the signifier into account and thereby reduce psychoanalysis to a relationship of duality.

Like the *Mirror Stage* essay, '*The Signification of the Phallus*' (abbreviated here as *Signification*) has had an impact on the reception of Jacques Lacan's thought that far outstrips its importance for that thought. While Lacan discusses the constitutive role of the signifier in subjectivity and its impact on the emergence of desire, he develops these ideas in more detail in other writings. What does stand out about *Signification* is that it marks the first time in his written work that Lacan distinguishes phallus from penis. Even though this essay proffers a defense of Freud's interpretation of sexuality against that of his followers, this distinction between phallus and penis is not one that Freud himself makes, and for many cultural theorists and feminists, it has the effect of creating a more politically palatable version of psychoanalysis, which is why the essay has the importance that it has on the cultural stage. The distinction between phallus and penis constitutes the essential contribution of the essay and contributes to the theory of the signifier that Lacan was developing at this stage of his teaching.

By insisting on the phallus as a signifier, Lacan offers an original interpretation of Freud's theory of sexual difference and of the essays where he develops that theory—for example, '*The Dissolution of the Oedipus Complex*' (Freud, 1924/1961), '*Some Psychic Consequences of the Anatomical Distinction*

Between the Sexes' (Freud, 1924/1961), and '*Female Sexuality*' (Freud, 1930/1964). Where Freud identifies the central role that the penis plays in the identity of both sexes, Lacan clarifies this role through understanding the penis as the phallus, which is to say, as a signifier rather than as an organ or an object. For those who think of Lacan primarily as the author of a structuralist reading of Freud, *Signification* provides strong evidence in support of this claim. In this essay, the assertion of the centrality of the signifier in the constitution of the desiring subject comes to the fore again and again. Lacan attacks other psychoanalytic theorists for failing to recognize that the phallus has the importance that it has in the psychic economy of both sexes because of its status as a privileged signifier, not because of any natural privilege that the penis as a sexual organ enjoys or because of any cultural investment in the penis.

The phallus plays a fundamental role in the structure of the symbolic order and subjectivity. It is the one signifier that signifies meaning as such. In *Seminar V*, Lacan calls it "the signifier of the signified in general" (S5, 1957–1958: 240). In this sense, all meaning (or every signified) involves an implicit reference to the phallus. One signifier must play this role, and the phallus has, as a result of the variegations and contingencies of history, come to do so. But if we recognize that the phallus is not the penis and thus has no natural privilege, we can relate to its privilege as structural rather than ontological.

Furthermore, as Lacan's analysis shows, the privilege of the phallus is illusory. If the phallus is just a signifier, its status is that of an imposter, and its bearer must have recourse to imposture in order to take on the position the phallus. If the phallus is ever forced to show itself, its imposture would become evident for everyone to see, which is why it can only play its role as the privileged signifier while veiled.

Imposture derives from the phallic signifier's relationship to the signified. Because the phallus signifies meaning as such, it does not have its own signified. The phallus means at once everything and nothing. Its privilege as a signifier is intrinsically linked to its lack of a proper signified. In *Signification*, Lacan sees the phallus as the meaningless signifier that anchors all meaning. Every other signified implicitly refers to it, and this is the basis of its privilege.

Signification is not a critique of the phallus or of phallic privilege, nor is it a work justifying this privilege. It is rather a description of the effect of the phallus and an account of why the phallus has the status that it has. Lacan devotes much of his time in the essay to the distortion in subjectivity that the phallus signifies. Because the human animal is subjected to the signifier, a passion emerges that has nothing to do with the nature of this animal. The signifier rips the human animal out of its animality and creates a desiring subject.

There is, as Lacan shows in the essay, a fundamental distinction between need and desire, and demand is the pathway leading from one to the other. The signifier always carries with it a demand, and this demand uproots the speaking being from its needs. Because the demand operates through the signifier, it is always a demand for love or recognition. For Lacan, the signifier's primary function is to indicate recognition. We respond to the demand by meeting the needs of the other—when the child cries, the parent provides it with food, for instance—but the demand seeks love, not the fulfillment of its needs. The result of this impasse is the emergence of desire, the desire that the phallus signifies.

Viewing the phallus as a signifier enables Lacan to avoid what he sees as the two basic psychoanalytic heresies. He denounces both in this essay. The first heresy understands the subject as a biological entity through and through and reduces the subject's desires to animal needs. The privileged role that the phallus plays in the subject's desire reveals the falsity of this position. The human animal's subjection to the signifier produces a distortion in human needs so that they cannot find direct satisfaction in an object. The fact that human animals don't directly pursue their needs gives the lie to the biological interpretation of subjectivity. The second heresy is what Lacan refers to as a culturalist position, a position that he associates with Karen Horney. The culturalist sees desire purely as the result of social forces and attempts to account for the privilege of the phallus in these terms. The culturalist that Lacan criticizes anticipates today's social constructionist—someone like Judith Butler (1990). Again, it is the distorting effects that the signifier has on the subject that renders this position untenable. One cannot trace an uninterrupted through-line from the dictates of the social order to the desires of individual subjects. Though Lacan doesn't mention him, one might say that this is the mistake that Michel Foucault makes in his critique of psychoanalysis in the first volume of the *History of Sexuality* (1976/1978). Desire emerges not directly through an ideological imperative given by culture but through the distorting effect that demand has on the human animal's needs. By theorizing the phallus as a signifier, Lacan can guide his thought between the Scylla of biologism and the Charybdis of culturalism. This strategy animates his conception of psychoanalysis from beginning to end, but it finds one of its most concise expressions in '*The Signification of the Phallus*.'

The place that the phallus has in Lacan's thought evolves during the course of his intellectual trajectory. Its importance is never greater than when Lacan writes *Signification*. The essay represents the summary or culmination of one period of his thought, and soon after he writes it, his thought moves in another direction, even though he doesn't abandon the central insights that he comes to here. In the years following the writing of this essay, Lacan's seminars and writings place less emphasis on the phallus. It has no role in the development of an ethics based on desire in *Seminar VII* (1959–1960), and Lacan makes only brief mentions of the phallus in his explanation of psychoanalysis to a general audience in his landmark *Seminar XI: The Four Fundamental Concepts of Psychoanalysis* (1964). In *Signification*, the phallus explains the structure of desire. In *Seminar XI* and subsequent seminars, it is the object *a* that takes on this function. Lacan arrives at the insight that the object *a* is the object-cause of desire and thus has more importance in the structure of desire than the phallus, which takes on a more secondary role in Lacan's thinking about desire. Lacan continues to view the phallus as the signifier of desire, but its importance for explaining desire diminishes. In sections of *Signification*, the phallus functions not just as the signifier of desire but also of what is desired. This function would soon disappear entirely, and the phallus would be restricted to being the signifier of desire. Toward the end of his intellectual trajectory, at the time of *Seminar XX* (1972–1973), the importance of the phallus returns to some extent as Lacan theorizes sexuation according to formulas that make use of both the phallus as a signifier and the phallic function as the mark of castration.

The formulations in *Signification* allow us to distinguish between the sexes in terms of two fundamental positions that they adopt relative to the signifier—masculine imposture and feminine masquerade. Lacan never mentions the term 'imposture' in the essay, but he does allude to it when he points out that the phallus "can play its role only when veiled" (581). This indicates that the phallus must hide itself through imposture in order to sustain its privileged position. There is a direct reference to masquerade, which Lacan associates with femininity. The distinction between imposture and masquerade is crucial for grasping how the phallus functions in sexual difference. Imposture involves feigning as if one has something that one doesn't have, while masquerade involves acting like what one is not. The imposter hides what he has because he doesn't have the secret power that he pretends to have, whereas the masquerading woman puts a secret on display so that she will be loved for it even though it has nothing to do with her. Imposture hides through hiding, and masquerade hides through showing, which is, as Lacan illustrates in his analysis of Edgar Allan Poe's *The Purloined Letter*, a more effective strategy.

Throughout Lacan's seminars and writings, he makes a distinction between the symbolic and imaginary phallus that he doesn't make in *Signification*. The symbolic phallus is the phallus as the privileged signifier, whereas the imaginary phallus is the object lost in symbolic castration. In his *Seminar IV* (1956–1957), Lacan provides his most detailed description of the imaginary phallus, and he links it to castration in order to indicate that castration involves the subject losing what it never had (which is why its object is imaginary and not real). This distinction between the symbolic and imaginary phallus does not appear in *Signification* because Lacan's concern in this essay is not so much an account of the forms of the phallus but the distortions created by signification. This absence itself signifies Lacan's aim here.

Of all Lacan's essays, none has been more important for feminism than '*The Signification of the Phallus*.' By separating the phallus from the penis, Lacan makes a decisive intervention against any patriarchal privilege. This is undoubtedly why when they constructed the first volume of Lacan's writing on female sexuality for the Anglophone world, Juliet Mitchell and Jacqueline Rose (1982) decided to include a translation of '*The Signification of the Phallus*' (which Rose translated as *The Meaning of the Phallus*). This collection, entitled *Female Sexuality: Jacques Lacan and the école freudienne*, asserts that both psychoanalysis in general and Lacan in specific have a vital role to play in feminist theorizing.

Both Mitchell and Rose write introductions to this collection in which they justify the idea of Lacan as a fellow traveler of feminist theory. Mitchell (1982) describes Lacan's insistence on sexual difference as the indication of the failure of ideological interpellation and thus the basis for any political activity. For Rose, Lacan's conception of the phallus as a signifier marks his most important contribution to feminism. This conception enables us to see that "the phallus stands at its own expense and any male privilege erected upon it is an imposture" (Rose, 1982: 44). As Lacan makes clear in this essay, the phallus is the privileged signifier, the signifier of all the signifieds, but this privilege doesn't betoken any ontological privilege for its bearer. The bearer of the phallus is always an imposter, and psychoanalysis exposes this imposture of the phallic signifier. For both Mitchell and Rose, *Signification* is a pillar in the assault on patriarchal society.

For some feminist critics of Lacan, however, the replacement of penis with phallus and the interpretation of the phallus as a signifier don't go far enough in combating the sexism inherent in Freud's account of subjectivity. The most prominent of these critics is Judith Butler, who claims in *Gender Trouble* that the physical organ functions as a hidden support for the authority of the phallic signifier. She writes, "the Phallus, though clearly not identical with the penis, nevertheless deploys the penis as its naturalized instrument and sign" (Butler, 1990: 106). Butler's critique of Lacan follows from her larger critique of sexual difference and its constitutive role within psychoanalytic theorizing. Claims about sexual identity, according to Butler, illicitly utilize biology even when they claim not to be doing so. Every discussion about sex is really a subterfuge in which gender characteristics are smuggled in. According to Butler, this is the case with Lacan: even when he insists that the phallus is just a signifier, his retention of the association with the bodily organ has the effect of giving a hidden authority to the phallus.

Followers of Lacan have vigorously stepped up to his defense against Butler's critique and other related feminist attacks on Lacan's supposed sexism. Joan Copjec (1994) offers the definitive response to Butler in the final chapter of *Read My Desire: Lacan Against the Historicists* entitled '*Sex and the Euthanasia of Reason.*' Contra Butler and following Lacan, Copjec insists that sexual difference is not a simple cultural construction but rather real. That is, sexual difference exists because cultural constructions fail to produce symbolic identities and because the symbolic order necessarily contradicts itself when it attempts to signify a whole. The phallus is the mark of this contradiction, and sexual difference is its result. According to Copjec, Butler's rejection of the phallic signifier and sexual difference indicates an abandonment or obscuring of contradiction rather than an argument against the inherent sexism of psychoanalysis and Lacan.

The most far-reaching development of the feminist implications inherent in Lacan's interpretation of the phallus appears buried in Alenka Zupančič's book on comedy, *Odd One In* (2008). In the midst of her discussion of the role that the phallus plays in ancient comedy, Zupančič includes an excursus on psychoanalysis, the phallus, and feminism. She argues that far from upholding the privilege of the phallus that undergirds patriarchal society, the project of psychoanalysis exposes the ultimate contingency of this privilege. According to Zupančič,

> By spelling out the link between the traditional almighty phallus (which, by the way, functioned symbolically, and as a symbolic power, long before Lacan came along) to an anatomical particularity, he (and psychoanalysis) made a crucial contribution to the removal of the phallus from the mode of necessity to that of contingency.
> (2008: 205)

By unpacking the mystery surrounding the phallus and revealing its essential contingency as a signifier, Lacan, though he never mounted the feminist barricades, contributes to the feminist effort to undermine the privilege of the phallus.

'*The Signification of the Phallus*' fully justifies Zupančič's claim that psychoanalysis works to unravel the mystery of the phallus rather than strengthen it. Toward the middle of the essay, Lacan makes clear that observing how the phallus functions in psychoanalysis may ultimately "lift the veil from the function it served in the mysteries" (579). If the phallus can only function while veiled, lifting the veil will undermine its privilege. But it is not a matter for Lacan of undermining the privilege of the phallus in order to replace it with another signifier of privilege.

There will always be one signifier that functions in the way that the phallus does, one signifier that signifies all meaning or all signifieds. Replacing this signifier would have no political effect at all because the structure would remain the same. This is the problem with traditional feminist critiques of the privilege invested in the phallus. One must give up the struggle against the phallus. What is necessary, instead, is altering the relationship to the phallus and recognizing its imposture. The privilege of the phallus is no privilege at all, though this is the most difficult recognition to accept. It requires one accepting the inescapable and fundamental stupidity that provides the foundation for all sense. But it is the political position that Lacan stakes out in '*The Signification of the Phallus*.'

Commentaries on the text

The essay begins (575, 1) with an examination of the castration complex and the power that this complex has for regulating both our symptoms and identifications. The decision to begin a discussion of the phallus with castration is telling: it indicates that even at this midpoint in his intellectual trajectory Lacan has already placed castration at the center of the Freudian doctrine. The castration complex is and remains much more important for Lacan than the Oedipus complex. He might have chosen to begin with the Oedipus complex and the role that the phallus plays in the child's Oedipal struggle, but he opts for castration as the starting point in order to suggest the decisiveness that castration has for subjectivity. Later in his thought, Lacan will align being subjected to castration with what he calls the phallic function, but even at this point it is clear that castration is the key term within the psychic economy.

Castration becomes central for Lacan but he understands the concept much differently than Freud. It isn't related to the fear of losing, or trauma of having lost, the penis but to the lack that every speaking subject endures as a result of its subjection to the signifier. The major reinterpretation of castration is one of the points of Lacan's originality as a thinker and also a reason for his attractiveness to feminism. It goes along with his reinterpretation of the phallus.

The connection between the signification of the phallus and castration is not immediately apparent in the essay, despite the fact that Lacan opens his essay on the phallus with an account of the effects of castration. The phallus is not, as we might suspect, the cause of castration but rather its signifier. That is to say, the phallus signifies what the desiring subject—the subject of the castration complex—has given up in order to exist as a desiring subject. But the reason Lacan can say that the phallus is a fraud or the badge of imposture is that even though the subject has given up a part of itself, this part exists only in being lost. Other psychoanalytic theorists who talk about the lost satisfaction of the original object thus completely miss the point. One has sacrificed nothing but an imaginary phallus (though Lacan doesn't explain this here). The (symbolic) phallus signifies what the subject lost but never actually had. This is why it is the signifier without a signified: its signified—what the subject has sacrificed in order to be a speaking being—doesn't exist.

Because castration plays the central role in the psyche, the relationship that the subject has to castration determines its symptoms and everything else that psychoanalysis can analyze (575, 2). It is decisive for neurosis, psychosis, and perversion. Castration or subjection to the signifier regulates the development of the subject and enables it to identify with the symbolic ideal of one of the sexes (575, 3). The loss that occurs with castration even permits the subject to meet its own basic needs through a desire that doesn't address them directly. Lacan begins the essay by placing castration on center stage, and he moves from this to a discussion of the difficulty that castration creates.

A central problem emerges that Lacan (575, 4) labels an "antinomy." This reference to Kant and the Transcendental Dialectic in the *Critique of Pure Reason* (Kant, 1781/1998) indicates an impossible alternative—an alternative in which either both solutions are false or both solutions are true. The antinomy here involves the position that the subject can take up relative to castration: it can either be a threat (for the male) or a deprivation (for the female). Much later in his thought, in *Séminaire XIX: … ou pire*, Lacan will change his mind about the deprivation of the female and insist that symbolic castration doesn't in fact apply to female subjects, indicating that "they are not castratable" (S19, 1971–1972: 47). But here, threat and deprivation represent two failed alternatives, which is why we can add a sexual antinomy to Kant's mathematical and dynamical antinomies. Castration is the foundation of subjectivity, and it leads inexorably to an antinomy.

Neither threat nor deprivation—neither the male version nor the female version of the castration complex—allows the subject to achieve a normal or well-adjusted sexuality. Instead, the choices that the subject has reveal that human sexuality goes awry not because of particular errors on the part of individual subjects but because of what Lacan calls "an essential disturbance" in its functioning that manifests itself through the options presented in castration (575, 4). In order to underscore Freud's insistence on this disturbance of sexuality, Lacan refers to two of Freud's works where it becomes most prominent—*Civilization and Its Discontents* (1927/1961) and *Analysis Terminable and Interminable* (1937/1964). He mentions without comment Freud's theorization of the castration complex in male subjectivity and *Penisneid* or penis envy in female subjectivity, though this latter is an idea that he would explicitly reject in his seminars. Neither side in this opposition has an enviable position, and the opposition itself bespeaks the fundamental failure of sexuality.

This failure extends into psychoanalytic practice. Lacan asserts the primacy of the problem that castration introduces into analytic experience, even as he allows that other problems also exist. Neither culture nor biology can explain the role of the castration complex. For Lacan, it is a result of the insertion of the biological entity into culture, which occurs through the signifier. Later in the essay he will reject the culturalist interpretation of castration, but first (575, 5) he dismisses the possibility of a biological explanation for the different relationships to castration in the masculine and feminine positions. The problem with the biological explanation is that it fails to take the necessary universality of the myth of the origin of castration into account (576, 1). If the different relationships to castration were biological, the myth of the origin of castration would not be universal but simply a contingent development in particular societies. This myth—the myth of the possibility of a full enjoyment of the mother accomplished through the murder of the father—develops out of the lack in signification.

It is on the question of the father's murder that Lacan offers an implicit critique of Freud. Freud locates the myth of a primal father and his murder as the substrate of the Oedipal myth. In his famous account of the murder of the primal father in the fourth section of *Totem and Taboo* (1913/1955), Freud turns to an inherited memory of this event in order to explain the structuring role of the castration complex. Lacan argues that this claim is obviously untenable (though without attributing it to Freud) not just on its scientific merits but on the basis of the impossibility of establishing a direct link between the memory of killing the primal father and respect for the castration threat, when this threat is precisely what one kills the father in order to sidestep. Freud's scientific error in *Totem and Taboo*—the belief in inherited memory—obscures a more significant logical one—the association of the murder of the father or even the desire for the murder of the father with the castration threat.

Instead of invoking the inherited memory of the experience of the father's murder to explain the castration complex, one must stick to clinical facts and the experience of the analyst (576, 3). In analysis, we see that the anatomical distinction between male and female does not play a determinative role in the relationship of the subject to the phallus. Anatomy is not destiny for Lacan. Even though the essay is entitled '*The Signification of the Phallus*,' this is the first time Lacan introduces the term 'phallus,' as he subtly turns from a focus on castration to a more direct focus on the phallus and the difficulties that inhere in the woman's relationship to the phallus. Concerning these difficulties, he raises four important questions. He wonders why the phallic mother is the agent of castration for the little girl (576, 4), why both boy and girl view the mother as a phallic figure (576, 5), why the discovery of the mother's castration is determinative for the subject's symptoms (576, 6), and why Freud theorizes a phallic phase in the subject's development (576, 7). These questions focus on the disturbance in the child's sexual development, especially that of the girl, introduced by the phallus. This marks a turning point in the essay, as the explanation of castration gives way to a discussion of the phallus. In a sense, the phallus is the answer to the question posed by castration.

Lacan's discussion of the phallus initially focuses on the theorization of the phallic phase. In the phallic phase, Freud attributes to both sexes an ignorance of the vagina as a site for sexuality. According to Lacan (576, 8), this ignorance is not the product of chance but a necessary misrecognition, a misrecognition of sexual difference. In order to explain the misrecognition, Lacan alludes to an ancient Greek romance by Longus, entitled *Daphnis and Chloe*, in which Lycaenion, whom Lacan refers to just as an old woman, explains the intricacies of lovemaking to Daphnis so that he can approach his beloved Chloe. Lacan likely knew of this romance due to the influential French translation by Jacques Amyot (1559/1947), who provided the first version of the romance in a modern language. This reference illustrates the lack of knowledge that both sexes have about the vagina in relation to enjoyment.

This ignorance of the vagina suggests repression, according to the thesis of certain psychoanalytic theorists, but Lacan (576, 9) quickly rejects this idea because of the immense confusion surrounding it. According to this reading, the phallic object is a symptom, but for some it is a symptom of phobia, for others a symptom of perversion, and for others a symptom of both phobia and perversion, which is manifestly untenable (577, 1). Phobia and perversion place the object in different structural positions and thus cannot possibly coincide. The problem with this interpretation of the phallus runs deep in the history of psychoanalysis. It stems from object relations theory and the concept of the part-object, introduced by Karl Abraham (1927) and then taken up by Melanie Klein and her followers. As long as psychoanalysts conceive of the phallus as a part-object, they fail to understand its role as a signifier, which is why Lacan so thoroughly rejects the interpretation of the phallus as a part-object, the dominant interpretation at the time when Lacan wrote this essay.

Though Lacan (577, 2) criticizes the theorization of the phallic phase by object relations psychoanalysts, he nonetheless celebrates the debate that circulated around this concept between 1928 and 1932 for the passion that animated it. But the debate didn't advance the understanding of the role that the phallus plays in subjectivity, which is why Lacan must write *Signification* in an attempt to revisit this question by focusing on the phallus as a signifier rather than as an object.

Returning to the debate about the phallic phase provides Lacan an opportunity to showcase the originality of his conception of the phallus. Lacan mentions the key contributors to the debate—Helene Deutsch (1930), Karen Horney (1932), and Ernest Jones (1933)—without describing their respective positions or taking sides (577, 2).

Though Lacan does not side with Jones, he singles out his contribution on the question of the phallic phase as significant (577, 3). The most important idea promulgated by Jones in his three essays on the phallic phase is that of 'aphanisis,' though Jones doesn't grasp the proper importance of his own concept. Jones introduces this concept in an essay entitled '*The Early Development of Female Sexuality*' (1927). For Jones, aphanisis signifies the absolute loss of the capacity for sexual enjoyment, the loss of desire itself. This is the fear that drives all neuroses, according to Jones. Lacan finds this theorization ridiculous, but he is nonetheless eager to borrow Jones's concept for his own ends. Interestingly, in his *Seminar IV* (1956–1957), just over a year prior to writing '*The Signification of the Phallus*,' Lacan cites Jones's concept without criticizing it and in fact seeming to invoke it. But now, for Lacan, aphanisis indicates something quite different from what Jones had in mind. It is the loss that must occur to constitute the desiring subject. Later, in *Seminar XI*, Lacan will turn to the concept of aphanisis to explain the central role that castration plays in the emergence of subjectivity. He claims there, "There is no subject without, somewhere, *aphanisis* of the subject, and it is in this alienation, in this fundamental division, that the dialectic of the subject is established" (S11, 1964: 221). Aphanisis is thus what leads to the castration complex. But despite the key term that Jones introduces, his own work completely ignores the relationship between castration and desire, which is the central problem for psychoanalysis.

Along these same lines, Jones completely misreads Freud's conception of the phallus (577, 5). He manages to discover in Freud a position that is precisely the opposite of what Freud advances—namely that both sexes have the same relationship to the phallus. Lacan ironically says that he appreciates the difficulty of this kind of extreme misreading.

Jones concludes his essay '*The Phallic Phase*' by citing the Bible (577, 6). He says, "Lastly I think we should do well to remind ourselves of a piece of wisdom whose source is more ancient than Plato: In the beginning ... male and female created He them" (Jones, 1933: 33). This is a failed attempt to forge equality between the sexes, and Jones attempts to do this by appealing to the phallus as an internal object in the mother's body, which Melanie Klein (1932/1975) discovered in the children's fantasies. The position of Jones and that of Klein on the question of the phallus are indistinguishable. Lacan insists that we must reject both if we want to grasp how the phallus actually functions.

As Lacan sees it, Freud himself had more insight than any of his followers (like Jones or Klein) into the question of the phallus and castration because he emphasized the unconscious in a way that they did not (577, 7). The followers strayed from locating castration in the unconscious and thus erred.

Freud's own thought leads Lacan to an understanding of the centrality of the signifier in the psyche (578, 1). Though he had no knowledge of modern linguistics, Freud reveals the psychic resonance of the division between the signifier and the signified that Ferdinand de Saussure (1915/1959) and other linguists insist on. Freud is the first to understand the active role that the signifier plays in producing the signified through the passion that it evokes.

The subject doesn't simply speak, but the passion of the signifier speaks through the subject (578, 2). Here, Lacan calls this passion 'it' [*ça*], which is also the French translation for Freud's concept of the id. This means that the relationship to the signifier has a more profound effect on the subject than the subject's ideas.

The effect of the signifier in the subject is unconscious, but there has been a general failure in analytic theory to recognize this effect (578, 3). Lacan's project is to restore the unconscious to its proper place in psychoanalytic theory. In analytic practice, on the other hand, Lacan observes the effect of the unconscious in his colleagues' flight from it, rather than in their attempt to actively engage it.

Though it seems like stressing signification is the same as stressing culture, Lacan (578, 4) claims that one must distinguish an emphasis on the signifier from the culturalist position associated with Karen Horney (1932). According to culturalism, the phallus plays the central role in the psychic economy due to its social privilege, and sexual difference is just an effect of social structure. The castration complex is ideological, according to this untenable and non-psychoanalytic line of thought. Lacan recognizes that he risks being mistaken as a culturalist or a constructionist, and he takes pains to make clear that there is a radical difference having to do with the distortion that Lacan sees the signifier producing in subjectivity. The signifier is not simply the straightforward manifestation of culture.

Instead of turning to culturalism, one must examine the effects of language in the unconscious (578, 5). This is done through the study of metonymy and metaphor, which are the two relations of the signifier that produce the signified and constitute the subject. The subject is constituted through a topology rather than through internalization, and understanding this topology enables us to analyze the formation of symptoms. The subject is a surface, not a depth. Here, Lacan identifies topology as a diagnostic tool. This privileging of topology follows directly from an understanding of the role that the signifier plays in subjectivity, and it allows Lacan to create diagnostic structures, such as the R Schema, that clarify the relationship that a particular clinical structure, such as psychosis, has to the signifier.

The priority of the signifier over the signified manifests itself in the subject having a location in the big Other prior to the subject viewing itself through the lens of meaning (579, 1). The subject is split by signification in the sense that the I that speaks is distinct from the I that is spoken. Or, in Lacan's own terms, the subject of the enunciation is not the same as the subject of the statement. This splitting forms the unconscious by separating the subject from itself. The emphasis on the signifier allows Lacan to recognize the subject as split, which is another way of describing castration.

When we grasp the role that the signifier plays in the formation of the subject, the function of the phallus becomes clear (579, 2). Lacan distinguishes the phallus from a fantasy, from a part-object, and from the penis. The phallus isn't the penis but instead symbolizes the penis. When he says this, Lacan marks his distance from any defense of patriarchy. Lacan's insistence that the phallus is a simulacrum rather than a substantial source of identity aligns him with the feminist project and not the patriarchal one.

This leads to the decisive paragraph in the essay (579, 3). Here, Lacan calls the phallus a signifier directly for the first time. By identifying the phallus as a signifier, it loses the aura of mystery that has always surrounded it. The phallus gains this aura of mystery because it is not just any signifier but the signifier that signifies signification itself. That is, the phallus brings the whole field of meaning into existence.

Indeed, the phallus signifies the distortion of human need through the effect of the signifier (579, 4). Needs are never just needs but must pass through the register of demand, which means that the subject always finds itself alienated from its own needs and must relate to its own needs rather than experience them directly. It is not as if subjects rely on signifiers actually to fulfill their needs—what Lacan dismisses as a "real dependence"—but that their needs must be articulated through signifiers. It is the form of the signifying demand that alienated the subject from the need that this demand expresses.

The problem is not just that need must be articulated in demand but that need cannot be articulated in demand even though this is the only vehicle for it (579, 5). This failure of demand or failure of the signifier constitutes what Freud calls primal repression, and it is the origin of desire. For the first time in this essay, Lacan deploys the three terms that underlie any attempt to understand the signification of the phallus—need, demand, and desire. One could conceive of the difference between the biological thinker, the culturalist, and Lacan in terms of this triad. We should align biology with need, culture with demand, and Lacan with desire. Desire is absolutely distinct from need, which analytic experience proves and moralists have always grasped. The problem is that, according to Lacan (579, 5), psychoanalysis itself is falling into obscurantism through its attempt to view desire as simply need. Lacan's essay is part of the effort to combat this reductionism.

Fighting this reduction of desire to need requires articulating the status of desire (579, 6). The idea of frustration, which psychoanalysts have used to theorize desire, is completely misleading, which is why Freud himself didn't employ it. Desire is lack, but it is a lack resulting from subjection to the signifier, not from the frustration of not obtaining one's object. Again, Lacan stresses the signifier at the expense of any direct relation to the object.

After showing the problems with theorizing the subject in terms of need, Lacan turns to demand. Demand is a demand for presence or absence, and it grants a power to satisfy or deny needs to the Other (579, 7). Lacan theorizes demand as a form of capitulation to the Other (580, 1). Elsewhere, he will claim that the neurotic places demand in the position of desire and thus believes that it can subvert the difficulty inhering in the confrontation with the Other's desire. Demand is always a demand for the Other's love, which is the one thing that the Other doesn't have. This is why demand cannot be satisfied: the Other doesn't have what the subject demands from it.

Demand occurs with subjection to the signifier, but it doesn't provide the key to the subject (580, 2). It has no concern for any particularity. Whatever particularity the Other gives becomes a proof of love. Even when demand manages to produce the satisfaction of need, the satisfaction has no value because it is not a sufficient proof of love, which is the sole concern—and thus, for Lacan, the limitation—of demand (and explanations that focus on it).

But particularity doesn't vanish altogether (580, 3). The destruction of particularity in the demand leaves a remainder in desire, and this remainder is a resurgence of particularity. Desire seeks out singularity, as it passes between need and demand. Desire results from the subtraction of need from demand. The splitting of these two functions produces desire. Here, Lacan presents one of his most famous formulas for desire, and it offers a way of distinguishing a desiring subject from both a biological entity and a cultural identity.

Lacan follows the discussion of need and demand with an explanation of desire, which is where his real concern lies (580, 4). Desire makes itself manifest in the contours of the sexual relationship. Each demands a proof of love from the other and the satisfaction of need, but the relationship is sustained not through either demand or need but through being the cause of the desire of each other. The sexual relationship requires that each partner occupy the place of the cause of desire for the other, and desire reveals how this relationship necessarily unfolds.

There is thus an irreducible gap in the relation of the subject to the Other in the sexual relationship (580, 5). This relationship will always have defects, and no genital stage or maturation will eliminate these defects. Lacan is harshly critical of attempts, especially by French analysts, to establish the notion of achieving the genital stage and thereby becoming capable of freely giving of oneself as the goal of analysis. This moralizing cuts against the fundamental insights of psychoanalysis and establishes a hypocritical and unrealizable ideal for the subject.

Maturation and achieving the genital stage fail because no one can become whole (581, 1). The insistence on a split subject is foundational in Lacan's theory. One cannot even try to become whole. The centrality of displacement and condensation—effects of the signifier—in the subject makes attempts at wholeness impossible.

Lacan moves to connect his earlier discussion of the phallus with what he is saying now about desire (581, 2). It is the phallus that plays the role of the privileged signifier and thus determines how the signifier gives birth to desire. The phallus is the signifier that orients the desiring of the subject. The subject desires according to the relation that it takes up to the phallus.

There are possible physiological justifications for the choice of the phallus as the privileged signifier (581, 3). During intercourse, the penis functions metaphorically as the copula that brings the sexes together, and the phallus signifies this connection. It is also possible to claim that the turgidity of the penis provides an image of vitality, and that is why the phallus is the privileged signifier. If one takes these claims as Lacan's own, it would provide ammunition to the charge that he is a thinker invested in patriarchal society, one who roots the privilege of the phallus as a signifier in nature itself. But the next paragraph gives the lie to this reading.

Any physiological justification for the role that the phallus plays in signification serves to hide the fact that the phallus functions only if veiled (581, 4). The fact that one cannot expose the phallus reveals that no physiological characteristic can actually be the basis for its privilege. If the turgidity of the penis were the characteristic that led to the privilege of the phallus, then the phallus wouldn't have to be veiled in order to function. It is functioning as the privileged signifier only when all its characteristics are hidden.

This implies that a subject acts in thrall to the phallus not when displaying what appears as clearly phallic behavior—like a muscled Arnold Schwarzenegger evincing indestructibility in *The Terminator* (James Cameron, 1984)—but instead when a seemingly innocuous figure exercises an authority that doesn't appear as authority. This is the case with all of the compassionate fathers in Steven Spielberg's films, including the hero of *Schindler's List*

(1994). The phallus is completely veiled with Oskar Schindler (Liam Neeson) because he simply wants to save endangered Jews, but the veil is precisely what enables the phallus to function through his acts, which, though they defy the Nazis, support a phallic regime. With this idea of the necessary imposture of the phallus, Lacan demystifies phallic privilege.

Though Lacan does not mention Hegel by name, he refers the phallus as a signifier to the concept most often associated with Hegel—*Aufhebung* or sublation (581, 5). The phallus has an effect not through its presence but through its disappearance, and this disappearance is a sublation. The phallus would not structure the desire of the subject if it did not disappear and thereby transcend its merely empirical being. It orients the subject's desire because it doesn't show itself. When the phallus is exposed, the subject experiences shame. Lacan alludes to the demon of Αἰδως, which is the demon of shame, and the painting in the Villa of the Mysteries in Pompeii, a painting in the ruins of a Roman villa that depicts a woman being initiated into the cult of Dionysus. In this fresco, the demon pops up because the phallus, which is hidden in the young woman's basket, is about to be unveiled. In this way, we see the effort to cover the phallus in these frescoes.

Lacan contends that the phallus must be veiled because it is the barrier to the meaningfulness of the signified (581, 6). The signified is nothing but the product of the signifying structure, and the phallus is the indication of this.

In the production of the subject by the signifier, a complementarity results (581, 7). This is the divide between signifier and signified. De Saussure and others theorize this, but Lacan is the first to place the emphasis entirely on the side of the signifier. As a result of this divide, there is a radical separation between the being of the subject and the signified existence of the subject (581, 8). The demand of love focuses on what one's being means for the other, but this is a mirage because meaning arises only through the signifier. This division between being and signified existence coheres with a primal repression. What is primally repressed in the formation of the subject is indicated by the repression of the phallus (581, 9). Along this way the role of the phallus in the economy of desire becomes clear (581, 10). It provides a ratio for desire that enables the subject to relate to desire. The phallus is not the object of desire but rather, as a signifier, its measure. The phallus as the ratio of desire functions like an algorithm (581, 11). We can think about the structure of desire in mathematical terms because it is a structure rather than an experience.

The subject must have access to the phallus in order to orient its desire, but the phallus is only present as a veiled entity at the level of the Other (581, 12). This means that the subject doesn't directly relate to the phallus but must do so through the recognition of the Other's desire (582, 1). The Other is an other divided by the signifier just as the subject is. Here, Lacan is silently alluding to Hegel's claim from the preface to the *Phenomenology of Spirit* (1807) that substance is also subject, that there is no undivided substance opposed to the subject. For Lacan, the Other is not an undivided authority but split just as the subject itself is. This idea will become increasingly prominent in the next few years of Lacan's intellectual career.

There is evidence in psychological development that attests to the role that the phallus plays as a privileged signifier (582, 2). Typically, Lacan takes a dismissive attitude toward developmental psychology, but he has recourse to it here only to show the problems with contending hypotheses about the phallus. If we examine this psychological development, we can reject Melanie Klein's hypothesis (1932/1975) that the phallus is an internal object within the mother (582, 3). This hypothesis fails to grasp the function that the phallus has as the signifier of the mother's desire. Lacan wants to rethink all development through the relation to the phallic signifier (282, 4). Development occurs through a dialectic of the demand for love, which involves the presence and absence of the signifier, and the desire that underlies this demand.

The problem with the demand for love is that the desire that underlies it has no signifier (282, 5). As Lacan says later in '*Kant with Sade*,' desire "cannot be indicated anywhere in a signifier of any demand whatsoever" (653). That is, the signifier, which is associated with demand, cannot satisfy desire. The child attempts to respond to the mother's desire by being the phallus, but this attempt always fails because the mother's desire is divided from itself. Nothing that the child does will satisfy this desire. The child will always fail to have the phallus for the mother.

The Other's desire doesn't inform the child about its own status relative to the phallus—whether the child has the phallus or not (282, 6). But the Other's desire does teach the subject that its mother does not have the phallus, and this is a key moment for the development of symptoms and for the structure of subjectivity based on the castration complex. The phallus, which signifies desire, shows that desire has a relation with an original not-having.

But the trajectory of desire will depend not just on its initial emergence but on the Law of the Father (582, 7). That is to say, desire is not just the product of the relation with the mother but with a third party in the form of the Law. One doesn't need this Law to see that the phallic function governs the relations between the sexes (582, 8). The overt presence of the Law of the Father merely makes the veiled role of the phallus explicit, Lacan contends.

When the phallus is a signifier, sexual difference takes on a less obscure form (582, 9). The relations between the sexes is a relation between having and not-having. The sexes either have or don't have the phallus, which is a signifier. Because sexual relations are constituted through the signifier, they have reality in the signifier but are unreal on the level of the signified. There are no relations on the level of the signified, an idea that anticipates Lacan's later celebrated formulation '*there is no sexual relationship*' (S19: 12).

Lacan introduces the term '*paraître*' or 'seeming' to indicate the attitude that both sexes take up relative to the phallus—the man in order to protect his having and the woman in order to mask her lack (582, 10). This seeming transforms the behavior of each sex into comedy because both sexes are constantly trying to project an ideal that neither can fully uphold. The masculine and feminine ideals are capable of satisfying the demand for love, which has the effect of strengthening their hold over the subjects attempting to project them (582, 11). But these ideals have the effect of reducing desire to demand, which is a neurotic reduction (583, 1). In other words, masculine and feminine ideals are ultimately unsatisfying for the subject.

The woman tries to be the phallus or the signifier of the Other's desire, and she does this through a masquerade (583, 2). This is a concept developed first by Joan Rivière, in her essay '*Womanliness as Masquerade*,' where she identifies "the eternal feminine" as a mask that the woman uses to make herself desirable (1929). Masquerade requires the woman to reject her femininity in order to be desired and loved for what she isn't rather than what she is. She has to find the signifier of her desire in the man, but his organ functions as a fetish for her, allowing her to disavow the absence of the phallus. That is to say, the actual male penis enables the woman to engage in a fetishistic disavowal of male castration. With this formulation, Lacan silently reverses Freud's understanding of fetishistic disavowal as relating to the absence of the penis on the female. In the encounter with the male organ, the woman's desire finds its signifier, which is an experience that the male subject does not have. But at the same time, the object that fulfills the demand for love doesn't function as an object but as a signifier. Lacan postulates that this coexistence of the fulfillment of the demand for love with the failure of desire leads to an acceptance of frigidity or the lack of sexual fulfillment in women. It also coincides with less displacement in the woman's desire than in the man's because the object that fails to satisfy the woman's desire nonetheless responds to her demand for love and also signifies that desire. The sexually dissatisfying object for the woman has other appeals that often outweigh this sexual dissatisfaction for her. This is Lacan's explanation for women's ability to accept frigidity, which contrasts with men's inability to accept impotence or a woman's frigidity.

For the man, no such trade-off exists (583, 3). The demand for love isn't satisfied where desire fails. As Freud shows in his essay '*On the Universal Tendency to Debasement in the Sphere of Love*' (1912/1957), the dialectic of demand and desire makes things more difficult for the man. He requires the debasement of the love object in order to desire it.

Because the woman gives what she doesn't have in the masquerade and the man seeks in this the phallic signifier of his desire, his desire is constantly disappointed (583, 4). He will continually seek the phallus in another woman, and this other woman signifies the phallus as either virgin or prostitute. Unlike the woman, the man finds impotence unbearable, and his desire undergoes a perpetual displacement toward other objects that appear to signify the phallus.

But we shouldn't see infidelity as the province of men alone (583, 5). The same split in the Other is operative for woman as well, though it takes on a different form. The man she loves always has behind him a Loving Other who is the source of her satisfaction. This is the source of woman's infidelity, which can be just as rampant as man's.

This preceding analysis allows us to understand the different structures of male and female homosexuality (583, 6). Male homosexuality is constituted through desire and thus involves the man in the game of perpetual displacements, whereas female homosexuality operates through the demand for love. The mask—or masquerade—provides the key to this demand by establishing a point of identification through which the subject can find a solution to the refusal of its demand for love.

Femininity manifests itself in the mask that is the phallus, and as a result, all displays of virility seem feminine in human beings (584, 1). This contrasts the human realm with the animal, where the display of virility is most often masculine. Once again, Lacan contends, the signifier completely distorts the sexual being of subjects, distancing them from their animality.

But the centrality of the phallus in the structure of desire also shows that Freud was right to claim that there was only one libido, as he does, for instance, at the end of '*Female Sexuality*' (1930/1964). This one libido is necessarily masculine. This leads Lacan to a conclusion from psychoanalysis that confirms ancient wisdom concerning the unity of Nous and Logos. The fact that there is only one libido becomes clear with the central role that the phallus as a signifier of desire plays for both sexes. This one libido reveals that there is no divide between Nous and Logos or between mind and word. The phallic signifier brings together mind and word. The signifier doesn't permit the mind to articulate the word that it aims to say in the way it aims to say it. Instead, the signifier produces a desire in the subject that inevitably leads to words that the subject doesn't mean. The phallus signifies the impossibility of the subject ever simply saying what it means.

References

Abraham, K. (1927) 'A Short Study of the Development of the Libido, Viewed in the Light of Mental Disorders, Part II: Origins and Growth of Object Love', in *Selected Papers*. London: Hogarth, pp. 480–501.

Butler, J. (1990) *Gender Trouble: Feminism and the Subversion of Identity*. New York: Routledge.

Copjec, J. (1994) *Read My Desire: Lacan Against the Historicists*. Cambridge, MA: MIT.

de Saussure, F. (1915/1959) *Course in General Linguistics*, C. Bally and A. Sechehaye (Eds.), trans. Wade Baskin. New York: Philosophical Library.

Deutsch, H. (1930) 'The Significance of Masochism in the Mental Life of Women', *International Journal of Psychoanalysis*, 11, pp. 48–60.

Foucault, M. (1976/1978) *The History of Sexuality, Volume I: An Introduction*, trans. Robert Hurley. New York: Random House.

Freud, S. (1912/1957) 'On the Universal Tendency to Debasement in the Sphere of Love (Contributions to the Psychology of Love II)', in J. Strachey (Ed.), *The*

Standard Edition of the Complete Psychological Works of Sigmund Freud, Vol. 11. London: The Hogarth Press and the Institute of Psycho-Analysis, pp. 177–190.

Freud, S. (1913/1955) 'Totem and Taboo', in J. Strachey (Ed.), *The Standard Edition of the Complete Psychological Works of Sigmund Freud*, Vol. 13. London: The Hogarth Press and the Institute of Psycho-Analysis, pp. 1–162.

Freud, S. (1924/1961) 'Some Psychic Consequences of the Anatomical Distinction Between the Sexes', in J. Strachey (Ed.), *The Standard Edition of the Complete Psychological Works of Sigmund Freud*, Vol. 19. London: The Hogarth Press and the Institute of Psycho-Analysis, pp. 241–260.

Freud, S. (1924/1961) 'The Dissolution of the Oedipus Complex', in J. Strachey (Ed.), *The Standard Edition of the Complete Psychological Works of Sigmund Freud*, Vol. 19. London: The Hogarth Press and the Institute of Psycho-Analysis, pp. 172–179.

Freud, S. (1930/1964) 'Analysis Terminable and Interminable', in J. Strachey (Ed.), *The Standard Edition of the Complete Psychological Works of Sigmund Freud*, Vol. 23. London: The Hogarth Press and the Institute of Psycho-Analysis, pp. 209–254.

Freud, S. (1930/1964) 'Civilization and Its Discontents', in J. Strachey (Ed.), *The Standard Edition of the Complete Psychological Works of Sigmund Freud*, Vol. 21. London: The Hogarth Press and the Institute of Psycho-Analysis, pp. 57–145.

Freud, S. (1930/1964) 'Female Sexuality', in J. Strachey (Ed.), *The Standard Edition of the Complete Psychological Works of Sigmund Freud*, Vol. 21. London: The Hogarth Press and the Institute of Psycho-Analysis, pp. 223–243.

Hegel, G. W. F. (1807/1977) *The Phenomenology of Spirit*, trans. A. V. Miller. Oxford: Oxford University Press.

Horney, K. (1932) 'The Dread of Women', *International Journal of Psychoanalysis*, 13, pp. 348–360.

Jones, E. (1927) 'The Early Development of Female Sexuality', *International Journal of Psychoanalysis*, 8, 459–472.

Jones, E. (1933) 'The Phallic Phase', *International Journal of Psychoanalysis*, 14, pp. 1–33.

Kant, I. (1781/1998) *Critique of Pure Reason*, trans. P. Guyer and A. Wood. Cambridge: Cambridge University Press.

Klein, M. (1932/1975) *The Psycho-Analysis of Children*, trans. Alix Strachey. New York: Delacorte.

Lacan, J. (1973/1994) *The Seminar. Book XI: The Four Fundamental Concepts of Psycho-Analysis* (1964), trans. A. Sheridan, ed. J.-A. Miller. New York: W. W. Norton & Company.

Lacan, J. (1986/1992) *The Seminar. Book VII: The Ethics of Psychoanalysis* (1959–1960), trans. D. Porter, ed. J.-A. Miller. New York/London: W. W. Norton & Company.

Lacan, J. (1994) *Le Séminaire. Livre IV: La relation d'objet* (1956–1957), texte établi par J.-A. Miller. Paris: Éditions du Seuil.

Lacan, J. (1998) *Le Séminaire. Livre V: Les formations de l'inconscient* (1957–1958), texte étabi par J.-A. Miller. Paris: Éditions du Seuil.

Lacan, J. (2011) *Le Séminaire. Livre XIX: … ou pire* (1971–1972), texte établi par J.-A. Miller. Paris: Éditions du Seuil.

Longus (1559/1947) *Les amours pastorales de Daphnis et Chloë*, trans. J. Amyot. Paris: Horizons de France.

Mitchell, J. (1982) 'Introduction—I', in J. Mitchell and J. Rose (Eds.), *Female Sexuality: Jacques Lacan and the École Freudienne*. New York: W. W. Norton & Company, pp. 1–26.

Rivière, J. (1929) 'Womanliness as Masquerade', *International Journal of Psychoanalysis*, 10, pp. 303–313.

Rose, J. (1982) 'Introduction—II', in J. Mitchell and J. Rose (Eds.), *Female Sexuality: Jacques Lacan and the École Freudienne*. New York: W. W. Norton & Company, pp. 27–57.

Zupančič, A. (2008) *The Odd One In: On Comedy*. Cambridge, MA: MIT Press.

2

IN MEMORY OF ERNEST JONES

On His Theory of Symbolism

Filip Geerardyn and Alain Pringels

Context

The reader is not just a passive receiver of meanings that are transferred by the text. Reading is an act, at its best a creative act. Marc-Alain Ouaknin is very convincing on this in his magnificent *Bibliothérapie.* Reading turns you into a subject *par excellence* (Ouaknin, 1994: 282–283). Reading Lacan puts this thesis at its limit. The text you're reading right now is the rewarding product of a close reading of Lacan's text '*In Memory of Ernest Jones: On His Theory of Symbolism*,' henceforth called *In Memory*, and '*Syllabary*' (which is commented on by Baldwin) in a cartel 'à trois' (the authors and David Schrans). Simultaneously we read some of the texts through which Lacan wrote his palimpsest, slowly, during a semester.

Lacan's *In memory* is a 'palimpsest' in the sense that – to a significant extent – it has been written on, or better yet, through Jones's text *The theory of symbolism*. This dense interweaving of both texts becomes clear while reading Jones's text. It remains to be seen whether or not this 'palimpsest' also indicates that Jones's text is of no value to Lacan, or has been disqualified by him, as is implied in the traditional use of the word palimpsest.

Ernest Jones died on the 11th of February 1958. Exactly one year later (February 11, 1959) Lacan completes a series of seminar sessions on Ella Sharpe, and during this period he also wrote *In Memory*. Actually, in *Seminar VI – Desire and its interpretation* – Lacan dedicates five lessons on a dream analyzed by Ella Sharpe, during the months of January and February 1959. The topic of these lessons is first the status of the signifier in the praxis of psychoanalysis as part of the transference relationship between the analyst and the analysand, and second the signifier as a symptom of the cure asking to be analyzed. In March 1959 Lacan started his lessons on Hamlet. Both Ella Sharpe (1875–1947) and Ernest Jones (1878–1958) were pioneers of psychoanalysis in the United Kingdom. Both were members of the British Psychoanalytical Society founded by Jones (30/10/1930). Sharpe became a member of the Society in 1921. In 1937 she wrote her major book *Dream Analysis: A Practical Handbook for Psychoanalysts.* Based on this book Lacan discusses a dream interpretation by Sharpe in his Seminar on desire. Lacan's *In Memory* and his lessons (on Sharpe's dream analysis) are dealing with the same concern: the danger of interpretation. The danger of considering the signifier as a skin filled with meaning, waiting to be discovered. At the beginning of 1959 Lacan was studying the status of the signifier in the actual praxis of psychoanalysis. Lacan was pleading for a signifier emerging in a discourse as a sort of revelation, retroactively carrying traces of desire, the phantasm and the subject. He resisted seeing the signifier as a symbol waiting for interpretation.

On a theoretical basis one could say that this text is about Lacan's research on the status of the signifier in the analytical praxis. But there is more to it. More even than an ode for a deceased person, the text is also a petition concerning the recognition of the IPA, founded in 1910 by Freud and of which Jones had been chairman. Since 1953 Lacan and, among others, Daniel Lagache and Françoise Dolto had left the *Société Psychanalytique de Paris* (SPP), that is, the French department of IPA. The major reason for the conflict was the educational or didactic analysis. The rebelling members took a stance against the orthodoxy of Sacha Nacht, the former chairman of the SPP. Lacan and his group immediately founded a new association: the *Société Française de Psychanalyse* (SFP) and they asked for official recognition from the IPA. It was important for this group that the new analysts in training would obtain international recognition as psychoanalysts. It was a problem for the IPA to recognize two psychoanalytical associations in France. At the time that Lacan is writing his text *In Memory*, the SFP had already existed for six years without the recognition of the IPA. The question of recognition resonates through *In memory* as a kind of appeal addressed to the dead founding fathers of the IPA, being Freud and Jones himself. In that sense the Shakespeare quote at the opening of the text is more than significant.

Lacan starts *In Memory* with a quote from one of the History plays: *Henry IV part 1.* In this play King Henry is compelled to deal with the rebellion of Glyndwr, a Welshman, and Hotspur, the nickname of Sir Harry Percy, who even dares to claim the throne. Glyndwr, leader of the Welsh rebels, is a believer of ancient pagan Welsh traditions. Hotspur makes fun of these beliefs and of Glyndwr's claims of magical power. Lacan quotes Glyndwr: "And bring him out that is but woman's son / Can trace me in the tedious ways of art / And hold me pace in deep experiments." Lacan seems to disclose a mirror palace here. Quoting a Shakespearean character, like Jones a Welshman, who claims to be the best "in the tedious ways of art." The art of magic for Glyndwr, the art of psychoanalysis for Jones. As biographer of Freud and chairman of the IPA, Jones was perceived as the true heir of Freudian psychoanalysis. But it happens to be Lacan who's quoting here, not the Welshman Jones. So it seems that in the mirror image it's Lacan himself who appears to be the true heir of psychoanalysis. The only one who returns to the Freudian text. Isn't Lacan here, tongue-in-cheek, claiming to be the best "in the tedious ways of" the art of psychoanalysis? Starting his text with a sort of *Witz* wherein Lacan's appeal for recognition by the IPA for his group and their "tedious ways of art" seems to be resonating.

In his text Lacan mentions a series of missed encounters between him and Jones. It's extraordinary and provocative to start an *In Memory of* by mentioning the three times you tried to encounter the person in question but failed to do so. Three attempts that all ended in disappointment. The first encounter was at the IPA congress in Marienbad. Lacan, young explorer of psychoanalysis, 35 years old, had prepared a contribution for this conference on his elaboration of the mirror stage. Due to a lack of time chairman Jones stopped Lacan's discourse. It was Lacan's first contribution at an international conference: "his unmitigated imperiousness toward the newcomer I was in Marienbad" (585, 3). Lacan, hurt and angry, left the conference. The saying goes he went to see the Olympic Games in Berlin. The second encounter was planned in 1950 in Elsted at the residence of Jones, a house rebuilt by the son of Freud, an architect. Jones stayed there during holidays but he was working on Freud's biography. Lacan met him "among the letters by Freud spread out on an immense table" (585, 3). But the meeting was quickly cut off because Jones had an appointment with one of his patients. Lacan calls this meeting "an indelible yoke" (585, 3). And lastly Lacan mentions the letter Jones wrote to him. The letter was Jones's "apology for not coming to see me at my house in the country" (585, 3). It's July 1957. Jones had cancer and had suffered two heart attacks. He was sick and wanted to spend all the energy he had left to finish Freud's biography (585, 3). It was the very same month of the IPA conference in Paris, with Chairman Heinz Hartmann. One of the topics of this congress was Lacan's request to acknowledge his group, the SFP, as a member of the IPA. Jones was in France for the conference. Yet he rejected Lacan's invitation to meet him. It's not clear whether Lacan was trying to lobby in favor of the recognition of his rebellious group of psychoanalysts. However, retroactively the missed encounters with Jones could be seen as a metaphor for the IPA's rejection.

In a way we have already started to comment on Lacan's text. Reading his text, one has to keep a few things in mind. First of all there is Lacan's struggle to get the IPA's recognition, both on a personal level and in relation to the SFP. This is about resisting the orthodoxy of psychoanalysis (of ego analysis), Lacan's rereading of Freud's texts and the influence of both linguistics (the linguistic turn) and structuralism (Lévi-Strauss) on Lacan's insights in psychoanalysis. These three perspectives are Lacan's major tools in writing *In Memory*. It is a very close reading of Jones's *The theory of symbolism*.

The thesis Lacan puts forward, as an answer to Jones, is the following: a signifier as such – Jones would talk about a symbol – does not refer to something that is concrete (an ontological being) or to something that is there, but is always a signifier of the lack. And the phallus as signifier teaches us about this, par excellence. What we can say about the phallus as a signifier can also be said about all other signifiers. It remains that the phallus as a signifier is a specific signifier. The phallus as signifier par excellence of the lack is (but) one aspect of Lacan's theoretical elaboration in that period – the period starting from 1953 – the period in which Lacan is inspired by linguistics and structuralism. One could ask: in what sense does this signifier of the phallus differ from other signifiers? In that matter it connects directly with the human condition, that is, as bodily and at the same time 'linguistic' creatures. What is Lacan's contribution to psychoanalytic theory in his text '*In memory of Ernest Jones: On his theory of symbolism*'? Asked in the context of a university discourse, our answer to that question could be written on a cigarette paper. That contribution consists in his theory of the phallus as signifier par excellence of the lack.

Commentaries on the text

Discord: This is what motivates Lacan in writing the text. Discord "in the art of psychoanalysis" (586, 3). Discord on how "an experience of truth" (586, 3) like psychoanalysis, in fact the experience of a cure, is seen. For Lacan this experience can only be seen as something "scandalous" (586, 3) and this is how it should be understood. Every attempt in trying to find the phenomena "to be most signifying" for "the ends of utility" could be called a "consideration of power" (586, 4). Because it will affect "the very purpose" (586, 4) of the practice, being the psychoanalytical practice of the talking cure. Of course this is the whole dilemma Lacan confronts in explicitly taking a stance against the psychoanalytical orthodoxy of the IPA. "This is why no consideration of power, even the most legitimate since it involves the professional building, can intervene in the analyst's discourse without affecting the very purpose of his practice at the same time as its medium" (586, 4). The question of the training of new psychoanalysts was the main issue of recognition between the SFP and the IPA. Lacan definitely gives Jones all the credit for ensuring that "analytic values" get "official standing" (586, 5). But he wonders if all these efforts to build a theoretical framework for psychoanalysis isn't, after all, just an "immense apology" (586, 5) for the scandalous experience of the psychoanalytic cure.

> While Jones is the one who did the most to ensure analytic values a certain official standing, and even a status recognized by the public authorities, can we not propose to question the immense apology his theoretical work constitutes in order to assess its dignity?
>
> (586, 5)

For this purpose Lacan chooses "a sample of his work" (586, 6), namely *On the theory of symbolism.* Lacan chooses "a sample," meaning he could have chosen other 'symptoms' of Jones's work.

One of the main characteristics of Lacan's education and writings is humor. So not coincidently Lacan refers to Freud's inner circle or Secret Committee (586, 9). This Committee was established in 1912 on the recommendation of Jones. In his biography on Freud, Jones refers to a letter he received from Freud written on August 1st of 1912:

> What took hold of my imagination immediately is your idea of a secret council of the best and most trustworthy among our men to take care of the further development of psychoanalysis and defend the cause against personalities and accidents when I am no more … I know there is a boyish and perhaps romantic element too in this conception, but perhaps it could be adapted to meet the necessities of reality. I will give my fancy free play and leave to you the part of censor.
>
> (1955: 153)

The Committee was formed as a reaction to the differences in opinion between Freud, Jung and Adler, the latter left Freud's group of psychoanalysts. The Secret Committee would, from then on, discuss any question of alienation from the fundamental tenets of psychoanalytic theory in private. Theoretical differences would undergo a close examination before public representation. This Committee consisted of five members: Jones, Sándor Ferenczi, Otto Rank, Hanns Sachs and Karl Abraham.[1] They had all received a golden ring. Since 1919, with membership of Max Eitingon, there were seven bearers of a ring, including Freud. Here Lacan refers with tongue-in-cheek to his own problems with the IPA. A ring as a symbol of power is precisely the example Jones uses in his article before he summons the common attributes of a symbol (Jones, 1918: 183). The example Jones uses could be seen as a metaphor for Lacan's position towards the IPA. Jones: "When, in 1469, Louis XI dispossessed his brother of Normandy he publicly broke the ducal ring; the act symbolized the complete destruction of his brother's authority" (Jones, 1918: 183). This was exactly the position of Lacan: a knight banished by the IPA.

It remains unclear, however, why Lacan refers specifically to Rank and Sachs as "these autodidacts" (587, 2) either because they did not receive a proper medical training, like the other members of the initial Committee (Ferenczi, Abraham, and Jones himself), or because they did not see any patients, or whether they were not analyzed themselves. In order to distinguish 'true' symbolism from Jung's conception of symbolism, Jones bases his text on the six characteristics of true symbolism put forward by Rank and Sachs. Among others he refers to their "constant meaning" and their "non-dependence on individual conditioning factors" which Jones regards as a major step towards a rationalization of a theory of symbolism. One could say that theorizing psychoanalysis was the quest of the seven ring bearers. This is the point where Lacan presents his one and only quote from Jones's text (587, 3). It's a quote from the opening of Jones's text on "the progress of the human mind" (Jones, 1918: 181–182). For Lacan this beginning can only lead towards a fundamental ambiguity of the project as such: "Such is the tone with which things begin and they advance by ever more closely closing in on the ambiguity this departure opens up" (587, 4).

For Jones the main issue at stake here is the schism between Freud and Jung concerning their ideas on symbolism: "Jung's fundamental divergence regarding symbolism, which Freud realized already in 1911, breaking with Jung in 1912" (587, 6). Actually this is a question of the power and authority of the Secret Committee. For Lacan the main issue of *In Memory* is of a totally different order: it's the praxis of the analytical experience. "The two different manners of utilizing symbolism in interpretation are decisive as to the direction they give analysis" (587, 7). In this way Lacan warns both parties: fighting as they are for a paranoiac truth on symbolism, both parties might end up as snakes biting their own tails. One merely has to read Jones's text (1918: 204–205) where he points out the differences between a Jungian interpretation and the one prescribed by the Secret Committee:

> By the psycho-analyst the symptom would be regarded as the result of the complex and, in certain circumstances, as a symbol for it; Jung, on the other hand, calls the complex the symbol of the symptom, i.e., according to him, an unconscious idea may be a symbol of a conscious one.

It looks as if Lacan wants to warn us against this kind of defensive theorization:

> A figuration of the libido—that is how a disciple of Jung's will interpret the appearance of a snake in a dream, vision, or drawing, manifesting, unbeknown to himself, that while its seductive power is eternal, it is also always the same. For here we see the subject about to be captured by an autistic eros which, however revamped its [theoretical] apparatus may be, seems like an Old Acquaintance.
>
> (588, 2)

The point is that Lacan is very consequent in the one perspective he values the most: every bit of his writings and teachings start with the praxis of the cure, the analytical experience comes first. An insight Lacan owes to a rereading of Freud.

Finally, the discoveries of Freud are what it is all about. Concerning the Freudian discoveries Lacan is very clear: "that there is no compromise possible with psychology" (588, 6). Jung's interpretation of the libido and the investigations of Brücke, Helmholtz and Du Bois-Reymond, his forerunners in psychology are, according to Lacan, no more than attempts to save the human soul.

> In other words, the soul, which is a lucid blind man, reads its own nature in the archetypes that the world echoes back to him: how could he not end up believing he is the world soul? What is strange is that in their haste to take this soul into account, Calvinist pastors were fooled.
>
> (588, 3–4)

It's in this context that Lacan mentions the name of Herbert Silberer for the first time.

The major discovery of Freud is of course the workings of the unconscious. This is what instigated a Copernican revolution, but still it is very difficult to grasp the impact of these insights. This is exactly the heart of Lacan's text: "Still it is not easy to grasp the cut so boldly traced by Freud in the theory of the revision [elaboration] of dreams" (588, 7). It is interesting to take a closer look at Silberer's role in this discussion. Herbert Silberer (1882–1923) was the son of Viktor Silberer, a very wealthy and successful entrepreneur in Vienna. His father wanted him to be a sports hero but he ended up as head of sports in a journal owned by his father. Silberer took an interest in psychoanalysis and joined the Freudian Viennese circle of psychoanalysis. That's where he met Jung. He published on dreams, hallucinations and on symbolism (Silberer, 1910, 1912, 1914). These writings inspired both Freud and Jung. In 1923 Silberer committed suicide by hanging. Was he crushed between two giants of psychoanalysis? Four works by Silberer are mentioned in the bibliography of *The interpretation of dreams*. Freud's quotations on these works have been added in additional texts and footnotes in 1911, 1914, 1919 and 1925. The first quotes are positive, but later on the remarks on Silberer's work become more critical. In a footnote, added in 1911, Freud writes: "Silberer (1909) has given some nice examples of the way in which, in a drowsy state, even abstract thought become converted into pictorial plastic images which seek to express the same meaning" (Freud, 1900/1982: 114). In 1925 Freud adds a reference to this footnote. A reference to a paragraph he added at the same time. It's a paragraph in what's perhaps the most important chapter of Freud's book: *The dream-work*. More specifically it's an addition to the section dealing with *Secondary revision*. It's specifically this chapter that Lacan pinpoints as a "cut," a fracture, which is "not easy to grasp" (588, 7). Things not even Silberer could grasp. We can read this in a footnote Freud added in 1911 and in an addition to this note he added in 1914. But more important is the paragraph Freud adds in 1924. Speaking on *Secondary revision* in *The dream-work* he marks the main difference between his own vision and

Silberer's. Grasping this point is precisely what Lacan devoted his life and work to. What exactly are the critical notes Freud has on Silberer? In an addition to *Secondary revision* that Freud adds in 1924: "The very interesting functional phenomenon of Silberer's has, through no fault of its discoverer's, led to many abuses; for it has been regarded as lending support to the old inclination to give abstract and symbolic interpretations to dreams" (Freud, 1900/1982: 648). And further on in the chapter named *The psychology of the dream-processes*, in the section on *The forgetting of dreams*, Freud adds in 1919:

> On the other hand, I cannot confirm the opinion, first stated by Silberer, that all dreams (or many dreams, or certain classes of dreams) require two different interpretations which are even stated to bear a fixed relation to each other. One of these interpretations, which Silberer calls the 'psychoanalytic' one, is said to give the dream some meaning or other, usually of an infantile-sexual kind; the other and more important interpretation which he calls 'anagogic', is said to reveal the more serious thoughts, often of profound import, which the dream-work has taken as its material. [...] As in the case of many other theories put forward in recent years, it is impossible to overlook the fact that Silberer's views are influenced to some extent by a purpose which seeks to disguise the fundamental circumstances in which dreams are formed and to divert interest from their instinctual roots.
>
> (1900/1982: 670)

Silberer seems to be at the focus of the struggle between the Secret Committee and dissident thinkers like Jung. We already mentioned that in 1911 Freud was rather positive about Silberer's discoveries. But he becomes critical on Silberer because his theories open the door for Jungian visions on the dream-work. Lacan, caught in a similar battle between orthodoxy and non-orthodoxy, is very clear on this:

> Let us bc glad that spiritual hierarchies—along with the materials, pneumatics, psychics, and all the rest—did not return through this door, but we see here the source of the infatuation of those who consider themselves to be 'natural born psychoanalysts.'
>
> (588, 8)

Instead of getting lost in translation, finding symbolic or mythic explanations of symbols in dreams, Lacan wants us to keep focusing on the signifier appearing in a dream. The signifier veils an emptiness and camouflages a revelation of instinctual forces at work, covered and caused by the most wanted and most feared object *a*.

Is it worth noting that Lacan only mentions Freud's 1914 additions to *The interpretation of dreams* concerning Silberer and not his additions in 1919 and in 1925.

Jones, in his text, warns against opening the doors of mysticism. Lacan:

> Regarding the snake, Jones rectifies [Jung's position by asserting] that it is the symbol not of libido—an energetic notion which, as an idea, can only be brought out at a high degree of abstraction—but of the phallus, insofar as the latter seems to him to be characteristic of a "more concrete idea," even concrete through and through.
>
> (589, 2)

Referring to Jones's text: "Hence the common mistaken view that symbolism in general represents the abstract in terms of the concrete" (Jones, 1918: 213). It's about literally looking at the signifier, listening to the concreteness of its gaze. "For this is the pathway Jones chooses with which to ward off the dangerous return to a kind of mysticism that symbolism seems to allow for" (589, 3). "True symbolism" (Jones, 1918: 213) is about taking the symbol seriously in accepting its concreteness as part of a given particularity. Silberer operates in the opposite direction. Silberer sees "symbolism as the presentation of the abstract in terms of the concrete" (Jones, 1918: 213). Lacan:

> The symbol is displaced from a more concrete idea (at least that is how he expresses himself on the subject), to which it primarily applies, to a more abstract idea, to which it relates secondarily, which means that this displacement can only take place in a single direction.
>
> (589, 4)

This displacement is part of *secondary revision*. Lacan: "this snake is the symbol of the phallus and of nothing else" (589, 6). Lacan is referring to the case of Anna O. (Freud and Breuer, 1893–1895/1983). The snakes in Anna's hallucinations are not symbols of an abstract idea you can explore through mythology or some kind of a collective unconscious. The snakes are a product of—to quote Freud—"a strong unanalysed positive transference of an unmistakably sexual nature" (1893–1895/1983: 95). The hallucinated snakes are, in a way of speaking, a gift of love towards her doctor Joseph Breuer. A phallus at its purest, symbolizing the lack Breuer was looking for. As if the snakes were masks hiding the question "is this what you're looking for, doctor?" Empty signifiers hiding an even more existential questioning of her being: "stop looking for an answer to the question 'who am I' doctor, just take me as I am." A questioning primordially aimed at Anna's own father.

Taking the symbol seriously in all its concreteness, means focusing on displacement, resistance and secondary revision. For Lacan some ways of the art of psychoanalysis are nothing more than overlooking this focus. Lacan: "But to whom this phallus belongs 'concretely' is what is less easy to determine in the register of contemporary psychoanalysis that is so nicely labeled by Raymond Queneau as the *liquette ninque*" (589, 6). Queneau's novel *Zazie in the subway* (1959) is about a young girl's first encounter with the big city. She has one dream: taking the Paris metro. But due to a strike in public traffic she has to move through Paris in taxis and by foot. Louis Malle adapted a very lighthearted movie based on this novel (1960). It's one of Queneau's most well-known writings. The "*liquette ninque*" is a hapax from Queneau's novel. He used it in the context of describing how difficult it is to do the laundry. They are talking about an upcoming product of the consumer society, namely the washing machine. One of the characters has an ad hoc problem: getting away with dirt. A nice example of the concreteness of the phallus: something that keeps on insisting in writing itself. Dirt's devilish emptiness. Something that never stops rewriting itself, such as getting rid of the dirt over and over again.

Jones in his text *On symbolism* proposes arguments against the anagogic interpretation of symbols. Jones: "Along this path the post-psycho-analytical school loses itself in a perfect maze of mysticism, occultism, and theosophy into which I do not propose to penetrate" (Jones, 1918: 222). As if speaking in the name of the Secret Committee, he continues:

> We are concerned with three groups of psychical material: (1) the unconscious complexes, (2) the inhibiting influences (Freud's ethical censor) that keep these in a state of repression, and (3) the sublimated tendencies derived from unconscious complexes. In my judgment, the relation of symbolism to these three groups is this. Like the third group, symbols are a product of intrapsychical conflict between the first two groups. The material of the symbol is taken from the third group. The second group, which prevents the first one from coming to direct expression, is to some extent represented in the formation of the symbol; but the dynamic force that creates the symbol, the meaning carried by the symbol, and the reason for the very existence of the symbol, are all derived from the first group, the unconscious complexes. The fundamental fallacy of Silberer's work, as it seems to me, is that he tends to confound the process of symbolic equivalency with that of symbolism itself, as was indicated above in regard to the relation between symbolism and mental progress.
>
> (1918: 223)

Analytical work means in the first place listening to the *secondary revision* at work. And these processes are always at work. Even in the development of a theoretical framework. So referring to Jones's later works on the phallic phase Lacan asks:

> does the phallus—if it is truly the object of phobia or of perversion, which he relates, first the one and then the other, to the phallic phase—remain in the state of a 'concrete idea'? In any case, he is forced to recognize that the phallus takes on a 'secondary' application here.
> (589, 7)

Jones's elaborations on the phallic phase are from the late twenties and the early thirties. Lacan adds an important note concerning the effects of these elaborations; they stop any thinking about symbolism in psychoanalysis until Lacan's paper '*The Function and Field of Speech and Language in Psychoanalysis*.' The point Lacan wants to make is very clear: "I am getting ahead of myself, as you see, regarding the only notion that allows us to conceive of the symbolism of the phallus: the particularity of its function as a signifier" (590, 1).

In his text *In Memory* it seems that Lacan wants his readers to keep something more important 'in memory' than the works of Ernest Jones. In his text he follows traces of Jones's and Silberer's thinking, both trying to find a theoretical framework on symbolism. The first, Jones, by closely relating to Freud's thinking (as Lacan also does), the latter, by adding new pathways to the art of psychoanalysis, being the 'anagogic' interpretation. Lacan shows us the pitfalls of both. First of all, he underlines that the work of Jones should be considered in view of the schism between Freud and Jung. The importance of Jones's critical thinking on Silberer's work is about opening paths to mysticism. But second, Lacan criticizes Jones's thinking in his persistence of elaborating a theoretical framework of psychoanalysis, in a kind of quest for an objective truth on psychoanalysis, most importantly where Jones neglects the primacy of the signifier, the logic of the signifier. With Slavoj Žižek we would like to emphasize the following: "Lacan rehabilitates a knowledge more radical than truth, a knowledge touching the real" (Žižek, 2016: 217). It's a knowledge following a different logic than the logic of truth. The logic of truth follows the logic of interpretation as in the case of a symptom. The logic touching the real follows the logic of construction as in the case of phantasm. Even though Jones "immediately realized that analytic symbolism is only conceivable if it is related to the linguistic fact of metaphor" (590, 2) he keeps on looking for a contingency between the symbol and "the primordial complexes displayed in symbolism" (590, 4). Jones, similar to Freud, rejects a mythological interpretation of symbols; the so-called 'anagogic' way of Silberer and Jung. But he continues to look for a theoretical contingency of symbols with some sort of archaic layers of the unconscious referring to a pre-language age. Jones:

> All psycho-analytical experience goes to show that the primary ideas of life, the only ones that can be symbolised – those namely, concerning the bodily self, the relation to the family, birth, love

> and death – retain in the unconscious throughout life their original importance, and that from them is derived a very large part of the more secondary interests of the conscious mind.
>
> (1918: 204)

Jones believes in a 'real' truth that is hidden behind symbols, a 'true symbolism,' originating in a primordial past. For Lacan the only source for the creation of symbols lies in the network of the signifier. Lacan:

> All of these are "ideas," the most concrete of which is the network of the signifier in which the subject must already be caught up in order to be able to constitute himself there as self, as part of a lineage, as existing, as the representative of a sex, and even as dead, for these ideas can only be passed off as primary if all parallelism with the development of needs is abandoned.
>
> (590, 7)

All that matters is the logic of the signifier. The field of the signifier was already there long before we were born. This is precisely the reason why we have to take those ideas seriously, as concretely as possible. The logic of the signifier is the only way of letting those ideas speak for themselves. Not by looking for a kind of mythical or past reality behind them but as a true revelation, a construction happening right now. An appearance shifting from one signifier to the other. It all comes down on Lacan's definition of the signifier as that which represents the subject for another signifier. The problem with Jones is that he didn't render the signifier "it's primacy" (591, 4). Lacan:

> Absent this step, he did not manage to formulate what analytic interpretation nevertheless makes almost obvious, which is that the relationship between reality [reel] and what is thought is not that between the signified and the signifies and that the primacy reality [reel] has over thought is reversed from the signifier to the signified.
>
> (591, 5)

The effects of meaning are created by "permutations of signifier" (591, 5). Reality loses its primacy over thought. The signifier determines reality as we see or think it.

For Jones, symbolism is constituted through "the memory of a metaphor" (591, 6). Jones calls this the evolution or decay of the metaphor in which he determines three stages. In the first we see a shift in the use of a word from its literal sense to a figurative sense. In the second stage both senses (literal and figurative) become so familiar that the difference between the two senses is blurred or unnoticed. In the third stage the figurative sense predominates and becomes the literal (usual) one (Jones, 1918: 185). For Lacan, analytic symbolism generates its meaning through the permutation of the signifier. It's the displacement of one signifier for another that constitutes meaning. Lacan gives two examples on pages 591 and 592: the roar of the lion of the media company Metro Goldwyn Mayer (MGM) and the creation of the 'new franc' by the government of General de Gaulle.

The logo of a company is a narcissistic representation of the "self-satisfied" ideals of that company (591, 6). In fact, up to now six different lions have been used in the history of the MGM logo. To position a lion in front of a camera is not an easy thing to do. Instead of going to Africa and hoping for the right camera shot, you use a domesticated or trained lion. So most of the MGM lions were circus lions. But even when you use a trained lion it takes a lot of patience and time before Mr. Lion does what the image of a logo requires. Those familiar with the training and handling of exotic animals know well how difficult it can be to get a creature such as a lion to roar on command. Even lions have personality, even more than some real actors have. So Jones "does not see that it is the lion as a signifier that has been abraded right to the yon, and even to the yon-yon, whose meek growl serves as an index of the self-satisfied ideals of Metro-Goldwyn" (591, 8). The roar of the MGM logo is a signifier which has nothing to do with the roar of the African lion in the bush.

The second example concerns the creation of the 'new franc' by the government of General de Gaulle. A few months before Lacan writes his *In Memory* the French government decided for a devaluation of the French franc. On the 27th of December 1958 the economic plan Pinay-Rueff was approved by president de Gaulle. It was part of an economic restructuring of post-war France. In practice it meant that one 'new franc' would be worth 100 'old francs.' So something you paid 318 old francs for, would now cost 3,18 new francs. The French called this new franc "le franc lourd," the heavy franc, meaning that every Frenchman would be "carrying a heavier [plus lourd] wallet when he has equally weighty bill denominations [poids des coupures" (592, 2). Exploring the metaphor of 'le franc lourd,' Lacan asks:

> But what can we say about the application that gave us this word, lourd – namely, the new unit of French monetary reform? What vertiginous or grave perspective will we open up, what trance of thickness will we resort to, to situate this new flapping of wings from the literal to the figurative? Would it not be simpler to accept here the obvious material fact that there is no other mainspring of metaphorical effect than the substitution of one signifier for another as such?
>
> (592, 2)

The relationship between signifier and signified is one of pure contingency. This doesn't mean that there is no effect of meaning.

In this regard we believe that it is important to read Lacan very slowly; not to find deeper and heavy-weight meaning in his text, but to be able to discover the playfulness with which he lets the signifier permutate as if it was in a carrousel, with a great talent for comedy. Reread, for example, paragraph 3 on page 592 and take your time to discover the associations it is pregnant with. After the devaluation of the French franc the Frenchman will be carrying a heavier wallet but he will not feel it because there will be fewer coins and less paper money in his wallet.

> And who can say how weighted [ponderation] his spending will become in his tourist peregrinations, but also the unforeseeable effects that the metaphorical sliding of his metal coin-related likings toward heavy [lourde] industry and heavy machinery will have on the El Dorados of his investments or his luxury utensils?
>
> (592, 3)

This 'economical metaphor' shows how the shift in the 'weight' of a signifier generates an effect of meaning. Lacan's paragraph, and indeed his writing and his spoken word, open up a rizomatic network of signifiers referring to other signifiers. In this particular case he pinpoints the added value of a signifier when he is tangled up in a metaphor disrupted by an alienating displacement. In this case the devaluation will have an effect on the Frenchman's "El Dorado of his investments of his luxury utensils." The devaluation of the French franc in 1959 created a boost in consumerism in the sixties. Not only Lacan foresaw this effect of meaning. Remember the paragraph where he refers to the novel of Queneau, more specifically to a dialogue on the usefulness of buying a washing machine. The El Dorado that Lacan is criticizing is the beginning of a mass consumption society in the fifties. Where an endless series of products as desirable objects will gradually empty out all of the subject's desire, reducing it to a wallet, an object with no ideas at all, filling and emptying his pockets endlessly.

The major point in this discussion between Freud, Silberer, Jones and Lacan is "whether or not a knowledge-value [valeur de connaissance] should be granted to symbolism" (592, 5). Even though symbolism "has the importance of informing us about a more primitive activity in being" (592, 5) one should not "fall into the sin of circular reasoning (…) to deduce from it that a more profound reality, even if qualified as psychical, is manifested in it" (593, 1). The importance of symbolism in the cure is not the discovery of a deeper level of reality, but the possibility it generates to add fluidity to the chain of signifiers. So the importance of symbolism is the discovery of the "structural function" (593, 2) of the signifier. And that point Jones misses completely:

> All of Jones' efforts are devoted to denying that an archaic symbolism can retain any value compared to a scientific apprehension of

> reality. But since he continues to refer symbols to ideas, understanding by ideas the concrete props that development is supposed to give symbols, he himself cannot help but maintain the notion of a negative conditioning of symbolism right to the bitter end, which stops him from grasping its structural function.
>
> (593, 2)

This is exactly the function that the signifier "quack" has for the child as Jones mentions in an example: "Darwin's oft quoted example of the child who, on first seeing a duck, onomatopoetically named it 'quack' and then later applied this word also to flies, wine, and even a sou" (Jones, 1918: 197). Lacan himself gives the example of "the child, who designates with a "bow-wow" what in certain cases we strove in front of him to call only by the name of "dog," assigns this "bow-wow" to just about anything" (593, 5). The signifier structures the reality of the child: "it is by the play of signifying substitution that the child rips things from their ingenuousness in subjecting them to his metaphors" (593, 7).

According to Jones, analytical symbolism has the same structure as the structural base that Freud assigns to symptoms and repression. He sets the same goals, namely "to repair the deviation the unconscious underwent" (594, 2). This reparation could be seen as a sort of translation of the unconscious value of the symbol. It is not the meaning nor the concreteness of the symbol which determines its unconscious effect, but its concrete impact "in repressing desire into the position of that which is misrecognized" (594, 6). Or "it is the signifier's concrete impact in submitting need to demand" (594, 6). The game with signifiers plays an active part in structuring the subject's reality. So the drive to kill or eat a duck or to run away from it in fear, is quickly run over with signifiers such as "quack" or "duck." Soon an army of signifiers will be framing and reframing the subject's desire, "repressing desire into the position of that which is misrecognized" (594, 6). Creating a sort of encyclopedic vocabulary of symbols is absurd. The creation of symbols is infinite because it is "open to individual invention" (594, 7). This "very enlightening remark" (594, 7) puts limits on any given ambition in creating an exhaustive catalogue of symbols. This confronts us with the kernel of the 'talking cure.' Any speaking subject "sustains himself there only on the basis of discourse" (594, 8). The "primary ideas" (ibid.) lurking behind the symbol are exactly the points "at which the subject disappears under the being of the signifier" (594, 8). Masking "the lack of being" (594, 9) is precisely the point where "phallic symbols" (594, 9) take their function. From the moment a child is born into language and discovers its existence in a field of signifiers, desire emerges. This is called the *Ürverdrängung* and is why desire is linked to the concept of castration. The lack-of-being will from now on be situated in the Other. Signifiers of the lack are the cause of "the subject's reduplication brought on by discourse" (595, 2). Lacan:

> It is thus clear that analysis reveals that the phallus serves the function of signifying the lack of being [*manque à être*] that is wrought in the subject by his relation to the signifier. This gives its full import to the fact that all the symbols highlighted in Jones' study are phallic symbols.
>
> (595, 1)

These "points of the subject's umbilication" (595, 2) refer to "the most fundamental of them being the *Urverdrängung* [primal repression]" (595, 2).

"Analysis has shown us that it is with images that captivate his eros as a living individual that the subject manages to ensure his implication in the signifying sequence" (595, 3). This is exactly what happens during what Lacan called 'the mirror stage.' In *The Mirror Stage* Lacan describes how an infant assumes a *Gestalt* of his body, his specular image, as a primordial *I*, while physically feeling as a '*corps morcelé*' (1949/2006: 75). A process of identification that is mediated through signifiers offered by the (m)Other. "For the total form of his body, by which the subject anticipates the maturation of his power in a mirage, is given to him only as a gestalt, that is, in an exteriority" (1949/2006: 76). The narcissistic form the implication of desire in the signifier assumes, is the '*deus ex machina*' in the play where '*corps morcelé*' and specular image are the protagonists. Drive will be articulated in repeatedly insisting structures and sequences of the signifier. Permutating endlessly.

> The function of the mirror stage thus turns out, in my view, to be a particular case of the function of imagos, which is to establish a relationship between an organism and its reality – or, as they say, between the *Innenwelt* and the *Umwelt*.
>
> (78, 4)

Desire becomes a sort of algorithm between drive (the Real), imago (the Imaginary) and the signifiers (the Symbolic). This is why human sexuality is not at play on the stage we biologically call the sexual organs. Language in its function always stumbles on its impossibility to symbolize sexuality. Lacan explores this in his *Seminar XVIII, D'un discours qui ne serait pas du semblant* (S18, 1971: 148). The subject is divided by the signifier through which it endlessly keeps permutating in order to pass the lack-of-being. An impossibility, knowing that the signifier is always mediated through the Other. Lacan calls this "the subject's reduplication by the signifier" (595, 8). This recalls what Lacan writes in '*The Signification of the Phallus*' (581, 12): "The fact that the phallus is a signifier requires that it be in the place of the Other that the subject have access to it". The phallic symbol is a structure that centers itself on a lack, and which gives the field or chain of signifiers its order or cohesion.

Jones is trying to grasp this "heterogeneity of the 'true symbolism'" (595, 10). However, it's impossible.

> A minimum composition of the battery of signifiers suffices to institute in the signifying chain a duplicity that re-covers his reduplication as a subject, and it is in this redoubling of the subject of speech that the unconscious as such finds a way to become articulated – namely, in a medium that is only apperceived by being perceived as just as stupid as a cryptography without a cipher.
>
> (595, 9)

In that sense the discourse of every speaking subject functions as an oracle of Delphi. It is a place where truth speaks without being expressed intentionally by the speaker. The "knowledge-value symbols have" (596, 2) "is considerable when it comes to praxis, is nil when it comes to reality [*réel*]" (596, 2). There is no absolute truth to be said on any symbol or signifier. The value of a symbol lies in its particularity as a creation during the praxis of the talking cure, as an event, a process of truth. What more can there be said of paragraph two on page 596. A paragraph in which the signifier 'members' turn up five times. This makes it a very enigmatic paragraph. This is Lacan at its best: the analyst hiding behind the mask of … Punchinello. Humorous and full of wit Lacan uses a word that in French (and in English) has a double meaning: 'member' ('membre' in French). Meaning 'being a member of a group' (re*member* Lacan's starting point in writing this text as an excluded *member* of the psychoanalytic group), and also meaning 'dick,' 'cock,' 'prick' or 'willy' (in French 'queue,' 'zizi,' 'bite'). So we can formulate the hypothesis that the signifier 'members' in this paragraph stands for the phallus as signifier of the lack, or the object, of desire. In this particular paragraph the value of the symbol 'members' lies in the praxis of reading with a double attention.

"It is very striking to see how much effort it takes Jones to establish this conclusion" Lacan argues (596, 3). Jones clearly tries to make a division in what he calls "true symbolism" as the producer of symbols, creation at its purest and "symbolic equivalents" which can be measured objectively in reality. But Jones's desire to formulate a scientific theory on symbolism makes it very difficult. To illustrate true symbolism Jones refers to a phallic symbol: Punchinello. An example of an empty signifier, impossible to interpret and escaping all definite forms of meaning. Very much like the 'Name-of-the-Father.' Here Jones is very close to Lacan. But what Jones calls the "symbolic equivalents" are indeed symbols ready to be interpreted or measured objectively. Precisely what Rank and Sachs are up to (see Rank and Sachs, 1913: 11). Jones quotes them:

> The symbol represents an almost ideal union of all these means of expression: it is a substitutive, perceptual replacement-expression for something hidden, with which it has evident characteristics in common or is coupled by internal associative connections. Its essence lies in its having two or more meanings, as indeed it originated itself in a

> kind of condensation, an amalgamation of individual characteristic elements.
>
> (1918: 188)

This is how Jones presents a theory of "true symbolism" to the world of science. Lacan believes this is a mistake, demonstrating that science is impossible without "the extermination of all symbolism" (596, 5). As the history of science clearly demonstrates: science is a gradually abolishing and counteracting of belief and superstition, of mythic and religious symbolism. Lacan:

> For the history of science alone can settle this matter and it brilliantly demonstrates, in the birth of the theory of gravitation, that it was only on the basis of the extermination of all symbolism of the heavens that the terrestrial foundations of modern physics could be established.
>
> (596, 5)

"Rediscovering the traces of a logical creation" (596, 6), is at stake. This is precisely what science does. So the history of physics as a science is a narrative of deconstructing and abolishing all possibilities of metaphysics and harmonic or religious images of the universe. Lacan takes the same route with psychoanalysis by stopping all mythological or metaphysical interpretations of symbols and studying them as empty signifiers. In this regard Lacan sees sublimation as a "detour": "the usual detour of all sublimation" (596, 6). A detour which will always be left incomplete. *Durcharbeiten* or working through is the message (596, 7). This is the most important argument of Freud's *The interpretation of dreams.* Psychoanalysis is not about interpreting symbols but about analyzing the primary process that creates symbols: "that analysis, in the case of dreams but of symptoms too, needs to highlight symbolism only as subordinate to the major mainsprings of the processes [elaboration] that structure the unconscious – namely, condensation and displacement first and foremost" (597, 94). The quest for the remains and signs of a presupposed identity that once existed between a symbol and a reality is not important. In psychoanalysis symbols exist by the grace of repression: "This is strictly correct insofar as symbolism is considered to be intimately related to repression" (597, 6). It's a kind of prohibition (a "no") that creates the circumstance by which a substituted operation "becomes truly symbolic" (597, 5) of an affect. The divergence between Jones and Lacan becomes very clear with Jones's example of agriculture as a form of sexualized tasks, becoming symbols of sexuality during the ages.

> It was just the way in which primitive man must have met the world, the desire for ease and pleasure struggling with the demands of necessity. He succeeded by making a compromise in which he sexualized

> his tasks. A few examples may be given from the vast subject of the associations between ploughing in particular, or agricultural in general, and sexual activities.
>
> (1918: 199)

For Lacan it is the mediation of the (phallic) signifier that sexualizes things. This is what he calls "a certain effect of the laws of marriage and kinship" (597, 5). It is this "operation substituted for the former operation" that "becomes truly symbolic of a sexual satisfaction" (597, 5). Lacan is amazed that Jones does not come to this conclusion because "he would have gained much in his quest to grasp the true place of symbolism had he remembered that it was granted no room at all in the first edition of the Traumdeutung" (597, 8). Reading this paragraph in Lacan should remind you of the Shakespeare quote with which he opens his *In memory.* It indicates a difference in view.

And what exactly makes this difference? Jones doesn't take Freud's warning seriously in believing "that what is repressed in symbolism's metaphorical retreat is affect" (598, 2). The result of this hypothesis is "an extraordinarily ambiguous exploration of the whole panoply of affects, insofar as they supposedly substitute for each other as such" (598, 2). Freud is not ambiguous on this at all. In his writings on the drive, on repression and on the unconscious (all written about 1915), Freud articulates unambiguously that "it is the signifier that is repressed, there being no other meaning that can be given in these texts to the word *Vorstellungsrepräsantanz*" (598, 3). Affects are not repressed. "Freud articulates that affects are simply displaced" (598, 3). The less an affect is justified, the more a subject is bound to 'understand' it. Silence is the *via regia* for such an 'understanding.' Silence is one of the hardest things to endure during the cure. Gradually the uncomfortable silence will make place for a comfortable silence. A silent silence with no tension, no expectations, except for one thing maybe … a smile. Silence opens up the doors of the real. Knowing when to make or create silence is crucial. But making silence is not the same as keeping quiet. Lacan makes this point in his Seminar *Crucial problems for psychoanalysis* (1964–1965), seminar of Wednesday 17th of March. But silence has nothing to do with the analyst keeping his mouth shut. Just keeping quiet is not silence.[2] The presence of a silence does not depend on two people who stop talking. It's silence as a creation. Exactly what God did on the seventh day … The Sabbatical rest is not an absence of work, but a real creation, the creation of "emptiness" or "the nothing" (Ouaknin, 1994: 67). The seventh day is the empty day. The day where time takes time to renew itself (Sibony, 1992: 150). Every creation is left radically unfinished if it doesn't create the emptiness as a suspension of time. A narrative suspension creating time for new creations to come. An emptiness that carries time further on, to a 'more' to come, "un encore à venir" (Ouaknin, 1994: 67). When Jones tries to describe the characteristics of true symbolism he writes that "an important characteristic of true symbolism is that the interpretation of the symbol usually evokes a reaction of surprise, incredulity, and repugnance on the part of those unfamiliar with it" (Jones, 1918: 186). Aren't these reactions always in a sense preceded by a silence? A small suspension of time followed by a creative breakthrough (associations) or by a resistance (repression). Silence convokes the proximity of the Thing or the absence of the Other. In a way silence is an indication of the joining of the Thing and the Other (Morin, 2009: 6).

Nothing creates a more baffling silence than homophonies – be it in a slip of the tongue, a joke or wordplay. Mostly the silence is almost immediately followed by laughter. A joyful affect as an effect "of the very loss the subject suffers due to the fragmentation brought on by the signifier" (599, 2). The signifier of this loss is what we call "the phallus." An empty signifier "by which an object is led into the subordination of desire to the symbolic dialectic" (599, 2). It's the empty signifier "dad" or "mum" that leads the objects representing them into a symbolic field, an endless play of signifiers representing one another, subordinating desire to the symbolic dialectic. "Mum" and "dad" as signifiers are empty. When you speak of your "mum" everybody knows who you're talking about, even though they haven't got a clue of the particular use the signifier has for the user. If there is any 'true symbolism' as Jones suggests, then it should be one that respects the particularity of its creation. Any scientific knowledge on symbols opens up doors to moralism.

The Italian *Pulchinello* became in England *Punchinello*. Lacan: "The Neapolitan *polecenella*, little turkey, *pulcinella*, little chicken, and *pullus*, a tender term bequeathed by Roman pederasty to the modest outpourings of romantic schoolgirls in my youth, are recovered here by the English "punch," in order, having become *punchinello*" (Lacan, 598, 3). Jones takes *Punchinello* as an example of a phallic symbol explaining it as a "conception of the male organ as a mannikin" (Jones, 1918: 186). He refers to "dwarfs and gnomes," "the long hooked nose, long chin, projecting hump on his back, prominent stomach, and pointed cap," "Priapus," "iconoclasms, seditions, and blasphemies" and "linguistic connections" (Jones, 1918: 186, 187, 190). Lacan's comment is sharp: "How can one fail to see the dominance of the signifier here, manifest in its most materially phonemic form?" (598, 4). And Lacan is right. There is more to be said to *Pulchinello* as a phallic symbol than to the references Jones is making. The figure of *Pulchinello* goes back further than the Renaissance. *Pulchinello* existed long before *Commedia dell'arte* was born. He was part of the jesters who took over the cities during *Carnival* or mid-winter festivities in the middle Ages. He acted in a group. A group of *Punchinellos* terrorizing the community with *lazzi*, sketches and jokes. Jones: "the modern Italian *pulcino* means pullet, *pulcinello* being its diminutive" (Jones, 1918: 190). From that point on Jones starts up a rather 'phallic' association naming "the turkey-cock," "the domestic cock," "the young of any animal," "the idea of a male child, a little boy or little man" (Jones, 1918: 190). An interpretation that brings the male organ into focus. But he misses a crucial point. The Italian philosopher Giorgio Agamben points out that the etymological meaning of *pulcino* is uncertain. According to Agamben there are indications that the diminutive *pulleciniello* seems in a strange way to refer to the female organ, or at least to an uncertain sex (Agamben, 2017: 37). Everyone who has bred chickens knows how difficult it is to determine the gender of a pullet. The real of a pullet is having an uncertain sex. Also, the mask of *Pulchinello* indicates the figure as an empty signifier. Compared with the other *Commedia dell'arte* masks *Pulchinello* is the only one with a black mask. A rather neutral mask with as a main characteristic a bowed nose. More likely a symbol of impotence than of an erect phallic member, which is reserved for the mask of *Il Capitano*, he has a long nose standing right up. Agamben (2017: 44) calls this the expressionlessness of the *Pulchinello*-mask. A *Pulchinello*-actor did not take off his mask to greet the public after his performance. Because in reality there was no face behind the mask. No face and even no voice. An actor impersonating *Pulchinello* was trained for years to be able to speak with what is called a *pivetta* or *swazzle*. A little device positioned between the tongue and the roof of the mouth, used to produce a distinctive harsh, rasping voice. The voice of *Pulchinello* is not a human voice, it is an artificial voice, a non-voice (Agamben, 2017: 100). This artificial voice is another charateristic which differentiates him from the other characters of *Commedia dell'arte* (Agamben, 2017: 99). It is with this artificial voice that *Pulchinello* speaks very rhythmically, exploring the limits of language and demonstrating the impossibility of communication. *Pulchinello* always understands the other in a wrong sense. So language is not fit to communicate, its only purpose is to make us laugh. This is what his *lazzis* or sketches are about. They suspend every action with nonsense, jokes and jests. Be it a dramatic action, in a play or our daily action when we meet a horde of *Pulchinellos* involved in a street act. And whatever his actions, he never has to take any responsibility for them. Even when he is put to justice by law, in the end he will escape punishment. Not because of his innocence in crime, but because of what he is: just a character you can't reproach, a mask with no morals, a voice with no personality, an empty shell who does tricks and *lazzis*. The *lazzi* makes us laugh because the action of which it consists is refuted or challenged by that action itself. Every action in a *lazzi* loses its political consistence. In this way *Pulchinello*'s actions not only demonstrate the impossibility to communicate, but also the impossibility to act. This doesn't mean *Pulchinello* is apolitical. He announces another way of politics: he shows what a body can do when every action has become impossible. In this way the law, confronted with *Pulchinello*, always shows its comical mask: a court room or a police arrest become a parody in no time (Agamben, 2017: 52). Jones was right after all: *Pulchinello* is a phallic symbol par excellence, an empty signifier, communicating nothing, doing nothing, but dominant in its most material form, a mask.

When Lacan points out Jones's major contribution to psychoanalysis as being "the elaboration of the phallic phase" (599, 3), he warns for "the dawn of the maze in which clinical work itself has gotten bogged down" (599, 3). Any phased elaboration heads towards a question of normalization and, as such, towards moralization. Focusing on developmental stages like the oral, the anal and the phallic phases opens the door for a standardization. This kind of focus creates a noise that interferes with an accurate listening in the cure. Lacan warns "for a greater misrecognition of the essential import of desire" (599, 3). These were major concerns of Freud's starting point. Initially Freud focused on the analysis of the primary process to highlight the dialectic in which "demand and desire become separate" (599, 3).

Lacan's moment of conclusion of *In memory* is definitely an appraisal:

> But I will not present any further my own contributions in a study that can but bow—in confining itself to the sole text it concerns—before the obstinate dialectical demands, the loftiness of perspective, the feeling for analytic experience, the grasp of the whole of it, the immense information, the inflexibility regarding goals, the faultless erudition, and, lastly, the weight [*poids*] that give Jones' work its exceptional place.
>
> (599, 4)

An appraisal because "this discussion of symbolism led us so close to this destiny of man to go toward being" (599, 5). Lacan refers to Heidegger's man as a "shepherd of being" (599, 5). In his *Letter on Humanism*, Heidegger writes:

> But for man it is ever a question of finding what is fitting in his essence that corresponds to such destiny; for in accord with this destiny man as ek-sisting has to guard the truth of Being. Man is the shepherd of Being.
>
> (1947/1977: 161–162)

Man stands outside himself. Lacan: "the destiny of man to go toward being since he cannot become one" (599, 5). Freud subjugated "the good subject of philosophical knowledge" into "the bad subject of desire and its impostures" (599, 5). This is the subject of desire, divided through the signifier. It's this "bad subject" that Jones tries to "advocate" in his conclusion on symbolism (599, 6). Jones writing on the difference between metaphor and symbolism:

> The circumstance that the same image can be employed for both of these functions should not blind us to the important differences between them. Of these the principal one is that with metaphor the feeling to be expressed is over sublimated, whereas with symbolism it is under-sublimated (sic); the one relates to an effort that has attempted something beyond its strength, the other to an effort that is prevented from accomplishing what it would.
>
> (1918: 229)

With tongue-in-cheek this reminds Lacan of Kierkegaard's "immortal division of human functions" (600, 2). This is a reference to Kierkegaard's *Repetition*:

> A wit has said that one might divide mankind into officers, serving-maids and chimney sweeps. To my mind this remark is not only witty but profound, and it would require a great speculative talent to devise a better classification. When a classification does not ideally exhaust its object, a haphazard classification is altogether preferable, because it sets imagination in motion. A tolerably true classification is not able to satisfy the understanding, it is nothing for the imagination, and hence it is to be totally rejected, even though for everyday use it enjoys much honor and repute for the reason that people are in part very stupid and in part have very little imagination.
>
> (1843/1941: 56)

Lacan is referring to Kierkegaard's ode to the imagination, to the power of metaphors. And in his conclusion Lacan goes even further associating on this, telling a Jewish story of "two men who exit one after the other from a chimney" (600, 4). "Wisdom settles the question here regarding all the subtleties that could be deduced from the darkness of the faces they present each other and the reflections which, in each of them, diverge, when it expressly concludes: when two men meet coming out of a chimney, they both have dirty faces" (600, 4). So, Lacan concludes, when the Welshman and the Frenchman come out of the chimney "they both have dirty faces" (600, 4).

Conclusion

A Shakespearian Welsh rebel challenges a hero with Royal ambitions. Lacan opens a palace of mirrors with a simple quote. He himself choosing voluntary exile and founding a new group, the *Société Française de Psychanalyse*; Undertaking vain attempts to acquire recognition from the IPA, in which Jones played an important 'royal' role; Alluding to three missed encounters with Master Jones, Freud's chosen prince of psychoanalysis; Mirroring Freud's closest circle, the bearers of the ring, and their controversial censorship towards dissident thinkers such as Jung and Adler. All battles to protect "the tedious ways of art" (Shakespeare). Exactly what Lacan does in his text on Jones. Doing this with the greatest respect for Jones's work (599, 4). Still defending his 'tedious way of art': being the signifier and desire. All circling around one major question, the heart and motor of the text: "How can one fail to see the dominance of the signifier here, manifest in its most materially phonemic form?" (598, 4). A question in which Lacan's mirror palace comes to a standstill right before our eyes. A question of the greatest importance for psychoanalytic practice, not only in the past (the Freud/Jung controversy), or in the time Lacan wrote this text (the schism in French psychoanalysis) but for everyone practicing psychoanalysis now and in the future. The clinical implications might best be illustrated with the example of the interpretation of *Pulchinello*. Remember how tempting the Jones associations are, even when they follow a scientific path: *Pulchinello*, a phallic symbol referring to a 'cock' and 'a male organ,' all in line with the dominance of the 'phallic phase.' Taking a closer look at the pure theatrical signifier *Pulchinello* enables you to discover a pure empty signifier, a phallic signifier at its purest, a mask hiding nothing but a void dressed in an artificial voice … the empty mirror of the Ego.

Notes

1 "The committee met for the first time in May 1913. Freud dissolved the group in April 1924, re-established it at the end of 1924, and finally disbanded it in 1927" (Rubin, 1998, p. 39).

2 "Le *se taire* n'est pas le silence." Séminaire XII, *Problèmes cruciaux pour la psychanalyse* (1964–1965).

References

Agamben G. (2017), *Polichinelle ou Divertissement pour les jeunes gens en quatre scénes*, Paris, Ëd. Macula.

Freud S. (1900/1982), *The Interpretation of Dreams*. London, Pelican Books.

Freud S. and Breuer J. (1893–1895/1983), *Studies on Hysteria*. London, Pelican Books.

Heidegger M. (1947/1977), 'Letter on Humanism', *Basic Writings*. London, Routledge.

Jones E. (1918), 'The Theory of Symbolism', in *British Journal of Psychology*, Vol. IX, pp. 181–229.

Jones E. (1953–1961), *Sigmund Freud: Life and Work*. London, Hogarth Press.

Kierkegaard S. (1843/1941), *Repetition*, translated by Walter Lowrie. Princeton, NJ, Princeton University Press.

Lacan, J. (1949/2006), 'The Mirror Stage as Formative of the Function of the I', in Écrits, ed. J. Lacan and J.-A. Miller. New York/London, W. W. Norton, pp. 75–81.

Lacan J. (1958/2013), *Le Séminaire. Livre VI. Le désir et son interprétation* (1958–1959). Paris, Éditions de la Martinière.

Lacan J. (1971/2006), *Le Séminaire. Livre XVIII. D'un discours qui ne serait pas du semblan*t. Paris, Éditions du Seuil.

Lacan J. (2000), *Problèmes cruciaux pour la psychanalyse, dit «Seminaire XII»* (1964–1965). Paris, Éditions du Seuil.

Morin I. (2009), 'Œuvre de Silence', in *Psychanalyse*, ERES, 2, 15, pp. 5–19.

Ouaknin M. A. (1994), *Bibliothérapie, Lire c'est guérir*. Paris, Seuil,

Queneau R. (1959), *Zazie dans le metro*, http://bmlettres.net/IMG/pdf/QUENEAU_Zazie-dans-le-metro_texte-integral.pdf.

Rank O. and Sachs H. (1913), 'Die Bedeutung der Psychoamalyse für die Geisteswissenschaften', in *Zentralblatt für Psychoanalyse und Psychotherapie*, p. 11.

Rubin J. (1998), *A Psychoanalysis of our Time: Exploring the Blindness of the Seeing*. New York, New York University Press.

Shakespeare W. (1997), *The Norton Shakespeare. Based on the Oxford Edition* (S. Greenblatt). New York, W. W. Norton & Company.

Sharpe E. F. (1937/1988), *Dream Analysis: A Practical Handbook of Psychoanalysis*. New York, Karnac Books.

Sibony D. (1992), *Les Trois Monothéismes*. Paris, Éditions du Seuil.

Silberer H. (1910), 'Phantasie und Mythos', in *Jahrbuch für psychoanalytiche und psychopathologische Forschungen*, 2, p. 513.

Silberer H. (1912), *Probleme der Mystik und Symbolik*. Wien, Heller.

Silberer H. (1912), 'Symbolik des Erwachens und Schwellensymbolik úberhaupt', in *Jahrbuch für psychoanalytische und psychopathologische Forschungen*, 3, pp. 645–648.

Žižek S. (2016), *Disparities*. London, Bloomsbury.

3

ON AN EX POST FACTO SYLLABARY

Yael Goldman Baldwin

Context

In the English version of the *Écrits*, '*On an ex post facto syllabary*' (which I will refer to as *Syllabary*) is granted stand-alone essay status, but in the original French, '*D'un syllabaire après coup*' is placed just below the preceding essay, '*Sur la théorie du symbolisme d'Ernest Jones.*' The French positioning highlights that Lacan wrote it for the 1966 publication as a postscript or addendum to his essay on Jones. The French *Syllabaire* also has wider margins than any other essay in *Écrits*, further indexing its postscript status.

Lacan says *Syllabary* is the 'note' readers may have expected alongside Herbert Silberer's name in the preceding text, '*In memory of Ernest Jones: On his theory of symbolism*' (on pages 588, 590, and 592). Lacan claims this 'note' is not truly missing if one reads *In memory* closely enough; nevertheless, with *Syllabary*, he provides more thoughts on Silberer by particularly addressing Jones's fourth section of his essay '*The theory of symbolism,*' entitled 'functional symbolism,' which specifically takes up Silberer's 'invention' of the 'functional phenomenon.' Lacan discusses the 'functional phenomenon' in order to clarify the role and importance of symbolism and the Symbolic in psychoanalysis. Thus, seven years later, Lacan fills out an ellipsis from *In Memory*.

It is worth noting Herbert Silberer's role in psychoanalytic history. Silberer (1882–1923) was an Austrian psychoanalyst. Referred to as a "mysterious sportsman, balloonist, mystic," and "fascinating and deeply neurotic polymath" by Peter Gay (1986: 47, 219), Silberer wrote on symbolism, dreams, imagery, introversion, mysticism, alchemy, Freudianism, and yoga, to name a few. His works include *Hidden Symbolism of Alchemy and the Occult Arts* and *Problems of Mysticism and its Symbolism.*[1] Carl Jung acknowledged his intellectual debt to Silberer and vice versa. In 1909, Freud wrote Jung saying Silberer's paper on dreams was "good and throws light on an aspect of dream work" (1909/1994: 242) and should be published.[2]

In '*On Narcissism,*' Freud (1914/1957: 97) calls Silberer's concept of the functional phenomenon "one of the few indisputably valuable additions to the theory of dreams." Freud added discussions of Silberer's work to his 1914 edition of the *Traumdeutung*.[3]

In 1910, Silberer joined the *Vienna Psychoanalytic Society*. But Silberer's relationship with Freud and the psychoanalytic community was rocky. While Jung always championed Silberer's work, Freud and Silberer eventually had a falling out. At the age of 40, in 1923, Silberer took his own life. There is debate whether his suicide was in response to a negative letter from Freud (see Roazen, 1976 and Nitzschke, 1989).

Lacan works with three main texts in *Syllabary*. The first is Silberer's work on dreams, which Jones (1916/1948: 160) states is actually "incorporated in a half a dozen essays".[4] For this chapter, I employ Silberer's *The Dream: Introduction to the psychology of dreams* (1918/1955), in which Silberer expands upon Freud's theory of dreams.

The second is Ernest Jones's '*The theory of symbolism*', a seminal text in which Jones strives to attain a "fuller understanding of the theoretical nature of symbolism" (Jones, 1916/1948: 129) and "the way in which it operates" (Jones, 1916/1948: 130). Jones critiques Jung and defends psychoanalysis as being more "scientific" in its approach to symbolism than Jungian theory. Jones (1879–1958) was a British psychoanalyst perhaps most famous not for his clinical practice or theories, for which he is indeed well known, but for being Freud's official biographer. He also played a prominent position in psychoanalytic politics as president of two important psychoanalytic establishments (the *International Psychoanalytic Association* and the *British Psycho-Analytical Society*). Lacan was stung by his interaction with Jones at the Marienbad conference in 1936, when Jones interrupted Lacan's "mirror phase" talk, and remarks on Jones's "imperiousness" and "unpleasant" character (*Mirror Stage*: 151; *In Memory*: 585). Lacan does not let Jones off the hook in *Syllabary*; Lacan agrees with many of Jones's conclusions, but ultimately not with the arguments Jones bases them on.

The third text, weaved throughout the discussion, inspired the other two: Freud's *Traumdeutung*.

In *Syllabary*, Lacan takes up Silberer's theory of symbolism, particularly functional symbolism and threshold symbolism, and juxtaposes it with his own understanding of the symbolic, which highlights the importance of the signifier in the formation of dreams and their interpretation. Lacan argues that Jones's critique of Silberer is apt, but not adequate because he lacks the necessary theoretical tools that would help his argument have veracity and clinical significance. Lacan's terminology, such as his term syllabary, is drawn from the new discipline of linguistics, whose discoveries were not available to Jones or Freud, although both instinctively understood the role of language in the unconscious.[5] *Syllabary* is concerned with giving "symbolism its proper place" (607), particularly dream symbolism, and like much of Lacan's work, articulates the symbolic's role in psychoanalysis.[6] Both Lacan and Jones criticize Silberer's understanding of dream symbolism for being too Jungian;

Jones calls it the "Jung-Silberer school" (1916/1948: 170), as will be discussed below. Lacan's exploration of the role of dream symbolism is language-based, which he argues can be found in Freud. Dreams must be viewed as signifiers; *Syllabary* is an addendum explaining how the three theorists (Silberer, Jung, and Jones *in his argument*) fail to grasp the "signifierness of dreams" (*Instance of the Letter*: 424) "at the crux" of Freud's dream theory.

Such arguments were not particularly new for Lacan. In 1954, over a decade before *Syllabary*, Lacan said the dream "has no value for [Freud] except as a vector of speech" (*Hyppolite*: 315). In 1957, Lacan was already discussing linguistic analysis in relation to dreams, stating "dream images are to be taken up only on the basis of their value as signifiers" and in the dream "we are dealing with writing" (*Instance of the Letter*: 424). In exploring the unconscious meanings of dreams, as with symptoms, fantasies, parapraxes, and jokes, Lacan is most interested in the "constitutive role of the signifier" (426). He also investigates what we do with syllables, the small literal components of language, and their relations to the functions and productions of the unconscious. As early as 1953, in discussing the "vanguard role" of linguistics, Lacan stated that the

> form of mathematicization in which the discovery of the *phoneme* is inscribed, as a function of pairs of positions formed by the smallest graspable discriminative semantic elements, leads us to the very foundations that Freud's final doctrine designates as the subjective sources of the symbolic function in a vocalic connotation of presence and absence.
>
> (*Function*: 235)

These thoughts are echoed and expanded upon in *Syllabary*.

How have other commentators taken up *Syllabary*? My research revealed very little commentary and no sustained discussion of it. It is very briefly mentioned in J.-A. Miller's (2003) '*Lacan's later teaching*,' Christian Demoulin's (2001) '*Enjeux de la théorie Lacanienne*,' Tom Eyers' (2012) *Lacan and the concept of the 'Real'*, and in a footnote in Alain Badiou's (1983/2013) *The Incident at Antioch: A tragedy in three acts*.[7]

Commentaries on the text

Syllabary's title speaks volumes. The translation's "ex post facto" refers to retrospective action or force, which highlights Lacan's retrospection on the essay's topic. *Syllabary's* eight pages were added seven years after the completion of the previous text. It is the only addition to a specific text in the entire *Écrits* collection—the other additions, such as '*Overture*' and '*On my Antecedents*,' punctuate the *Écrits* as introductory and biographical notes, respectively. Thus *Syllabary* is *après coup*, 'after the event' of the initial essay.

The *après coup*, of the French title (*D'un syllabaire après coup*), can also be translated as deferred action. Bruce Fink's translator's endnote mentions *après coup* is used to translate *Nachträglichkeit*, the idea of retroactive understanding manifested following further events. These further events might be Lacan's work on psychoanalysis's relationship to science; when writing *Syllabary*, Lacan was thinking about this topic. In December of 1965, with '*La science et la vérité*,' he juxtaposes both Freud and Jung's relationship to science, and linguistics versus psychology. The *syllabary* part of the title is a pun and homophone—the first syllable of both syllabary and Silberer (syll and sil) share a group of letters that, although spelled differently, share the same pronunciation. And in the French pronunciation, the second parts of both words also share strong similarities: the last syllables, 'aire' and 'er' sound the same; what differs is the 'ab' versus the 'ber'. That Lacan uses a homophone here will prove instructive; it emphasizes the role of the signifier, the importance of which will become clear as we analyze the text. A syllabary refers to the written symbols, or syllabic representations, available to construct the words of certain languages. Syllabaries are how syllables are expressed in written characters or marks—how discrete units of sound are represented; they are a writing system. Sounds for things we are trying to depict can be written in the form of an alphabet (as in English) or a syllabary. The Cherokee language uses a syllabary in its script. Japanese uses two syllabaries. Thus, the title is a characteristic Lacanian play on words, referring to syllabaries, syllables, syllables' relations to unconscious formations,[8] particularly dreams, and Herbert Silberer's last name. The point being the letters, the phonemes that make up words, really count! They count enough for Lacan to put syllabary in the title, even though we do *not* see the word appear anywhere in the rest of the essay. Employing the syllabary term, Lacan emphasizes how symbolism in dreams must be understood as (phonematic) signifying material.

Lacan (602, 1) begins by saying this postscript is the note on Herbert Silberer that readers may have expected to find in the preceding '*In memory of Ernest Jones: On his theory of symbolism*' (abbreviated here as *In Memory*). Lacan claims the information about Silberer's "invention," which I take to mean "functional phenomenon," *is* in the preceding chapter in a "dissolved form". Yet, clearly Lacan believes there is still a lack in the preceding text and feels a need to speak more, particularly on Jones's discussion of "functional symbolism," which is the title of the fourth chapter of his essay, '*The theory of symbolism*.' Much that is in *Syllabary* can indeed be found in *In Memory*: Lacan does critique Jones for missing how "meaning effects are created by permutations of signifiers" (*In Memory*: 591), the way the phallus signifies lack, for giving primacy to the concrete, and comes closest to his *Syllabary* argument when he touches upon how Jones's discussion of Punchinello fails to reveal "the dominance of the signifier … in its most materially phonemic form" (598). But only in *Syllabary* does Lacan specifically elaborate on the role of functional phenomena. If it was important enough for Jones to devote an entire chapter, then, Lacan claims, he too should take it up more extensively.

In paragraph two (602, 2), Lacan says Jones's "functional symbolism" chapter "redoubles … his argumentation," that is, recaps the ideas he made in the preceding three chapters, and, furthermore, that his "argumentation" is an example of the problem to be found in Jones's work in general. Lacan calls Jones's argument "lame" and a "symptom (among others) of the problem found in [Jones's] theory." This symptom will prove to be an inattention to the role of the signifier and the lack of the necessary theoretical tools to make proper arguments.

Lacan (603, 3) claims he will also redouble his own text, *In memory*, and not get far with the inherent problem, except to clarify how it can only be redoubled, but that there is indeed "value" in doing so.

Silberer "intends to trace what becomes of the symbol's (historic)[9] impact" (602, 4) as it moves from material to functional phenomena. He divides the "phenomena of symbolization" into three classes: First, *material phenomena*—"contents are transformed into symbols" (1918/1955: 366), where the visual image of the dream represents the thought content, object, or ideas; second, *functional phenomena*, where dream images represent how the psyche is functioning, the dreamer's subjective state; and third, *somatic phenomena* ("somatic occurrences and [bodily] states of all kinds are reflected symbolically" 366). Silberer (1918/1955: 375) claims all three classes of symbolism occur, but Freud's theory highlights material phenomena.

Lacan (602, 5), following Freud, refers to the "functional phenomenon" by name. This dream symbolism represents or "symbolizes" an elaborate psychic structure—*how* the mind is functioning, what is going on in the psyche of the dreamer. Silberer explores what happens to symbols when we move from material phenomena to functional phenomena, from the contents of symbols to what they say about our psychic state or functioning.

One might rightly think the "it" of Silberer's "notorious illustration of it," refers to "functional phenomenon" given Lacan's wording in this paragraph (602, 6; 603, 1). Already in *In Memory* (588), Lacan referred to how "Silberer asks us to recognize the 'functional symbolism' of the layers of the psyche in a cake knife cutting through a puff pastry". However, regarding Silberer's three classes of symbolization phenomena, Silberer actually gives the cake/pie[10] example to illustrate the first kind of symbolism—material phenomenon. Here is Silberer's example:

> I try to assess to myself the benefits to be gained from certain metaphysical studies I intend to make. The aim of such studies seems to me to be that while in search of the essence of existence, one works one's way through to higher forms of consciousness or levels of existence. In the hallucination scene I see the following: I slide a long knife under a pie in order to take a piece of it. The interpretation is: My handling of the knife is that 'working through' mentioned. In

> this seemingly silly symbol is nevertheless expressed the care necessary for the operation. The neat lifting of the cut piece with a knife demands accurate preparation. It reminds one of the clean separation of concepts in philosophy.
>
> (1918/1955: 367)

This is Silberer's last example of the material class. He then gives examples of the functional class and the somatic class. As I read the example, clean cut as a 'clean separation of concepts in philosophy' can be viewed as the material symbol or phenomenon—the object of thought, whereas the 'working through' and the 'care' can be seen as representative of the functional class—the subjective states of the dreamer. To be sure, Silberer discusses simultaneous functional and material images in dreams. He also distinguishes the above example as a hallucination scene and earlier in the piece declares that "hypnogogic hallucinations are those dream-like images which appear to many people in somnolescence" (Silberer, 1918/1955: 364) hence Lacan mentions the transition to sleep in this paragraph. The illustration is "notorious" because Freud (1900/1953: 344–345) used it.

The layer cake is a material phenomenon for the "psychical strata … evoked" (603, 2). Lacan's mention of "a possible endoscopy of the depths that verge on the sublime" may refer to Freud's 1914 *Traumdeutung* comment that Silberer's contributions on functional phenomenon, particularly on 'threshold symbolism,' highlight

> the fact that in certain circumstances a species of self-observation plays a part in this and makes a contribution to the content of the dream. The probable relations of the self-observing agency, which may be particularly prominent in philosophical minds, to endopsychic perception, to delusions of observation, to conscience and to the censor of dreams can be more appropriately treated elsewhere.
>
> (Freud, 1900/1953: 506)

Lacan may likely be criticizing the notion that the "depths" (*profondeurs*) of the unconscious are "sublime," as opposed to sexual and aggressive in nature, and critiquing even the notion that the unconscious lies in the "depths" (the term "depth psychology" not being among his favorites).

When Lacan (603, 3) says, "the phenomenon is indisputable," he is referring to the "functional phenomenon."[11] Importantly, Lacan concedes that the functional phenomenon does exist in reality, and it is because it is "indisputable" that Freud "made room for it" in his 1914 *Traumdeutung* note. Freud (1900/1953: 344) says Silberer "pointed out a good way of directly observing the transformations of thoughts into pictures in the process of forming dreams". Freud further takes up Silberer while discussing the secondary revision of dream work, saying Silberer aptly notes that some dream elements or images "sometimes represented something other than the thought that was being dealt with—namely, the fatigue itself, the difficulty involved in the work. It represented, that is to say, the subjective states and mode of functioning of the person making the effort instead of the object of his efforts. Silberer described occurrences of this kind, which were frequent in his case, as a 'functional phenomenon,' in contrast to the 'material phenomenon,' which would have been expected" (Freud, 1900/1953: 503). Lacan (603, 3) adds that the phenomenon is "most striking" in Silberer's "symbolism of the threshold." Freud took up the "threshold phenomenon" in his 1914 note:

> Silberer has given examples which show convincingly that in many dreams the last pieces of the manifest content, which are immediately followed by waking, represent nothing more nor less than an intention to wake or the process of waking. The representation may be in terms of such images as crossing a threshold ('threshold symbolism'), leaving one room and entering another, departure, home-coming, parting with a companion, diving into water, etc.
>
> (1900/1953: 504)

The functional or subjective state symbolized in threshold symbolism is the falling asleep or waking. Illustrating "the symbolism of the threshold," Silberer (1918/1955: 368) presents examples of common images during the transitory states:

> I was on the point of departing from the waking state. The following image appeared to me: I am putting on my coat as if preparing to go out with another person who comes to call for me. The sleep appears here as a person who comes to call for me.

This person may be the "guardian of the threshold," who Lacan (having some fun) says, "possibly enriched" the symbolism. The point of the paragraph is that the existence of the functional phenomenon is "indisputable" and Lacan, like Freud and Jones before him, accepts the reality of Silberer's observation and contribution.

Lacan (603, 4) claims this phenomenon "seduces us." After discussing the value of Silberer's invention, Freud (1900/1953: 505) warns us that the "very interesting functional phenomenon" has led to "many abuses" of dream interpretations, at no fault of its inventor. It is seductive because it harkens back to a pre-psychoanalytic psychology, and as we shall see, is also situated in the imaginary realm. Thus Lacan says the true letter of Freud must be "resuscitate[d]." Silberer *might have* used the still new ("green") springboard ("trampoline") of Freud's inventions to jump off of and make further advances, but instead he resuscitates pre-Freudian psychology. We must thus be wary of its seduction.

Next, Lacan (603, 5) explicitly turns his attention to Jones's essay, praising Jones for "championing Freud," in his intention to slam on the brakes of a misdirected movement. Jones is working during "the germination stage of psychoanalysis" (*ab ovo*, from the egg), when some of Freud's colleagues (like Jung and Silberer) take dream symbolism in the wrong direction. Lacan is working some fifty years later, but states that Jones, via his critiques of Silberer and Jung and his reliance on Freud's texts, "confirms ... the position I [Lacan] adopt in my teaching"—the position of embracing the radicalness inherent to Freud's work. Lacan thus expresses solidarity with Jones.

Lacan (603, 6) employs Jones's criticism of Jung to highlight what is and is not psychoanalysis, according to Lacan, and more particularly, it is not just that there are differences, but Lacan says "Jones explicitly goes so far here as to enunciate the principle with which Jung excluded himself from psychoanalysis". This principle is likely the principle of hermeneuticization, which Lacan (603, 4) invokes in the next paragraph, that is, a principle based on a focus on meaning rather than a focus on signifiers, a principle that differentiates Jung from Freud. Lacan will take up the question of the principle of demarcation. Lacan may also be referring to Jones's criticism of Jung's notion of an anthropological "inheritance of ideas" (1916/1948: 140) as a means to explaining more stereotypical symbols. Jones states,

> I adhere to the contrary view [from Jung] that symbolism has to be re-created afresh out of individual material, and that the stereotypy is due to the uniformity of the human mind in regard to the particular tendencies that furnish the source of symbolism—*i.e.*, to the uniformity of the fundamental and perennial interests of mankind.
> (1916/1948: 140, emphasis in original)

Jung over-generalizes and thus loses psychoanalytic specificity, particularly with his 'Libido-symbol' (Jones, 1916/1948: 159). Jones (1916/1948: 159) says Jung "does not hesitate to use the term 'symbol' in precisely the reverse sense from that in which it is used in psycho-analysis" and that Jung loses the sense of the unconscious processes at work and relies too much on conscious processes. Jones levels a similar criticism at Silberer for tending "to leave out of account the real reason for the whole symbolism—namely, the unconscious, positive affects that are not allowed to appear in consciousness" (Jones, 1916/1948: 166). Jones later calls this kind of understanding and interpreting of dream symbolism "defensive"—"every boat-race becomes the ambition to succeed on the river of life"—and as such is a "resistance to the unconscious" (Jones, 1916/1948: 167). Jones argues that this defensive treatment of symbolism, as it relates to functional symbolism, "reaches once more the popular conception of symbolism as the presentation of the abstract in terms of the concrete" (Jones, 1916/1948: 169).

The problem with the Jungian take and those like it, says Lacan (603, 7), "can be summarized in a word": the "hermeneuticization" of psychoanalysis, which Lacan and Jones are adamantly against. When Lacan cries "hermeneutics," he is usually objecting to a search for hidden meanings, rather than focusing on the effects of the signifiers. That is likely the case here.[12]

Lacan (603, 8) juxtaposes Jones's "true symbol" with "the commonsense meaning of symbolism." Jones (1916/1948: 132) devotes section II of his fourth chapter, to his thesis that "true symbolism, in the strict sense, is to be distinguished from other forms of indirect representation." He holds we must be stricter and restrict our use of the term "symbolism" to avoid a pre-psychoanalytic psychology, claiming part of our difficulty in theorizing how psychoanalysis uses symbolism is because the "term 'symbolism' has been used to denote very many different things, some of them quite unconnected with one another" (Jones, 1916/1948: 130). Too many different phenomena are encompassed by a loose definition of the term. Jones offers an array of phenomena that fall under the term symbolism, all of which are quite different. He asks "amid this maze of meanings what attributes in common can be found between the various ideas and acts denoted by the word 'symbol' or 'symbolic'?" (Jones, 1916/1948: 131). He lays out six main characteristics and says "true symbols" also have six more characteristics. Lacan says Jones's "true" symbol is the one "Freud isolated" and this symbol "does not 'symbolize' in the sense in which the figures of the Old Testament symbolize on the basis of what becomes of them in the New Testament."[13] Lacan tends to reference Biblical studies when speaking on hermeneutics, and here again he differentiates between hermeneutics and psychoanalysis.

Subsequently, Lacan (603, 9) takes up the "slippage that occurs in Silberer's work," which "aligns him with Jung". For example, Silberer (1918/1955: 369) quotes Nietzsche that "in sleep and in the dream we cover the whole course of human history ... the dream takes us far back into past ages of culture." Jones (1916/1948: 170) refers to the "Jung-Silberer School" take on dreams, and Lacan agrees. Lacan is still distinguishing the commonsense symbol and the "true" symbol, which is independent of what it figures and its object (so a threshold in a dream does not necessarily mean crossing from one state to another). The symbol, as Lacan discusses in '*The Instance of the letter*,' is rather to be understood in relation to other signifiers.

Lacan (603, 10) says that once the symbol is "surpassed" by (or gives precedence to) what is symbolized, and symbols then come merely to stand in for what they symbolize (as in the hermeneutic tradition), it follows that they stand for what is hidden, invisible. When speaking of "invisible realities," Lacan may be referencing Silberer's interest in the occult, mysticism, and alchemy.[14] These "invisible realities" may refer to angels, sprites, demons, etc. Lacan may also be saying, with the "veil," which has been placed over these shadowy creatures "for quite a while," that we no longer take them seriously. The point is that these are all imaginary.

Lacan (603, 11) mentions that Freud deems functional phenomena as part of the "secondary revision of the dream," the stage of dream formation that gives dreams their sense of narrative coherence. Lacan (604, 1) places the secondary revision work in the realm of the "Imaginary." The dream is filled with gaps and narrative fractions, but secondary revisions allow us to make more sense of them as a whole, even if the whole is a fiction. Lacan says Freud himself designates the phenomenon as imaginary. Lacan claims later in the piece that his categories of RSI are inherent to Freud, and here provides an example. The fact that functional phenomena are imaginary "says it all" (603, 11); they are not in the realm of the symbolic, not formations of the unconscious, and hence are not as important to Freud's understanding of dream phenomena.

In the following paragraph, Lacan (604, 2) points to the parts in Freud's 1914 edition of *Traumdeutung* that take up the functional phenomenon and also to Jones's personal communication with Freud.[15]

Next, Lacan (604, 3) again points to Freud's 1914 comment that functional phenomena highlight "that in certain circumstances a species of self-observation plays a part in this and makes a contribution to the content of the dream. The probable relations of the self-observing agency, which may be particularly prominent in philosophical minds, to endopsychic perception, to delusions of observation, to conscience and to the censor of dreams can be more appropriately treated elsewhere" (Freud, 1900/1953: 505–506), and the reader is guided to '*On Narcissism*,' where Freud (1914/1957: 97) states, "Probably the reason why I overlooked it [functional phenomenon] is because it does not play any great part in my own dreams; in persons who are gifted philosophically and accustomed to introspection it may become very evident". Oh Freud!

"Which is laughable" Lacan (604, 4) says, and of course Freud's referencing his own mind as less introspective or gifted than others is simply laughable, as is the idea that philosophers are less affected by the unconscious. Furthermore, there is a "question ... echoed" regarding the functional phenomenon and its relation to "desire as sexual" and libido. Functional phenomena "come up short;" they are not the effects of desire and libido, do not have a sexual or libidinal component, which for Lacan must differentiate them from what is truly of interest to psychoanalysis: the status of the formations of the unconscious. For Lacan, following Freud, the role that desire plays, and the transformations of unconscious desire into signifiers in dreams, signifiers that are not tied to the initial concrete meaning, is of foremost importance. It is the dream work that symbolically transforms desire that is key.

Silberer attempts to observe "certain laws" (1918/1955: 363) regarding dream work. Lacan (604, 5) rhetorically asks, "Are there two different laws of sleep?" He answers, in the next paragraph, with an emphatic "no."

Lacan (604, 6) provides a rationale for why Freud did not initially take up functional phenomena. Lacan hypothesizes that Freud "rejected" a certain level of experience, and was "justified" in doing so because Freud was taking an "inaugural step of science." Freud's main focus was unconscious formations, in this case dreams. He could not take everything into account regarding dreams, but rather focused on dreams as the "royal road to the unconscious." He did not focus on the functional phenomenon until Silberer brought it to his attention.

Lacan (604, 7) argues we need theoretical apparatuses, "theoretical edifice," in science, to decipher the investigated phenomenon, and claims his registers of the Real, Symbolic, and Imaginary (RSI), and the relationships between them, are an important step in science and that the registers' distinctions derived specifically from psychoanalytic practice (a claim Freud often makes about his theoretical edifices). Lacan's RSI apparatus "proves to be eristic," that is, some people argue about and against this "theoretical edifice."

Somewhat explicating his RSI apparatus, Lacan (604, 8) plays on the word "threshold" (Silberer's "threshold symbolism"), while speaking of the Symbolic's relationship to the Imaginary and the Real. He introduces the role of the signifier, specifically "the signifier's relation to the subject". In the subject's life the Symbolic "forces the imaginary to decline," and in this way, rules over the Imaginary. The Symbolic's restructuring tendencies and how the subject is an effect of the signifier is a main current that runs through Lacan's oeuvre.

Tipping his hat to his theoretical edifice, Lacan (604, 9) says that once the distinction between Symbolic, Imaginary, and Real was solidly in place, he was able, in a "second retreat" from immediate experience, to introduce the object *a* as a second "knot". Although not stated here explicitly, the "first knot" is the division introduced into the subject by the signifier, as Lacan states later in the piece (608, 11). Note the knots here are *not* the knots of knot theory because in 1966, Lacan was not yet working on knot theory.[16] So while a rigorous approach would take into account object *a*, Lacan says he will "confine" his argument (605, 1), and returns to how Jones "fails" in his attempt to rescue symbolism because he does not have the RSI categories and "badly … needs" them. Lacan does not take up object *a* any further, although knots return at the end of *Syllabary*.

Lacan (605, 2) assigns himself the task of showing how he grasps his RSI categories from Freud's work—they are already there in Freud's work.[17] Part of Lacan's work in general is to illuminate these categories as they arise in clinical practice and from Freud's work.

Indeed, Lacan (605, 3) claims Freud's "attachment to science" contributed to his reluctance to venture into the exploratory field of the unconscious,[18] and that theoretical edifices like RSI are a "*vade mecum*," a useful manual or object, to have with us at all times, which we can use to do so.

Claiming it would be better to call Silberer's "threshold symbol" a *signifier* rather than a symbol, Lacan (605, 4) argues something is *not* a threshold because of a natural, physical, or 'real' resemblance—not a threshold because it is a "flat field stone," for example—but because it is a signifier. His larger argument in *Syllabary* is that Silberer makes the mistake of interpreting dreams as if they were based on a symbolism that is real and natural versus symbolic as signifiers. I like Bruce Fink's (2004: 98) example of how signifiers are the "motor force behind [dreams]. An image of a man standing under a line may have nothing to do with the idea of being below a certain standard, but everything to do with 'understanding'". The letters, the phonemes, matter.

In critiquing Silberer's threshold and functional phenomena for being based on natural, physical qualities, Lacan (605, 5) points to gravitational theory, invoking Alexandre Koyré's work, to exemplify borrowing signifiers from one realm to understand another. Lacan invoked the history of science and how we evolve our understandings via different theoretical apparatuses, in a proto-Kuhnian move, in *In memory*. The realm Lacan references, from which the theory of gravitation borrowed signifiers, is probably mathematics. It is a rich example as the history of gravitational theory's evolution can be traced to ancient Greece. Galileo produced some early equations for the law of gravitation, but it took Newton to introduce a mathematical formula, signifiers in the form of mathematical formula, to explain a natural phenomenon, and then Einstein to come up with his elegant equations (which was in 1916, the year Jones published his symbolism essay).[19] Lacan's use of "heavy" here may be a nod to how he used the example of the word "heavy" [lourd], in *In memory* (591–592) to demonstrate how Jones "loses his way".

Lacan (605, 6) aligns himself with Jones, saying they both consider the argument "relevant," but questions whether Jones grasps the shift of employing mathematics and mathematization, and how the Symbolic reigns over the Imaginary in terms of our relationship not just to science as stated above, but also to knowledge in general. With the advent of mathematical science, knowledge (*savoir*) sloughed off the Imaginary. Prior to this shift, knowledge (*connaissance)* was fettered by putting meaning into nature. Lacan also refers to Jones's recourse to the decency of psychoanalysis. The French "décence" can mean good manners, and also respecting social norms, particularly sexual, in word and deed, which is *not* what psychoanalysis should strive for, according to Lacan—just the opposite.

Next, Lacan (605, 7) criticizes Jones for weakening his argument by giving higher status to what is "concrete in symbolism" versus the arbitrary relationship the signifier has with the thing, object, or idea it is representing. For Lacan, Jones (a) does not get this important distinction between symbol and signifier, and (b) gives higher status to the concrete than to the abstract realms of the signifier/Symbolic and thus (c) loses his way, just as Silberer did because he lacked the needed theoretical tools.

What you end up with, regarding symbolism (including "true symbolism"), is a "fiction (607, 8)," it is *not* true because it is based on the concrete and also on Jones's (1916/1948: 131) *false* idea of a "primitiveness," the idea that the primary idea—which is sensorial and concrete—holds more significance than the less essential "secondary," condensed and abstract symbol. Jones (1916/1948: 132) says, "symbolic modes of thought are more primitive," more simple, and a reversion to an earlier mental development; Lacan (606, 1) calls this an "error." He rejects the idea of the unconscious being primitive.[20]

Lacan (606, 2) praises Jones for trying, but by falling prey to this fiction/error, and by appealing to characteristics like "primitiveness," Jones ultimately fails to "ward off ... *psychologization.*" Lacan sees symbols as operating by the same mechanisms as metaphor; for him, a symbol is a metaphor. And psychologization stands in "opposition to Freud's discovery"; this is a battle psychoanalysis continues to fight, one could argue, even today, almost fifty years after Lacan wrote *Syllabary*. Some psychoanalytic schools, by emphasizing consciousness and insight into the psychological mechanisms and feelings that affect one over and above the role of the signifier in formations of the unconscious, still fall prey to the traps and pitfalls that Lacan is criticizing here.

Tongue in cheek, Lacan (606, 3) admits the lure of psychologization given practitioners' role in society. But he does not demur, and argues that psychoanalysis "withered" after Freud's radical discovery because it "forgets that its first responsibility is to language" (a statement which is *key* to the essay), as opposed to say alchemy (Jung and Silberer are guilty as charged). Lacan made it his life's work to bring language back to psychoanalysis.

Furthermore, Lacan (606, 4) lays into Jones for being "too weak" to argue against Anna Freud's theories, which Lacan calls "Anafreudianism," even though Jones was more sympathetic to Melanie Klein than to Anna. Lacan claims "Anafreudianism" is "reduced for use as an *ana*"; the homophone, Fink notes, in French is a "collection of miscellaneous information, anecdotes, or sayings" about something or someone (826). In other words, Anna Freud's theoretical edifices are neither very useful nor instructive.

During the 1940s debates, Jones aligned himself with Melanie Klein over Anna Freud. Lacan (606, 5) takes this feud up in detail in his first Seminar (S1, 1953–1954) and in *Signification of the Phallus*. Lacan thinks Klein did not get it right, but her reading of Freud was more correct than Anna Freud's. That Jones felt the same way showed his "faithfulness to a truly psychoanalytic approach," which likely means an approach that stays with the importance of the unconscious (versus the ego and consciousness) and its symbolic basis. Ultimately for Lacan, a truly psychoanalytic approach is also one that stays true to the *importance of the signifier* in the formations of the unconscious (this last point Jones misses).

Lacan (606, 6) mentions Jones's "phallic phase in women" and the 1920s–1930s debates on female sexuality. In 1962, in *Guiding remarks for a convention on female sexuality*, Lacan criticized Jones's work on female sexuality. He says he will clarify his points in this arena.

Lacan (606, 7) highlights how Jones's "primary ideas" are falsely grounded, which he also stated in *In Memory*. It is not because they are grounded in concrete, natural, experience that they are primary, as Jones argues. Rather they must be understood as signifiers. Lacan says Jones's argument belies itself, since the examples Jones gives are actually "lacking in the concrete" and "stand up in the real only thanks to the signifier." Furthermore, these signifiers relate to the subjects' relationships to key signifiers in their life: "death, desire, and the name of the father,"[21] versus Jones's (1916/1948: 145) argument that "all symbols represent ideas of the self and the immediate blood relatives, or of the phenomena of birth, love, and death ... the most primitive ideas and interests imaginable". Lacan's work, in general, highlights the role of desire and the name of the father as a symbolic function.

Jones does not recognize the symbolic function of the role of the Name of the Father—the "nodal point"—that Lacan emphasizes in his work, and misses the import and working of the place of the signifier (607, 1).

For example, Jones situates the phallus in the Imaginary, which has the fiction of the whole, covering over the lack (607, 2). Lacan employs the snake symbol in the case of Anna O., which Jones employs at length, as an example of how Jones fails to understand that the symbol is not concrete—the snake is not the penis because of its resemblance, but rather is "the symbol of the place where the penis is missing." Lacan criticizes Jones for mistaking the phallus as a concrete thing, as opposed to a signifier. This seems in line with Jones's "symptom," which Lacan refers to at the beginning of *Syllabary.*

Next Lacan (607, 3) rationalizes that he did not force this argument in *In Memory* because his audience was not "prepared" to hear it. He says his aim is to train analysts (607, 4), and his difficult, complex, and evocative style of speaking and writing is in that service. Yet, even those "best prepared" to understand him failed to do so, (607, 5) and instead defensively focused on his style or form.

Lacan (607, 6) returns to the "function of place in symbolism" providing the Red Donkey game[22] as an example and reminder that we should be grappling with the "practice of the combinatory" and the sliding and resistances at work in signification or symbolism. Lacan (607, 7) states resistance is found in the Imaginary, and highlights how he began his theoretical apparatus articulating the Imaginary (the mirror stage), which then allowed him to articulate the role of the Symbolic and "give symbolism its proper place." "Confusions in the symbolic stem from the imaginary," and Jones confused the Imaginary with the Symbolic by defining the symbol as an image or figure (607, 8).

Lacan (607, 9) calls Jones "Baconian," meaning Jones follows the empirical epistemological theories of seventeenth-century British philosopher Francis Bacon as if all ideas ultimately arise from concrete experience and physical data. Jones also thinks of ideas and concepts as originating in sensory impressions, in line with Hume (hence the "recourse to the *sensorium*").

Lacan (607, 10) distinguishes the Imaginary (that which has actual effects, has "its function as real") from the illusory (that which does not exist), as he did in 1936 in *Beyond the 'reality principle'*. He indexes the imago and IRM (which likely refers to Konrad Lorenz's "innate releasing mechanisms") (608, 1). IRM is the hypothesis that animals have a pre-determined innate capacity to behave in certain ways to certain stimuli. Lacan referenced this, though not by name, in his mirror phase, with his discussion of the importance of the image, even a mirror image, for the female pigeon to get a pre-programmed process (gonad maturation) started, illustrating how the image/imago relates to and profoundly effects biology. There is an "innate effect of the imago which manifests in all forms of display," which Lacan referenced in *Seminar I* (1953–1954), with the role of homeomorphic identifications in the stickleback, which also indexed the intersection of the lure or seduction of the image and biology.

Lacan (608, 2) recognizes the nature-nurture or biology-culturalism debate, and psychology's broader tendency to biologize without recognizing the role of image and signifier upon that biology. So there is (a) the biological, (b) the cultural, and (c) the Imaginary and its effects. Lacan (608, 3) believes that to misrecognize this profound role of image and signifier, to think of the body as a biological entity divorced from image and signification, is a "delusion." Ethology does have biological meaning, but when we are speaking of instincts and drives, particularly sexual ones, we must also recognize the profound role of image and signifier upon the body (608, 4). The image and the signifier will always interact, intersect, and affect our bodily drives—RSI intersect.

How should we situate symbolic thought in relationship to science? Lacan (608, 5) locates the answer not in the "potential" but in the "actual." Lacan seems to be saying that symbolic thought—which is a pleonasm, as all thought is symbolic thought—cannot be studied "scientifically" *if* we think of thought in terms of its "potential" or "virtual" properties. To think of it in these terms leads to false assumptions (607, 9), or to those that resort to spurious biological explanation (608, 2). Symbolic thought is not an impoverished, confused, or depreciated form of thought (608, 8), but an "actual" form of thought, the study of which is part of the discipline—"science"—of linguistics. This is Lacan the structuralist. The relationship between symbolic thought and science should be viewed as "actual" because the scientific study of language (modern linguistics) explains "symbolic" thought; one cannot explain things without using the resources of language itself. Hence, Lacan (608, 6) firmly situates thought in the actual, symbolic realm. A very Lacan-like phrase announces, "There has never been any other thought than symbolic thought" (608, 7). J.-A. Miller (2003: 12) says Lacan, at this point in his teachings, could "then consider that thought itself anticipated science, because thought is the symbolic already present in the real."

Lacan again indexes mathematics, and denounces the idea that symbolic thought is somehow depreciated, or archaic, as if there are two different types—primitive, symbolic thought and mature, rational (or scientific) thought (608, 8).[23] Rather there is only one.

Conversely, if one says there are two types of thought, primitive-symbolic and rational-scientific, one cannot also maintain that the latter is imminent in the former; that would be having it both ways (608, 9). The "historical casuistry" probably refers to the unsound tendency to give a diachronic explanation for the synchronic features of a language (where *this* is a symbol for *that* because of the word's history), and is another dig at Jones. This line of thought, and this essay as a whole, particularly illuminates Lacan's structuralist tendencies.

Lacan (608,10) here explores the connection between symbolic thought and knowledge. Psychoanalysis is different from alchemy, mysticism, or psychology, in terms of where it finds its "truth effect," which for Lacan is in the letter. In psychoanalysis, symbolism[24] is reduced to "the truth effect". In 1957, Lacan emphasized that the letter "produces all its truth effects in man without the spirit having to intervene at all" (*Instance of the Letter*: 424). "Pathetic" is likely being used in the Kantian sense, as a synonym for affect and emotion. Lacan may be saying it is somewhat irrelevant whether the effect of psychoanalysis is experienced affectively (in its "pathetic forms"). Knowledge here is "*savoir*," distinct from the earlier "*connaissance*." Symbols constitute a kind of knot, or nodal point of knowledge (*savoir*) in the subject that we need to decipher in order to grasp the meaning of unconscious formations (here Lacan is still working with a model of the unconscious based on the deciphering of meaning). The important point, I think, is that the "truth effect" operates as a "knot," the knot as the Spaltung or division in subjectivity that is at once *produced by* the signifier and that *produces* truth effects as a result of the unanticipated signifiers that pop up in one's speech. These concluding paragraphs hearken back to paragraph 24 above.

The truth effect of psychoanalysis, the "true knot," divides the subject (608, 11). This division is the effect of language—the signifier and the automaticity of the signifying chain—and has ramifications in all three dimensions. Lacan reminds us that language, the signifier, "the symbol," introduces a twist—like in the Möbius strip—such that the human being is never the same, post language instantiation, and this twist cannot again be flattened.[25] Lacan employs topology, here, to highlight the importance of the *simultaneity* of the three registers. He already outlined above how we are particularly vulnerable to captivation in the Imaginary, at the expense of the Symbolic (and that Jung and Silberer fall prey to this in particular).[26]

Based on "this criterion," Lacan (608, 12) distinguishes between this "true knot," and the "knot of the functional phenomenon," which he says is a "false knot," because it does not engender a division in the subject, via a language effect. I think Lacan is again emphasizing that the functional phenomenon is thus not an "actual" formation of the unconscious, and it is a mistake to think so. Jones, in his fourth chapter, attempts to right a wrong by fleshing out his argument (he flattens the knot), but merely redoubles it (609, 1), and thus Lacan reiterates what he said at the beginning of *Syllabary*.

Lacan (609, 2) ends by stating positively what the structure of the symbol is: It is a "knot that one cannot flatten out," because, like the Möbius strip, which cannot be flattened without losing its particular topology, it takes into account the specific import of the signifier. In other words, language is the difference that makes the difference. This is what Silberer and Jones missed because they did not have the RSI tools. In the closing line—one of the most difficult of the essay—Lacan introduces identification. He seems to be adding, at the very end, that because the true symbol has this structure, something needs to be added, in order for the true (Gordian) knot of the symbol to be cut,[27] especially if one is to "found an identification." Perhaps Lacan is referencing that even identification, which often is placed on the imaginary realm, also takes place with signifiers—the Symbolic must be included here as well.[28] Or, perhaps, Lacan is implicitly referencing the Möbius strip, as he does in *Seminar XI* (1964), in speaking of the interior 8,[29] to remind us that identification with the ego (of the subject or analyst) and staying on the level of the Imaginary and consciousness (versus working at the level of language, the specificity of the signifier, *the symbolic*, unconscious, and even unconscious desire), is what we want to avoid in psychoanalysis, and why, if the functional phenomenon is not a true symbol, it is missing something, and is not the "true" concern, interest, and work of psychoanalysis (or the work of "true" psychoanalysis).

Notes

1 In 1957, Lacan mentioned Silberer's *Chance and Impish Pranks of the Unconscious* in a footnote (*Instance of the Letter*: 441).

2 Jung, in his return letter to Freud, indicates that Eugen Bleuler disagreed with Freud about publishing Silberer (1909/1994: 181).

3 On pages 344–345 and 503–506 in the Standard Edition. Strachey translates *Traumdeutung* as *The Interpretation of Dreams*; Lacan (1966) refers to *La signifiance des rêves* and to *La science des rêves*, which was the title of the standard French translation published by Presses Universitaires de France.

4 Jones lists the following essays as his references: Silberer, 'Bericht über eine Methode, gewisse symbolische Halluzinations-Erscheinungen hervorzurufen und zu beobachten,' *Jahrbuch der Psychoanalyse*, 1909, Bd. i. S. 513; 'Von den Kategorien der Symbolik,' *Zentralblatt f*ür Psychoanalyse, *Jahrg.* ii., S. 177; *'Phantasie und Mythos,' Jahrbuch, Bd. Ii*, S. 541; 'Symbolik des Erwachens und Schwellensymbolik überhaupt,' *Jahrbuch*, Bd. iii, S. 621; 'Über die Symbolbildung,' *Jahrbuch*, Bd. iii, S. 661; 'Zur Symbolbildung,' *Jahrbuch*, Bd. iv., S. 607.

5 Lacan states, "when the *Traumdeutung* was published it was way ahead of the formalizations of linguistics for which one could no doubt show that it paved the way by the sheer weight of its truth" (*Instance of the Letter*: 426).

6 Lacan believes other analysts, here Jones and Silberer specifically, confuse the imaginary and symbolic registers and their relationship to the real. In 1953, in *Seminar I*, Lacan argues Melanie Klein at least shows a greater understanding of the symbolic register, whereas Anna Freud gets stuck in the imaginary. Lacan indexes this feud again and Jones's role in it in *Syllabary*.

7 Fink (1995: 103) also mentions the text, although not by name (rather as the 1996 afterword to the preceding article), when discussing the phallus as signifier of lack.

8 On what we do with syllables, I remind the reader that Lacan employs Freud's example of the syllables involved in "Signorelli" and their relation to the workings of the unconscious in *Seminar III* (1955–1956), and in *Psychoanalysis and its teaching*, Lacan also discusses the important relationship between the signifier and the symptom: "recall the broken tip of the memory's sword: the *signor* of the name Signorelli that Freud could not recall" (*Teaching*: 373). In discussing this memory lapse, Freud goes beyond words and breaks things down into syllables—"Bo" and "Herr"—highlighting their "signifierness" rather than meanings.

9 Perhaps the "historic" parentheses refers to Silberer's discussion of symbolism's history: the Romanticists versus the "sober realists," the believers versus the skeptics, and Scherner's "attempt to create a complete system of dream symbolism" as the "first approach to scientific dream interpretation" (1918/1955: 363). Scherner's dream symbolism connects imagery with "the realistic basis of body stimulation" (which Silberer connects to somatic phenomenon). The symbolic representations found in dreams, as such, are stimulated by bodily sensations.

> In dreams which are stimulated by sensations in the teeth, for example, the mouth corresponds to a high vaulted hall, and the passage from the throat to the esophagus is a staircase. The dream prefers to depict the human body as a house and the individual organs as parts of the house.
>
> (1918/1955: 363)

Silberer relays that for Scherner, if the dream is symbolizing a headache, a ceiling will be portrayed; "the image of a cat expresses an angry temper"; the bladder is "round, or pouch-like, or just a hollow object" (363). Silberer says Freud brought this history of extremes to a "happy medium."

10 Lacan uses the term *millefeuille*, which Fink translates as layer cake and in his translator's note, says in English this is a "Napoleon." Jacob Blauner (1955) translates Silberer's example as pie. The point, for Lacan, is that there are many layers, which "pie" does not conjure. Lacan, says he "forces" the example, and it seems he does.

11 Even though Silberer was referring (in the cake example) to material phenomenon.

12 Lacan makes this case in *The Freudian Thing* (362). And, in other places, Lacan references the "primacy of the signifier over the signified" (*Situation*, 391). These are all ways of stating this "principle" that differentiates Freud and Jung.

13 Jones discusses how symbols can be found across time, place, and cultures, throughout world history; he offers the figures in the Old Testament as an example and traces the king and queen symbols as they relate to fathers and mothers in the Old Testament and then can be traced forward to the symbol for the ruler of the Catholic Church 'The Holy Father' (143).

14 See Silberer, Herbert. *The Hidden Symbolism of Alchemy and the Occult Arts.* New York: Dover Books, 1971 (Originally published in 1914).

15 The correspondence may refer to when Jones writes to Freud:

> *Re* your passage on S. 338, Vierte Folge der *Sammlung*, it has doubtless occurred to you what a pretty confirmation lies in our view that all *unconscious symbolism* is *concrete*, which I emphasised in my essay on symbolism. (By the way, I have never heard if you have read this, and if you agree with my criticism of Silberer therein).
>
> (1993: 367)

16 While Lacan's discussion of knots in the *Syllabary* do *not* refer to knot theory as Lacan will later use it, the comments do seem to interestingly foreshadow Lacan's later discussion and development of knot theory as found in, for example, *Seminar XX, Encore* (1972–1973).

17 Freud just did not have access to the works that Lacan did. Elsewhere, Lacan discusses the history of modern linguistics, being traced to "Geneva 1910 and Petrograd 1920" to "explain why Freud did not have this particular instrument at his disposal" (*Subversion*, 676).

18 It is rather interesting, given Lacan's take on science (he does not think of psychoanalysis as a science), that he here endorses Freud's commitment to science. Freud's commitment may have helped him navigate this difficult terrain that was still haunted by "invisible realities."

19 On the 'mathematization of nature,' the 'subversive weight of Newton's formula,' and the turn of the supremacy of the symbolic over the imaginary in the theory of science at play in Lacan's work see Russell Grigg's (2008) '*Descartes and the subject of science*.'

20 Lacan was influenced here by Claude Lévi-Strauss's (1962/1966) *La pensée sauvage*.

21 Lacan had connected the importance of the subject, the signifier, the unconscious, and death, in 1957, when speaking of the role of syllables in relation to Freud's forgetting of Signorelli because of the "death for which one has assumed responsibility" (*Teaching*: 373), and in 1954 as well discussing the name Signorelli in light of having "signifying material at [Freud's] disposal," in terms of its "repressed signification" and its relationship to death (*Hyppolite*: 316).

22 In France the game *L'âne rouge* is a block puzzle game in which the largest or special block has a picture of a red donkey and the goal is to *slide* the block pieces around (without removing them from the game board) in order to get the red donkey piece to its desired location on the board.

23 This is likely also a reference to Lévi-Strauss's work.

24 There is an ambiguity from this point on in the essay between "symbolism" in the narrow sense in which Freud understood the term, and the "symbolic" in the specific sense Lacan gives the term.

25 "True knot" is perhaps also a word play on Jones's concept of the "true symbol."

26 In myriad places, including *Les Noms-du-Père*, Lacan discusses the "inadequacy" of our thought in relation to the real, because we remain captive to the imaginary. Because of this tendency, we tend to think in two dimensions (on the imaginary), having trouble thinking in three-dimensional space (the symbolic). One difficulty is that we "write" topological objects in two dimensions when we need three. The three dimensional knots, which Lacan brings into his psychoanalytic theorization, help to right this wrong.

27 In English, the "structure is such that one cannot found an identification unless something serves as the support to cut it," and in French "quelque chose fasse l'appoint pour en trancher." The expression "faire l'appoint," can mean give the exact change or add coins such that the salesperson will give you back a dollar/note rather than cents. And "trancher le noeud," evokes "cut the (Gordian) knot."

28 A patient says her "big" boyfriend is the one, and we see that all her boyfriends are "big" men, the same word or signifier she uses to describe her father. Here we have a series of identifications based on the *signifier* big.

29 See *Seminar XI* on the Möbius strip in relation to working at the level of unconscious desire and the signifier, rather than on the imaginary axis (S11, 1964: 155–156 and 235). Perhaps the something missing is the analyst's desire? That the

analyst's desire is the needed support. In June 1964, Lacan says "it is in as much as the analyst's desire … tends in a direction that is the exact opposite of identification, that the crossing of the plane of identification is possible" (ibid: 274).

References

Badiou, A. (1983/2013) *The Incident at Antioch*. New York: Columbia University Press.

Demoulin, C. (2001) 'Enjeux de la théorie Lacanienne', *Psychoanalytische Perspectieven*, 46, pp. 7–18.

Eyers, T. (2012) *Lacan and the Concept of the 'Real'*. New York: Palgrave Macmillan.

Fink, B. (1995) *The Lacanian Subject: Between Language and Jouissance*. Princeton, NJ: Princeton University Press.

Fink, B. (2004) *Lacan to the Letter: Reading Écrits Closely*. Minneapolis, MN: University of Minnesota Press.

Freud, S. (1900/1953) 'The Interpretation of Dreams', in J. Strachey (Ed.), *The Standard Edition of the Complete Psychological Works of Sigmund Freud*, Vols. 4/5. London: The Hogarth Press and the Institute of Psycho-Analysis.

Freud, S. (1914/1957) 'On Narcissism: An Introduction', in J. Strachey (Ed.), *The Standard Edition of the Complete Psychological Works of Sigmund Freud*, Vol. 14. London: The Hogarth Press and the Institute of Psycho-Analysis, pp. 67–102.

Freud, S. and Jones, E. (1993) *The Complete Correspondence of Sigmund Freud and Ernest Jones, 1908–1939*. Cambridge, MA: Harvard University Press.

Freud, S. and Jung, C.G. (1994) *The Freud-Jung Letters: The Correspondence between Sigmund Freud and C. G. Jung*. Princeton, NJ: Princeton University Press.

Gay, P. (1986) *Freud for Historians*. New York: Oxford University Press.

Grigg, R. (2008) 'Descartes and the Subject of Science', *Lacan, Language and Philosophy*. Albany, NY: State University of New York Press.

Jones, E. (1916/1948) 'The Theory of Symbolism', in *Papers on Psychoanalysis*. London: Balliere, Tindall and Cox, pp. 129–186.

Lacan, J. (1973/1994) *The Seminar. Book XI: The Four Fundamental Concepts of Psycho-Analysis* (1964), trans. A. Sheridan, ed. J.-A. Miller. Harmondsworth: Penguin.

Lacan, J. (1975/1988) *The Seminar. Book I: Freud's Papers on Technique* (1953–1954), trans. J. Forrester, ed. J.-A. Miller. Cambridge: Cambridge University Press.

Lacan, J. (1975/1998) *Book XX: Encore, On Femininity, Love and the Limits of Knowledge* (1972–1973), trans. B. Fink, ed. J.-A. Miller. London: W. W. Norton.

Lacan, J. (1981/1993) *The Seminar. Book III: The Psychoses* (1955–1956), trans. R. Grigg. New York, NY: W. W. Norton & Company.

Lévi-Strauss, C. (1962/1966) *The Savage Mind*. Chicago, IL: University of Chicago Press.

Miller, J.-A. (2003) 'Lacan's Later Teaching', *Lacanian Ink*, 21, pp. 4–41.

Nitzschke, B. (1989) 'Freud et Herbert Silberer. Hypothèses concernant les destinataire d'une lettre de Freud de 1922', *Revue Internationale d'Histoire de la Psychanalyse*, 2, pp. 267–277.

Roazen, P. (1976) *Freud and his Followers*. New York: Alfred A. Knopf.

Silberer, H. (1914/1971) *The Hidden Symbolism of Alchemy and the Occult Arts*. New York: Dover Books.

Silberer, H. (1918/1955) 'The Dream: Introduction to the Psychology of Dreams', *Psychoanalytic Review*, 42, pp. 361–387.

4

SOME GUIDING REMARKS FOR A CONVENTION ON FEMALE SEXUALITY

Eve Watson

Context

'*Some Guiding Remarks for a Convention on Female Sexuality*' (1958) is an intriguing treatise on Lacan's thinking on sexual difference and female sexuality in the late fifties. It takes up points of controversy on the specific issue of feminine sexuality as it appears in clinical practice as well as asking key questions about the role and status of women in the social arena and considering how female sexuality has been defined by psychoanalytic doctrine. Written two years before a conference on feminine sexuality, organised by the *Société Française de Psychanalyse*, which took place at the *Municipal University of Amsterdam* in September 1960, the text is a complement to '*The Signification of the Phallus*' (1958), '*On a Question Preliminary to Any Possible Treatment of Psychosis*' (1958) and '*The Instance of the Letter in the Unconscious*' (1957) in addition to Lacan's fourth and fifth seminars on *Object Relations* (1956–1957) and the *Formations of the Unconscious* (1957–1958) respectively, these texts being part of a larger project of promoting a rational and scientific re-reading and interpretation of Freud's work by ascribing a linguistic structure to the unconscious. This linguistic structure, based on a post-Saussurian theory of the signifier and the designation of a symbolic function, principally derived from the work of linguist Roman Jakobson and his theory of metaphor and metonymy, is evoked throughout the text as a backdrop to a highly sophisticated and 'early' consideration of female sexuality, its 'early' status being relative to Lacan's later work in the seventies explicitly devoted to the theme.

Although the text is one of Lacan's lengthiest accounts of female sexuality, it is as the title sets out, a set of 'guiding remarks' about a constellation of themes pertaining to female sexuality. It seems likely that Lacan was influenced by Simone de Beauvoir, whose ground-breaking work, *The Second Sex* (1949), elaborated the feminine as a social construct, as well as by his close colleagues Francoise Dolto and Jenny Aubry, influential child analysts whose pioneering work was greatly admired by Lacan and who were supporters and confidantes of his. Stylistically, the text is densely packed with ideas that are little explained, requiring the reader to contextualise them, and knowledge of other texts such as '*The Signification of the Phallus*' is essential. There are few exegeses of the text but there are several excellent short commentaries by Genevieve Morel (2002) and Colette Soler (2002, 2006) and aspects of those are included here. In broad terms, female sexuality is developed throughout the text in terms of the sexual relation and the female body within a framework of feminine love and desire.

An important aspect of the text is its hinge-point status. Lacan in the late fifties was beginning to delineate the feminine relation as dual, that is to say, to the phallus and to the Other. This double orientation, which can also be described as woman's tendency towards 'bisexuality,' is propitiated throughout as crucial in approaching the symptomatic manifestations of the libidinal economy and Oedipal trajectory of woman. Lacan's analysis of the theory and clinical relevance of femininity, while elaborated with the 'paternal function' and the delimitation of the phallus, does, as the text shows, foreshadow his work almost twenty years later in his twentieth seminar *Encore* where he elaborates feminine structure in terms of a supplementary *jouissance* that a woman doesn't know about and cannot speak of. According to Roudinesco (1997: 365), the notion of femininity as supplement was mooted by Lacan, Wladamir Granoff and Francois Perrier at the 1960 convention. There are indications in *Guiding Remarks* that Lacan was already thinking of femininity beyond the feminism of phallic logic and the phallic realm of language, even if he was some way from fully defining the *objet petit a* and masculine and feminine structure in terms of the type of *jouissance* obtained.

The text can first be situated in relation to '*The Signification of the Phallus*' and Lacan's re-designation there of the phallus as a signifier in the linguistic sense, its role in the symbolic and in the sexual dialectic. *Guiding Remarks* in turn explores the implications of the phallus for female psychology. These implications are invariably linked to the 'phallocentric' nature of the symbolic which Lacan throughout his work upholds as a given and essential to his reframing of Freud's sexual binary of having/not-having, in his terms, as a non-symmetrical binary of masculine having/feminine being. The text develops the significance and the possibilities afforded by the position of 'being' the phallus on the side of woman in terms of her desire and '*jouissance*' and it is an appraisal of woman's relationship to language. Lacan's unabashedly 'phallocentric' stance has meant that he has been no friend to feminist models of sexual and political identities. His non-contestation of the phallic as symbolic has led to accusations of sexism by feminists and phallocentrism by psychoanalytic commentators such as Luce Irigaray in texts such as *Speculum of the Other Woman* (1974) and *This Sex Which is Not One* (1985) and Elizabeth Grosz in *Jacques Lacan: A Feminist Introduction* (1990). Conversely, Lacanian-inspired feminists such as Juliet Mitchell and Jacqueline Rose (1982: 86) assert the importance of *Guiding Remarks* in critiquing psychoanalytic ideological accounts that characterise femininity in terms of "mistake, omission and prejudice" and the importance of the text in indicating that the problem of femininity "is unequivocally the problem of the symbolic articulation of its forms."

Guiding Remarks continues a number of crucial themes developed in Lacan's fourth seminar on *Object Relations* (1956–1957), in particular a reconsideration of 'the object' of psychoanalysis and as such, the text is heavily pitched against developments in psychoanalysis that for Lacan had reduced the subversiveness of Freud's teaching. These developments include the near elimination of the role of the unconscious and its related fantasies, the rendering of psychic reality equivalent to external reality and the role of psychoanalysis in conspiring to become an agent of the adaptation of the subject to society. Another essential theme is Lacan's re-evaluation of the Freudian Oedipus complex. Modern civilisation, marked by the decline of the ideals of the paternalistic family, made Lacan's re-reading of the Freudian Oedipus complex not only essential but also necessary to differentiating his psychoanalytic method from that of the Anglo-American-dominated International Psychoanalytic Association and its French counterpart, the Société Française de Psychanalyse, which favoured standardised treatment and the universality of training methodology. His sustained intention to resuscitate psychoanalysis from what he describes as the fate that has befallen psychoanalytic doctrine and practice by attending too closely to the Freudian 'myth' and in particular how this had structured the elaboration of female sexuality is reinforced again at the end of the text with his rhetorical question asking if the "analytic myth of the prohibition of incest between father and daughter" fails to do justice to female sexuality (Guiding Remarks, 619, 10). This fate is set out by Lacan as the shift from the Freudian paternal castration complex grounded "in repression brought on by the father" to the maternal body and the linking of real defects in mothering to developmental problems and "affective deficiency" and this has led to misguided emphases that have become rife in designating woman's sexuality (610, 1–3). This shift has culminated in the assertion of the role of the natural order and the belief in a "fantastic phallophagy" of the mother (614, 1).

The text is nonetheless Freudian in that it remains close to many of the fundamental axioms of Freud's theorisations of women, and re-situates the Freudian father complex and the castration complex at the centre of subjectivity and in the role and function of female sexuality. It also elaborates three configurations of female sexuality – frigidity, heterosexual femininity and homosexuality – which closely echoes Freud's famous three lines of femininity in his femininity papers, the revulsion of sexuality, normative femininity and homosexuality (1931/2001: 229–230). In re-elaborating both the Freudian father complex and the castration complex, the text returns to Freud but with the crucial addition of the theory of the phallus as the dynamic factor not only in structuring the desiring economy of men and women, but as necessary to reclaiming psychoanalysis from the conceptual slippage that has led to "the lifelessness of analytic experience" since Freud (612, 5). The text's orientation to this reclamation is underpinned by a blazing commentary on the misrecognitions and biases inherent in thinking female sexuality in terms of "the female part" [*partie*] (610, 4), that is, as based in a female corporal bodily specificity that is purportedly indicative of female sexuality. This approach, that had become rampant in psychoanalysis and in other fields and would become the backbone of mainstream feminism, is behind many of the great disagreements and crises in psychoanalysis since the late twenties and is a repeated area of elaboration by Lacan in the text. For Lacan, these developments remain rooted in elaborating a differential feminine sphere in terms of phallic equivalence. He takes particular issue with the notion of phallic equivalence, which he argues fails to properly account for the feminine as properly distinct and ultimately renders the two sides of the sexual dialectic as opposing sides of the same coin. By contrast, Lacan affirms female sexuality as having a specificity of its own insofar as "phallic mediation" does not account for everything drive-related in a woman (614, 9) and this has implications in the consideration of feminine frigidity, feminine heterosexuality and feminine homosexuality.

In interpreting why contemporary psychoanalytic doctrine had gone so awry in the theorisation of female sexuality, Lacan takes no prisoners, including women and the 'myths' of women. He provocatively proposes that no-one, including women themselves, has lifted the veil of mystery ascribed to female sexuality (612, 11). He structures his unveiling of the 'mystery' via a trinity of questions posed at the very beginning of the text and in a section titled "Review of the Facts": what women actually say in their analyses regarding sex that confirms or fails to confirm the biological-scientific discourses on women's sexuality; second, to what extent are sex and love, as well as their transmitted consequences to children, subordinated to desire and its unconscious formations; third, what are the implications of Freud's conception of psychical bisexuality in subjective formation, first asserted in terms of anatomical duplication but progressively transferred to "personological" identifications that have taken its place? (611, a, b and c). Each of these questions is addressed in the text as Lacan situates women not as counterparts to men but as having a different relation to the phallus that has precise effects not only in the structuration of feminine subjectivity but as consequential to psychoanalytic technique.

Commentaries on the text

"The Shine [Éclat] of Absences": The 'Object' and 'the Object Relation'

The first sections of *Guiding Remarks* (Sections I–VI) set out in various ways Lacan's critique of the psychoanalysis of his time, in particular the growing emphasis on 'the object' and 'the object relation' and the ensuing consequences for female psychology in psychoanalytic doctrine. He focuses on two growing trends: one, the emphasis on the anatomical specificity of the female organ, linked to both essentialism and scientism and the elaboration of female psychology in developmental and teleological terms; and the other is the rise to prominence of 'the object relation' in the sexual relationship. To begin with, it is helpful to consider Lacan's critique of 'the object' in his 1956–1957 seminar on *Object Relations*. He takes up the object in strictly Freudian terms, which is that there is no object but a lacking object and every object is a substitute object that can also be hallucinated and dreamt (1895/2001: 366–367), with the result that the finding of an object is always its re-finding (1905/2001: 222). Thus, what is at stake in the field of an object relation is not an objectifiable object within a dual relation, as any notion resting on the supposed 'objectality' of the object misunderstands the Freudian object as essentially lacking (Lacan, S4, 1956–1957: 6–9). The lacking object can be traced to a gap opening up in the mother–child relation that the child attempts to make good by making itself the object of love for the mother and wedging itself between the desire of the mother and the imaginary object, which is the phallus (Lacan, S4, 1956–1957: 289). What counts, Lacan writes, "are the deficiencies, the disappointments which touch upon the mother's omnipotence" (Lacan, S4, 1956–1957: 70). The child invokes the symbolic order in a system of exchanges to address this lacking object but this inevitably disappoints, as the symbolic order cannot redress, reparate or make good the frustration and dissatisfaction in losing the object. This directly critiques the work of Melanie Klein, for whom the Oedipal trajectory is one in which the partial object relation is transformed into a full object relation through the exchange of a good object for a bad object (1935/1986: 118).

In effect, there is an insurmountable gap between subject and object as there is no object that can satisfy either the drive or the desire of the subject. Human relations are not between two subjects but between a subject and a partial object that stands in and gives the lost object an image. Consequently, the rise to prominence of 'the object relation' and the specification of the object relation as an anticipated reciprocity between subject and other introduces a new aim into psychoanalysis oriented to an ideal object and the normalisation of the subject (Lacan, S4, 1956–1957: 10). The notion of the ideal object, intrinsic to 'the object relation' is premised on a notion of a conflict-free and harmonious rapport between the ego and the object and such an object relation would correspond to a subject who has, as Lacan sarcastically puts it, perfectly liquidated the structuring conflicts of childhood (Lacan, S4, 1956–1957: 13). This has affected not just the conception and treatment of the sexual relation in psychoanalysis but the theorisation of women, and explains why Karen Horney, for example, writes, "for the one sex always seeks in the other that which is complementary to it or of a nature different to its own" (1932/1999: 247).

These critiques underpin Lacan's rebuke early in *Guiding Remarks* of contemporary psychoanalysis for promising to bring the "whole secret of sexuality to light" (612, 7), a rebuke that he harks back to in his seminar on *The Psychoses* (S3, 1955–1956) where he writes that "… the great secret of psychoanalysis is that there is no psychogenesis" and furthermore that

> if that is what psychoanalysis is, there is precisely nothing that could be further from psychoanalysis in its whole development, its entire inspiration and its mainspring, in everything it has contributed, everything it has been able to confirm for us in anything we have established.
>
> (S3, 1955–1956: 7)

In this, Lacan is taking aim at the psychoanalytic field's increasing emphasis on biology and anatomy in specifying sexual difference and in the application of a developmental telos in framing the subject. The result of these developments is that the unconscious is eliminated and the subject, he writes, fails to be taken as "the subject of a combinatory" which is what gives the unconscious its meaning (612, 1). This refers to the superior position Lacan gives to the signifier over the signified, the word over meaning, based on his reversal of the Saussurian algorithm and the juxtaposition of the ego to the unconscious. Lacan's work throughout the fifties, in particular in his analyses in Poe's purloined letter and in '*The Instance of the Letter in the Unconscious*' (1957) where he attests that the material basis of the unconscious is the signifier and its pathway is metonymic as he demonstrates in his study of the purloined letter – "a letter always arrives at its destination" (*Purloined Letter*, 30, 2). The signifier-to-signifier connection elides the relation to the real by inscribing it in a symbolic system that instates lack of being in the object relation (*Instance of the Letter*, 428, 5) and the enigmas of desire "are based on no other derangement of instinct than the fact that it is caught in the rails of metonymy, eternally extending towards a desire for something else" (*Instance of the Letter*, 431, 5).

Returning to *Guiding Remarks*, at the beginning of Section VI, Lacan states that the current state of affairs in theorising the feminine "betrays a scientific impasse in approaching reality ['*reel*']," but psychoanalysis "was born of a similar impasse" (613, 3).[1] While it is crucial to know the effect and scope of dominant paradigms, which are indubitably scientific, rational and cognitive, the manifold aporias of sexuality cannot be resolved by reducing them either to hermeneutical and biological data, notwithstanding that the cogito and the body are supremely implicated in the field of human sexuality. The adoption by psychoanalysis of scientific notions such as anatomical determination and genetic and endocrinal factors had become popular in the fifties. At that time, physiological and hormone-based therapies were a favoured form of treatment for homosexuality (lesbians for example were treated with hysterectomies and oestrogen treatments) and psychosis and mental ill-health were treated with lobotomies and electric shock therapy. As a brilliant counter-argument against the scientific turn in psychoanalysis, Lacan poses the new physiological findings in genetics and endocrinology that found clinical interpretation in psychoanalysis against their non-adoption by the scientific field, a field that readily bases its findings on what he describes as the "... messianic access to decisive chemisms" (611, 6). Quite likely here he is referring to developments such as the Meselson-Stahl experiment in 1958 that showed that when the double-stranded DNA helix is replicated, each of the two new double-stranded DNA helixes consists of one strand from the original helix and one newly synthesised. This shows a semi-conservative predictive sequencing formula and thus the outcome cannot be absolutely predicted. Perhaps too, Lacan is inflecting the tone in the medical literature about hormone replacement therapies that turned from enthusiastic to cautious in the fifties.

The problem for Lacan is where the dividing line ["*coupure*"] comes in (611, 7). If the psychoanalytic field is unwilling to draw a line between the psychical and the somatic and distinguish between organism and subject, it will be forced to draw on the scientific discourse to account for the inexplicable in the field of inter-subjectivity. The "lofty biological landmarks with which we continue to be content" (610, 5) and the anatomically visible "signs" of sexual differentiation, Lacan argues, are indicative of the "imaginary hold" that symbols have on the subject (613, 3), a process not helped by the insistence by Freud himself on what Lacan calls "Freud's paradox" (613, 7), on women's "primal ignorance of their sexual organ" (613, 6) that Jones attempted to resolve by appealing to the dominance of the natural order.[2] Jones in his address to the Vienna Psychoanalytic Society in 1935 describes the importance of a girl's relation to the "inside" of the mother's body which he attests successfully fills her with "pleasant material of both a solid and liquid kind" (Jones, 1935/1999: 278). Moreover, a girl's deepest anxieties are linked to the vagina (Jones, 1935/1999: 280) and to both the obscurity of this organ in childhood (Jones, 1935/1999: 279) as well as a girl's presumed "penis-wish" which is her wish to substitute the clitoris for the penis (Jones, 1935/1999: 280). This wish is evidenced, according to Jones, and taking his cues from Helene Deutsch and Karen Horney, in the association between penis envy and actual urethral activities (Jones, 1935/1999: 281). The part-object in this case is equivalent to the biological object. In practical terms, to presume that girls feel nothing vaginally is one-sided and if the phallic period is the period of the awakening of the genital region, it is so for both boys and girls. That is why Lacan references Josine Muller's work (1925/1999: 122–128), which speaks to the girl child's knowledge of the vagina (615, 1).

In this respect, in Section V, the section entitled "The Darkness Cast Upon the Vaginal Organ," Lacan notes the difficulty in separating images and symbols "in" women from images and symbols "of" women (613, 4). It is the Other of discourse that knots the norms, models, obligations and the interdictions of discourse to anatomical identity. Lacan is at pains to point out in the text that this process is inextricable from all representations of women, including psychoanalytic ones. He writes that:

> The representation (*Vorstellung* in the sense in which Freud uses the term when he notes that it is what is repressed) of female sexuality, whether it is repressed or not, conditions its implementation, and its displaced emerges (in which the therapist's doctrine may turn out to be an interested party) seal the fate of the tendencies, however naturally refined [*dégrossies*] one assumes them to be.
>
> (613, 5)

Women's articulations, including their analytic ones, do not support their supposed biologically essential nature, even if they haven't, as Lacan dryly puts it, lifted the nature of vaginal orgasm from its "obscurity inviolate" (612, 9). In effect, the "darkness" cast upon the vaginal organ stems from "metaphors whose loftiness in the ideal signifies nothing preferable to what the hoi polloi give us by way of a less intentioned poetry" (613, 1). In metaphoric terms, the route to female sexuality is thus not to be found in the fate of Tiresias from the Sophoclean myth of Oedipus Rex whose change of sex from man to woman entailed a bodily process, as if the route to understanding female sexuality is via the corporeal sphere (613, 2). The debates on the female genital part-object and the supposed opposition between clitoridal and vaginal satisfaction – debates that are premised on the "female part" (*partie*) (610, 4) have invoked notions as varied as the sensitivity of the cervix, the posterior wall of the vagina, clitoral versus vaginal *jouissance* and rectal dependence (612, 8–10, 12) – is an apportioning of sexuality into a distinct feminine physiological sphere, which is inextricably linked to the field of genital relations. The problem is that it is impossible to think of anatomy as a stable referent given the indissolubility of the psychic and the physical. Descriptions of the body are always physically and phantasmatically invested and psychic projection confers a bodily boundary and a unity, as Lacan demonstrates in *The Mirror-Stage*. Thus, Freud's sexed binary, "... between having a male genital and being castrated" (1925/2001: 145) and his insistence that in all of this the vagina is "virtually non-existent" (1931/2001: 228) is ultimately not a question of what signifies lack and difference but what causes the question of difference to emerge.[3] Consequently, 'organ-dominated' thinking introduces a conceptual impasse and a partial and ineffectual binary when as yet none exists and it easily lends itself to thinking that sexual difference is caused by anatomical distinction when it merely comes to be partially figured by it.

A belief in the natural order is behind the emphasis on what Lacan describes as "anatomical duplications" and "'personological' identifications" (611, c).

Such an emphasis on character markers or flaws as indicative of the subject, especially in the field of sexuality, which is arguably one precursor to the personality disorders taken up comprehensively in the *Diagnostic and Statistical Manual of Mental Disorders* (DSM), is linked by Lacan in *Guiding Remarks* to the repression of Freud's originary bisexual schematic, that is, the notion that the protean bisexuality and polymorphous perversity of the inchoate subject is rechanneled by Oedipalisation, which redirects the orientation of infantile desire to multiple love objects and inscribes the component drives in a socially sanctioned dialectic that overwrites, although it does not eliminate, the originary bisexual disposition. This repression of originary bisexuality is interpretable as re-emerging in the new duality of the "phallic equivalence" of the sexes and in the nomination of new 'perverse' identities, including homosexuality. The framing of women's sexuality in terms of phallic equivalence, and Lacan singles out Klein and Jones in particular,[4] categorically ignores "Freud's oft-repeated advice not to reduce the supplement of the feminine with respect to the masculine to the complement of the passive with respect to the active" (615, 9; Freud, 1931/2001: 258). For Lacan, this equivalence has resulted in the conceptual slippage that has mired psychoanalysis in questions about essentialism and development (612, 5).

In Section VII, "Misrecognitions and Biases," Lacan militates against this slippage and what he describes as the " 'legendary' fabulation" (614, 5) of the girl's organ and other objects that are fantasised as good and bad (614, 6). Instead what is required is a theory of the phallus that "explains the equivalence function [*function d'équivalence*] served by the phallus in the advent of any object of desire, the simple mention of its 'partial' character not sufficing" (614, 6). It's not that phallic equivalence isn't a factor in sexual difference but it is a factor of effect. Lacan explains that it is a synchrony in which the relation of non-being [*manque à ètre*] symbolised by the phallus is established as a diversion to the not-having [*manque à avoir*] that has its basis in the frustration of demand (614, 7).[5] The dialectic of frustration arises when the object is lacking. This leads to a substitution of the symbolic phallus rooted in language and the signifier, for the imaginary phallus, which is the child's sense of being the object that will satisfy the mother whose lack of object of satisfaction has been discerned by the child. For Lacan, the constituting factor in terms of the subject is less a question of what is imaged by the phallus than what is symbolised by it. Lacan's theory explaining the function of the phallus provides a "fundamental synchrony" in which any questions about development can by posed (614, 7).

This is the "fundamental synchrony" that reframes the pre-Oedipal, along with regression and idealisation, as the reduction of the symbolic to the imaginary and the reduction of the real to the imaginary respectively, this is the "imaginary complex." Klein's pre-Oedipal theatre, ranging from the maternal body to passive genital female maturity, is better understood as a pre-Oedipal reality delimited by the Name-of-the-Father (613, 6). Helpful here, as

Lacan writes in his seminar on object relations, is that "there is an anteriority of maternal castration, and paternal castration is its substitute" (S4, 1956–1957: 433). Consequently, the notion of the maternal body as a container is a phantasmagoria of the drama and conflict arising from the imposition of the Other as a third element into the dual relation, an imposition that causes the mother to appear omnipotent to her child. The child's sense of its own frustration and powerlessness in the face of the mother's omnipotence is thus the depressive position. In effect, the re-designation of the phallic object into its real, imaginary and symbolic aspects "assigns a limit to questions about development" (614, 8).

Misrecognitions and biases: castration and phallic non-equivalence

In Section VII, Lacan takes on a number of biases and misunderstandings arising from the repression of paternal castration and the promotion of a real object to the status of 'proper' object, which in his opinion has enmeshed the field with value-laden ideology (scientism, moralism, humanism, sexism, homophobia), a process that Lacan scathingly refers to as psychoanalysis having "degenerated to the point of swallowing its own vomit" (615, 7). It is, he argues, the misappropriation and the ignorance of castration that is responsible for the characterisation of women in biased and reductive ways. Against Jones's assertion in 'The Early Development of Female Sexuality' that castration is a partial threat (1927/1999: 135), Lacan posits that castration, which is the prohibition and repression of the pre-Oedipal relation to the mother, occurs when the symbolic father, as bearer of the phallus intrudes, prohibits and inaugurates the repressed unconscious of both sexes by positing the cultural implications of sexed difference. While the two sexes enter the symbolic order as castrated, as the symbolic is phallic in its constitution, identity is constructed within the realm of the masculine, as either 'having' or 'being' the phallus as indicated by him in '*The Signification of the Phallus*' (582, 9). On one side, there is a having to be protected, and on the other, a masking of lack and this is aided on the masculine side by dominant phallic models.

The non-symmetry of the sexes goes further in that, while both man and woman undergo frustration and castration, a woman additionally undergoes privation as there is no symbolisation of woman's sex (1956–1957: 441). Lacan in this way takes up Freud's idea of the 'non-existence' of the feminine organ as a problem of symbolisation. This is a lack of symbolisation of her real organ, which puts in her a position of 'not-having' in relation to the phallic 'plus' on the father's side. This causes the little girl to identify with the 'minus' side insofar as she does not have the phallus and her sexual organ is placed, as Lacan puts it in *Guiding Remarks*, "under the sign of an organic minus-value" (614, 4). The notion of phallic equivalence in men and women misses not only the function of castration as structuring men and women differently in relation to the phallus but it misses the crucial point that women, in their privation, relate to the phallus, which they do not have, and identify with the hole or 'minus' in the Other. In being already deprived and embodying lack in phallic terms, a woman is not fully encapsulated by the signifier. In terms of symbolic differentiation, her status as 'minus' means she has to relate to a phallus she does not have. In effect, she approaches having through 'not-having,' hence Lacan's idea that symbolic castration is "a castration that does not really concern her" (617, 6).

It is in this light that Lacan takes up women's supposedly natural inclination towards passivity and masochism (615, 2–3). Such ideas are proposed by both Helene Deutsch (1930/1999: 192–193; 1932/1999: 235) and Karen Horney (1932/1999: 248–249). Lacan argues that this is the promotion of masochism from the status of the Freudian partial drive to that of full post-Oedipal genital maturity (615, 2) and rhetorically asks, "can we rely on what masochistic perversion owes to male invention and conclude that female masochism is a fantasy of male desire" (615, 4)? The lack of cognisance of the symbolic role of the phallus in castration and its subsequent reappearance as a real object is behind various fantasies based on Freud's analysis of the taboo of virginity about the importance of the breaking of corporeal boundaries and the rupture of the hymen (615, 5).[6] These fantasies are representative of a masculinised viewpoint filtered through the prism of the real of a woman's body and thus "female masochism is a fantasy of male desire" 615,4). We must "distinguish between unconscious and bias regarding the signifier's effects" (615, 7) and this is ultimately what helps the analyst "to recognise, simultaneously, that the analyst is just as liable as anyone else to have a bias regarding sex, above and beyond [*passé*] what the unconscious reveals to him" (615, 8).

Moreover, Lacan argues, the misapprehension of the real object in its imaginary and symbolic forms is what is at stake in confusing anxiety and fear (615, 7). Klein, for example, writes in this vein that "the girl's very intense anxiety about her womanhood can be shown to be analogous to the boy's dread of castration" (1927/1986: 155). This is a limited description as castration anxiety is a permanent remnant of the castrating effects of the Oedipus complex and its forms are varied – it isn't just about the *fear* of the loss of sexual desire as Jones's aphanisis-theory proposes.[7] Freud's case of Little Hans, a four-and-a-half-year-old boy with a horse phobia shows major differences between anxiety and fear and the role and function of the *lacking* object. As the mother's imaginary phallus, he is delimited to a particular element of his being as opposed to his whole being that is taken as the desired object. He doesn't know this and mistakes his penis (*wiwimacher*) for the imaginary phallus, which is rejected by his mother (Freud, 1909/2001: 19). This presents him with a crisis and the exacerbation of his already-heightened anxiety. For Hans, this coincides with the arrival of his little sister Hannah and what this *wiwimacher*-less being means for his active little *wiwimacher*. The actions of his mother, notably her frequent trips out in pursuit of a new object and her unwillingness to allow authority to reside in Hans' father, leave the paternal agency degraded as authority and symbolic intercession. Hans' solution to the enigma of the void in the Other is to posit a phallus in everyone, especially his sister and his mother (Freud, 1909/2001: 106). Significantly, his relation to the anal object, his '*lumf*' as he calls it, is a reduction of the real object to an imaginary one which can fall and therefore it presents him with a hole, a gap that his succession of fantasies having to do with unscrewing help him to confront. This is necessary because the symbolic plane available to Hans does not support a virile identification and the right to the phallus that is available normatively to a boy and the phobia gives him the signifier 'horse' as a signifying place for his anxiety, what Lacan describes as a 'protection' (S4, 1955–1956: 16) against the failure of the symbolic system when confronted with the enigma of his sex and existence. The horse-phobia allowed him to substitute fear of the biting falling-down horse for his anxiety, that is, to substitute a real object for the missing symbolic one.

Frigidity and feminine subjective structure

> Castration cannot be deduced from development because it implicates the Other, in that it presupposes the subjectivity of the Other as a locus of its law.
>
> (616, 3)

In section VIII, "Frigidity and Subjective Structure," Lacan explores a number of themes, notably the relation between woman and man, the role and nature of feminine frigidity and what he terms as the "monstrous" conceptualisation of woman generated by the phallic dialectic. In order to explore the remarks in this and the remaining sections, which contain some of the text's densest and most difficult passages, a further explication of Lacan's conception of castration is necessary. His notion of castration expands upon Freud's castration theory and enlarges the scope of sexual difference as a process of inscription and re-inscription of preceding losses that are retroactively rewritten within a languaging and symbolising framework, principally driven by the phallic signifier, a signifier that names the Other's desire. In its symbolic form, Lacan formulises the phallus in *The Signification of the Phallus* as a "privileged signifier" in that it governs the relations between the sexes, its 'privileged' status accruing because it cannot as a signifier ultimately unveil what is signified (581, 2). In both his fourth and fifth seminars, he specifies three Oedipal moments of crisis – frustration, privation and castration, that involve three different lacking objects – symbolic, real and imaginary. Phallic castration is the third stage and is the resolution of the Oedipus complex and it is the precondition for the subject's active entry into the symbolic order through symbolic identification with the father and the internalisation of the law. But a woman does not altogether identify with the father, given her 'minus-value' status in phallic terms and therefore she is less inscribed by the castration process. This is what is at stake in Lacan's remark: "At this same point, it is appropriate to investigate whether phallic mediation exhaustively accounts for everything drive-related that can manifest itself in women, especially the whole current of the maternal instinct" (614, 9).

As a languaging operation, castration cannot be based on either the Freudian real or the Kleinian 'split' or 'partial' object but is based on the 'lacking' object. Lacan points out that the "splitting of the object," intrinsic to the field of object relations, is a confusion of Freud's splitting of the ego and the fading of the subject (616, 9). Freud posits that the ego splits in order to defend against a conflict between the drive and the demands of reality and this highlights the lack of unity and the non-'synthetic' nature of the ego. He imputes splitting as a defence against the fright of castration that can cause a regression to the oral phase and the fear of being eaten by the father.[8] The splitting of the object into 'good' and 'bad' is therefore a misunderstanding of the function of the ego and treats the ego as the place of the subject. Another misunderstanding of the object singled out by Lacan is Jones's "false and dangerous" idea that conflates perversion and phobia in female homosexuality (616, 6–7). Jones argues that in women there is sometimes a phobic reaction to the penis and a 'penis-identification,' making them both 'phobic' and perverse, that is, homosexual (Jones, 1927/1999: 139–142). Phobia for both Freud and Lacan is the cornerstone of neurosis and as the case of Little Hans demonstrates, is about turning objects into signifiers (*Instance of the Letter*, 432, 4) and is not, as Jones argues, about turning objects into fetish-objects. Jones's conflation of phobia and perversion in female homosexuality is for Lacan a misunderstanding of the status of the object insofar as the phobic object stands in place of the phallic signifier and the fetish-object fills the disavowed gap in the Other. "I mean that the defence here can be conceptualized, firstly, in the dimension of mascarade that the presence of the Other liberates in the sexual role" (616, 5).

To turn to the phallocentric sexual dialectic and the relation between man and woman brokered by the phallus, Lacan asserts that "a man serves here as a relay so that a woman becomes this Other to herself, as she is to him" (616, 3). The non-correspondence of the two desiring positions lies in the different relations to the Other and masquerade functions by adjusting to the Other's desire and by seeking to captivate it and make it less unconscious and enigmatic. In masquerading femininity, a woman takes up being what a man lacks. This means that in her dividedness, in not 'having' the phallus, a woman is attractive to a man who on one level 'has' it, but on another level doesn't have it insofar as he is a subject who desires. In effect, a woman comes to the sexual couple as a fantasy-object and she is desired insofar as she meets with the coordinates of a man's fantasy. 'Being' the phallus, being what a man lacks is, in effect, the only way that a woman can relate to a man. As a result, masquerade takes on an especially powerful resonance for a woman as it is a defence against not-having and, furthermore, in 'being' the phallus, love takes on a special significance in that a woman's demand for love can take on an erotomaniacal character where "we find the most salient features in the most ordinary lived experience" (617, 2). The erotomaniacal character, as Morel (2002: 81) explains, arises from women's "overestimation of love that can almost be absolute" and in aiming at a point beyond the partner "presupposes that the initiative comes from the Other." It is erotomaniacal in its belief in the absolute nature of her partner's love.

On the side of man, a woman is desirable as a 'phallus-girl,' which for Lacan is "[a desire for] the phallus that was desired by the Mother" (617, 3). In this regard, a woman functions as the phallus to a man through what Morel (2002: 79) describes as an agalmic or phallic brilliance that operates as a "phallic veil," covering over the unbearable castration that the sexual act brokers. A man's satisfaction is tempered by the anxiety that even though he gets off, he can never gain or attain the *jouissance* that is hers (Morel, 2002). The desire of the masculine subject, modelled on the mother's desire that undergoes signification via the paternal metaphor, is later reframed in *Encore* as what causes a man to desire "*quoad matrem*" (Lacan, S19, 1971–1972: 35). To desire *quoad matrem* is to desire qua that mother's desire, which acquired phallic signification due to the paternal metaphor (Morel, 2002: 79). To desire qua the mother's desire organises the phallic significance of the man's partner according to the vicissitudes of the mother's desire. This is what causes in the masculine subject a split between love and desire, which Lacan draws out in *The Signification of the Phallus*. Here, Lacan outlines that a man loves one woman and desires another and this causes a persistent divergence towards "another woman" who can signify the phallus under various guises either as a virgin or prostitute (583, 3). A man's love is thus 'fetishistic' in that a woman is loved for being the object that he lacks and insofar as she embodies the missing maternal phallus.

If a woman wants to have a relation with a man, she must accept both her relation to the phallic function and her partner as subject to castration and the symbolic law of the phallus. Lacan remarks in this respect that "there is no virility that castration does not consecrate" (617, 6). Thus, a woman relates to a man qua his 'having' the phallus and qua his masculine function. He must also meet with the coordinates of her fundamental phantasy. There can be a fetish aspect to her desire in as much as she finds the signifier of her desire in her partner's organ, which thereby takes on the value of a fetish. On the woman's side, love and desire often reside in the same object and this can lead, as already noted, to a demand that the partner be faithful in absolute, unmediated and erotomaniacal forms.

This is, however, a displacement of her true partner to whom she is ultimately faithful. This true partner with whom she is ultimately monogamous is "a castrated lover or a dead man or the two in one" (617, 6). Moreover, this partner "hides behind the veil in order to call her adoration to it" (ibid). What is indicated here by Lacan is that behind a woman's not infrequent demand that the Other be faithful, which is often accompanied by the assertion of her own fidelity, is her own infidelity as her true partner is located "behind the veil" who is "a castrated lover or dead man." In addition, "it is because of this ideal incubus that an embrace-like receptivity must be displaced in a sheath-like sensitivity onto the penis" (617, 7). The "ideal incubus," an incubus being a sucking nightmarish creature, suggests a demonic nightmare, something, Morel (2002: 87) notes, that comes in the middle of the night and is on the side of *jouissance*. It is a representative of the Name-of-the-Father and is linked to the origin of the law in the unconscious. Thus a woman aims at the origin of the law in the unconscious in the ideal incubus and which is not reducible to the fundamental phantasy. In other words, a woman cheats on her partner with her "ideal incubus" in her unconscious and this is masked by the feminine masquerade that places a "veil" between her and the Other. She gains her *jouissance* thus with "a dead father or a castrated man," that is, from the Other, from the guardian of castration, the Name-of-the-Father, of which the dead father, including the figure of Christ (617, 11) is a representative. In this, "the duplicity of the subject is masked in women, all the more so in that the partner's servitude makes him especially apt to represent the victim of castration" (618, 1). This is the problematic of the woman's partner in trying to be all things to her and, as Morel (2002: 82) puts it, of having her all to himself.

The frigid woman is therefore faithful to the Other by refusing it in the actions of her partner. Her frigidity arises because she loses herself too much in the masquerade, which is by definition phallic as it veils the Otherness of the feminine unconscious in its orientation to an enjoyment at a point beyond the phallus. By wanting to be the phallus too much, she risks imaginarily saturating the lack that it covers over and ignoring the calls of the ideal incubus and losing all of her sexual satisfaction (Morel, 2002: 83). A solution comprised of the sexual act is therefore not going to be the answer for the frigid woman.[9] Thus it is that in the frigid woman, it is not a castrating phantasy (a man to be killed) that is at work, but the Other who mobilises her idealising love for a man already dead or castrated and her orientation is to a point behind the veil which is tied to the origin of the Name-of-the-Father and forbids maternal *jouissance*. That is why in a love relation, a woman will always be Other to herself because there is a *jouissance* that exceeds her and falls on the side of the Other.

Feminine frigidity is a symptom that emanates from feminine identification and is linked, as Lacan puts it, to the "phallic standard that props up fantasy" (617, 8). A woman's imaginary identification as the phallus moulds her to the coordinates of masculine desire and in order to go beyond the frigidity of this position, frigidity in terms of her own desire, a woman must, as Soler (2002: 102) puts it, go beyond her phallic identification to have her own *jouissance*. In other words, she must go beyond her constitution as fantasy-object, as one of her partner's 'phallus-girls' and not limit herself entirely to the coordinates of masculine desire. The problem for the woman-hysteric, as Dora demonstrates, is that she remains tethered to the phallic standard and this is augmented by posing her desire via the desire of the other. In both her aim at getting the Other to produce his castration and in her identification with the phallus, she pushes the place of both desire and *jouissance* to the side of the partner.

Lacan remarks that woman's 'Otherness' in the sexual dialectic arises through representing "the absolute Other in the phallocentric dialectic" (616, 6) and it leads to her conception as "monstrous." This is one effect of castration. Castration in this sense is the displacement via the agency of the paternal metaphor of the proximity to the real, the *jouissance* of the drives and the 'Thing' of the body, that is, the time before the child recognises its body as an entity and as separate from the Other.[10] The Thing is what comes in place of the traumatic void, that is, the real without lack and it is a radical, absolute, inscrutable Otherness that is often conferred with an uncanny monstrous character. Femininity in the sense that Lacan refers to it here is a designation of the 'Other-Thing,' phantasmatically reconfigured as a horror of women that is the result of an encounter with a void, with a limit of symbolisation. This is linked to the unknowability of the mother's body, which takes place because the sex of the mother, and indeed sexual difference in general, is unthinkable to a child, as it was to Little Hans whose anxiety is linked to the enigma of the mother's sex transformed into a monstrous anxiety.[11] The feminine is left behind, situated as a negative and as bodily exclusion outside of representation and culture. When it is included, it is as a monstrosity and representational forms include the vagina dentate, the preying mantis, Medusa's head, the biting horse and the big giraffe. For Little Hans, the woman's Otherness is represented not in a vagina dentate but in a 'phallus dentate' – not only the big giraffe but also the biting horse with the giant *wiwimacher* (Lacan, S4, 1956–1957: 398). Every time that Little Hans thinks he is going to be bitten by a horse, a horse that will fall and bite, it is the surging of something that happens each time the mother's love is lacking (Lacan, S4, 1956–1957: 408). When she is about to fall, the biting horse helps Hans to represent her privation. This also explains feminine passivity, which Lacan takes up in *Guiding Remarks* as "already metaphorical" (615, 3). This means that passivity is "the inverse of its regressive aspect," a turning around into its opposite "of castrating and devouring, dislocating and stupefying effects in feminine activity" (ibid). Therefore, feminine 'passivity' is a transformation of the Other-Thing into an idealised feminine positive attribute.

Female homosexuality and ideal love

In Section IX, Lacan formulates another perspective on feminine desire in the context of female homosexuality. He proposes that "in all forms of female homosexuality, even unconscious, the supreme interest is in femininity" (619,

4). The operation in question is "a sublation [*relève*] of the object; one might say that a challenge that is accepted [*défi relevé*]" (618, 8). It is not that a homosexual woman chooses the mother at the expense of her own femininity, in contrast to Jones's assertion that a homosexual woman chooses to identify with the phallus over her sex, what Lacan describes as Jones's "reliance upon the overly convenient prop of identification" (618, 7). It is rather that "what she does not accept is that this object only assumes [*assume*] his sex at the cost of castration" (619, 3). This doesn't mean that she renounces her own castration but that she renounces man, or rather a desire for him. This sublimating process has the effect of causing her relationship to the Other to constitute a link to men which is an idealised one, a point that is often missed but it is not, as Soler (2006: 186) notes, a point of sexual desire.

The idealised link to men refers to the adoption of the position of the imaginary phallus in a love relation, insofar as, as Lacan puts it, "what the homosexual excels in doing regarding what she is missing" (619, 2). Aided by the fact that she does not 'have' the phallus, she 'excels' in exploiting her condition of not-having in order to promote an Eros of the Other, a love of Woman. In this, the demand for love exceeds its more usual imaginary coordinates and aims at the real of feminine desire, a point 'beyond' the phallus. Lacan adds to this, "perhaps we see thereby the doorway that leads from female sexuality to desire itself" (619, 6). The courtly love aspect of Freud's young homosexual patient noted by Lacan (619, 1) indicates that her love is aiming at something else.

While Freud (1920/2001: 154) had noted "the sublime over-valuation of the sexual object so characteristic of the male lover" in his young patient, Lacan reframes this in terms of a sublimated relation to the phallus which causes her desire to be premised not on lack but on desire itself, on the virtue of lack, as Lacan puts it, "to be realised in competition with the desire that castration liberates in the male by giving him the phallus as its signifier" (619, 7). The sublimation of the phallic signifier means that the link to the Other is not completely overlaid with an idealised phallic function, which would cause the function of the mask to dominate the relations between the sexes. Lacan's characterisation of "the natural ease with which such women invoke their quality as men" (619, 5) has therefore nothing to do with a wish to actually 'be' a man (what the literature has despised her for!), nor does it refer to Freud's masculinity complex, nor as Lacan puts it, does it have to do "with the delusional style of the male transsexualist" (619, 5). While some women may identify with the desire of a man, this has to do with gaining *jouissance* as a man does.

A homosexual woman's secret link to man, in Lacan's assertion of "the fantasy of man, as invisible witness" (619, 4) is linked to Jones's (1927/1999: 141) assertion that "their aim is to vicariously enjoy the gratification of this at the hand of an unseen man the father incorporated in themselves." This refers to the phantasy of a paternal figure as witness that they seek to incorporate within themselves. Leader (1996: 66) notes that the presence of the third party is frequently discernible in the figure of a man who is actually present, or even in the form of a photograph or piece of furniture associated with the paternal register. It doesn't, he states, "have to be a real man and certainly not the real father." The link with the paternal field discerned by Lacan in female homosexuality is crucial in distinguishing a characteristic of female homosexuality. Homosexual women can be as oriented to the Other as heterosexual women and may be less encumbered by the phallic masquerade and their mode of love aimed at *jouissance* is indicative of the "doorway" that leads from feminine love to feminine desire.

Female homosexuality thus involves a link to the paternal register that is different to that of a woman whose *jouissance*-effects are oriented by an ideal incubus as represented by the Name-of-the-Father. Lacan's remark about "the care taken by the subject in giving her partner jouissance" (619, 7) is what, as Soler (2006: 186) puts it, "makes room for the Other of sex" without eliminating a secret link to man. She poses that this is a response that has a relation to the real, to the Other, as opposed to the devotion of certain hysterical women to the Woman who can guarantee what a woman is. This was the hysterical aim of Freud's young homosexual patient, whose adoration of the older woman constituted an effort at ascertaining the secret to femininity.

Female sexuality and society

In Section X, Lacan concludes the text with a consideration of the impact of female sexuality on society and poses three questions. First he asks "why does the analytic myth come up short concerning the prohibition of incest between father and daughter?" (619, 10). His answer interspersed throughout the text is linked to the idea that the signifier does not altogether account for the drive in women and this arises because the symbolic lacks a corresponding female equivalent to the phallus. Symbolic forms of womanhood and the phallic masquerade do not fully subsume the link to the maternal phallus, which proffers a real link to the Other at the place that is the Name-of-the-Father and represented by a dead father or castrated lover. Female homosexuality is also another mode of approach to the Other and it further develops the idea that Freud's single libido theory inflects the phallic nature of the symbolic, which, far from making man and woman relationally suited, engenders a dissymmetry between the sexes caused by different non-symmetrical modes of relating to the lack in the subject orchestrated by language.

Lacan's question about the shortcomings of analytic myth can also be linked to two different formulations of feminine Oedipalisation discernible in his fourth and fifth seminars respectively, a point discerned by Chiesa (2007: 87). In *Seminar IV*, he takes a distinctly Freudian position and asserts that castration is essential for every subject to be fully Oedipalised and Oedipal attachment is synonymous with successful heterosexual symbolic sexuation. He writes,

> the father is first of all for her an object of love … this object of love then becomes the one who gives the object of satisfaction, the object of the natural relation of childbirth. After that, she needs only a bit of patience until there will finally come, as a substitute for the father, one who will fill exactly the same role of the father, by effectively giving her a child.
>
> (S4, 1956–1957: 232)

Similarly, in his seminar on *The Psychoses* a year earlier, he asserts that woman re-creates with man her primordial attachment to her father just as man recreates his maternal attachment with a woman (S3, 1955–1956: 176). By contrast, a year later in *Seminar V*, he finds that the function of the castration complex is asymmetrical for the boy and the girl. She does not have to identify with her father and "a true femininity always has also a little dimension of alibi, real women always have something a little bit astray (*égare*) about them" (S5, 1957–1958, session of 22 January 1958).

This recalls what Lacan had just written in '*The Signification of the Phallus*,' that "the *Verdrängung* inherent in his desire is greater" (583, 4), meaning that woman's relation to repression and to the desire afforded by it is less. With this, Lacan is moving from an earlier Freudian stance to one that is making room for the feminine real beyond the phallus. This is how Lacan begins to go beyond Freud.

The question of love has an important bearing on Lacan's second question, which asks "how are we to situate the social effects of female homosexuality" (619, 11) as distinct to male homosexuality and he offers an interesting answer. Referring to the movement of the *Precieuses*, he writes "if we consider the Eros of female sexuality in the more accessible movement of the *Precieuses*, grasp what it conveys by way of information as running counter to social entropy" (620, 2). The *Precieuses* was an exclusive Parisian upper-class literary and social circle of ladies in the seventeenth century, comprised of women who preferred their own company and companionship. Much like the eighteenth-century English bluestockings, they were renowned for their culture, refinement and use of language. They tended to be married, even though they had a clear homosocial bond.[12] Thus, in contrast to the Cathars invoked by Lacan, the *Precieuses* kept a symbolic link to men open about the operation of the social world and the shortcomings of the phallic realm. The point thus is that the enjoyment of the *Precieuses* is primarily in each other and it is not directed at the unravelling of society or as Lacan puts it "a sort of entropy moving in the direction of a degrading of the community" (620, 1). As well as engaging in procuring a more stimulating feminine place in it, such a homosexual community is founded on the bond of love. Framed as "the doorway from female sexuality to desire itself" (619, 6), homosexuality and the Eros of woman also entails desire that transcends the phallic function that a woman's call to love engenders.

And the question of love is relevant to Lacan's third question which asks "why does the social instance of women remain transcendent to the contractual order propagated by labour?" and further, "is the status of marriage maintained by its effect, despite the decline of paternalism" (620, 3). Mythically woman enters culture and furthers the preservation of the species. If she revokes castration and privation, she will pull out of culture. The social instance of the woman transcending the contractual order is perhaps Lacan's clearest statement that a woman is not necessarily confined or delimited to her social and symbolic role, including marriage and motherhood, even if that's what women often do. The symbolic value of marriage remains in vogue today as it did in 1958 and now encompasses homosexual couples. While women's social and political autonomy has played a role in the rupture of marriages, their commitment to finding a partner and getting married continues.[13] The necessity of love for a woman and her tendency towards monogamy and her 'true partner,' as well as the heightened value of love in today's fragmentary social bonds, continues to result in women dedicating themselves to marriage in spite of the decline of paternalism. Women's monogamy and their faithfulness to the Other thus works in favour of marriage and the conjugal couple.

Marriages are unions that bear not only the mark of castration but the incest relation also, that is, the fixation on the mother and the father that is substituted par force into symbolically acceptable modes of relation (S4, 1956–1957: 244). If the ideal of the conjugal conjunction is monogamous for woman, it is "because she wants the phallus for herself alone" and aims in love at what is beyond the choice authorised by the Oedipal dialectic and the satisfaction of the object (S4, 1956–1957: 244–245). As Lacan indicates in *Guiding Remarks*, she aims at 'being,' at a point beyond the phallus, her 'true partner' represented by a dead father or castrated lover. In effect, the idea that women are interested in marriage is the result of their call to love and to being the phallus to the Other which, as Soler (2006: 199) puts it, "delivers her from the solitude of her *jouissance* and knots what cannot be identified – the Other that she is for herself." Love thus goes far beyond simply the register of object relations and in its many forms represents and makes up for a disjunction between imaginary and symbolic experiences and what the subject experiences as ultimately what is beyond the mother – that the human being is, as Lacan puts it, "deprived and forlorn" (S4, 1956–1957: 245).

Conclusion

As indicated at the outset, some important lines of connectivity can be drawn between component features of *Guiding Remarks* and Lacan's later work on femininity. Much of *Guiding Remarks* is given over to critiquing simplistic, naturalistic and sociological notions of feminine difference based on feminine anatomical distinction as well as a sustained critique of contemporary 1950s psychoanalytic formulations of femininity rooted in normative notions of womanhood, passivity and maternity. Throughout the text, Lacan distinguishes feminine sexuality as distinct to masculinity in its relationship to the phallus and he privileges feminine desire in different forms such as erotomaniacal love, frigidity and homosexuality. This is crucial to differentiating a specificity of feminine sexuality and desire in terms of the unconscious. However, with the formulation of *petit object a* in the early sixties as the crucial factor in desire and with his increasing emphasis on the role and forms of *jouissance* that are extralinguistic throughout the sixties, Lacan returns to feminine sexuality in the early seventies and re-formulates it, notably in his twentieth seminar, *Encore: On Feminine Sexuality, The Limits of Love and Knowledge* (1972–1973). There he distinguishes 'feminine structure' in his graph of sexuation that once and for all differentiates femininity in terms of both desire and *jouissance* and unhooks it from the female body.

While in *Guiding Remarks* Lacan asks "whether phallic mediation drains off the whole force of the drives in the woman, and notably the whole current of the maternal instinct," in *Encore*, Lacan takes this further and specifies that "being not-whole, she has a supplementary *jouissance* compared to what the phallic function designates by way of *jouissance*" (S20, 1972–1973: 73). In the year preceding this, in his nineteenth seminar *Ou Pire* (1971–1972), Lacan returns to evaluating femininity properly-speaking, writing there that "it is not true that castration dominates everything" (session of 15 December 1971) and the "essence of woman is not castration" (session of 12 January 1972). A woman's different relation to castration means that she is 'not-all' subject to the dynamic of phallic castration and she supplements her accession to the phallic-symbolic realm with a special enjoyment, a specifically feminine *jouissance* that is not commensurate with the order of language and meaning. This definition of woman, which designates the dual fields of her *jouissance*, phallic and supplementary, also demonstrates that the question of her 'being' and her specifically feminine desire is unanswered by her phallic coordinates and its attendant *jouissance*.

The centrality of the role of phallus in masculinity and femininity in terms of 'having' and 'being' the phallus explains the phallocentrism of the unconscious and how the phallus becomes the referent for 'all' to the exclusion of the feminine. In *Guiding Remarks*, Lacan shows how this exclusion is symptomatically revealed in the framing of femininity either within phallic masculinist terms (i.e. Ernest Jones) or in the reduction of femininity to female bodily specificity (i.e. Helene Deutsch, bio-scientific and bio-social models). His specification of feminine desire as operating in both frigidity and homosexuality implicitly indicates that no phallic model is sufficient to explain such desires, even though he specifies the 'dead father' or symbolic father as the referent in each. In *Encore*, Lacan goes much further and explicitly delineates femininity in terms of a special signifier S(Ⱥ) which constitutes a woman's non-dialectical Other partner, as well as a field of special supplementary *jouissance* that is 'not-all' in relation to the *jouissance* engendered by the domain of phallic relations, that is, between those subjects who 'have' the phallus and those who are constituted by 'being' the phallus. There is in this sense, Lacan says, "no such thing as a sexual relationship" (S20, 1972–1973: 12). In this, Lacan elaborates femininity in terms of the problematic of a being who is not entirely subject to the Oedipus complex and the law of castration and instead her Other partner, S(Ⱥ), can function just as well as the phallic signifier and it is more closely connected to her 'being' that is elided by the effects of phallic identification. Thus in feminine structure, it is the void in the Other which is supposed to be full of meaning that becomes the referent of all meaning and knowledge. A woman therefore has an ethical complaint against the symbolic order as she can expose its lack and demand the recognition of her real subjectivity. She can do so by means of unmasking the 'masquerade,' that is, the parade of metaphoric displacements, noted so carefully by Lacan in *Guiding Remarks*, that fails to capture or assimilate her Other subjectivity. S(Ⱥ) is not a signifier that exists but it implies a relation that has yet to be put into a signifier.

'Masculine structure' is described by Lacan in *Encore* as dominated by the phallic signifier and sexual partners are approached as phantasy-objects as the cause of desire (S20, 1972–1973: 80). To enjoy in the manner of someone characterised by masculine structure is to reduce the partner to the *petit object a*, whereby a phantasy part-object stands for the whole in setting desire in motion.[14] As well as entailing an identification with the 'all' of knowledge, the masculine position endows and amplifies the illusion of masculine virility and it depends intrinsically on its differentiation from the feminine 'not-all.' This *jouissance* is susceptible to failure because it misses the 'being' of a partner and as such it does not relate to the Other. It does not make up for the failure of the sexual relation as it is limited to the symbolic yield of the phallic signifier. It is essentially masturbatory and Lacan refers to it unflatteringly as "the *jouissance* of the idiot" (S20, 1972–1973: 81). In this respect, Lacan writes that, "phallic *jouissance* is an obstacle owing to which man does not come (*n'arrive pas*), I would say, to enjoy a woman's body, precisely because what he enjoys is the *jouissance* of the organ" (S20, 1972–1973: 7).

Throughout his work, Lacan does not set up an alternative 'essence' of woman that operates as a closed set in opposition to another closed set that is masculine sexuality. But in *Guiding Remarks*, Lacan clarifies that there is a specificity to femininity. It is because the symbolic is phallic that identity is constructed within the realm of the masculine, as either 'having' or 'being' the phallus. The feminine is left behind, situated as a negative, unconscious and as bodily exclusion outside of representation and culture. There is, in this sense, no essence of femininity that can encompass what womanhood or the multiplicity of women is. Rather, the existence of feminine *jouissance* is tantamount to a belief in an enjoyment outside of language, a hypothetical enjoyment beyond the inherently limited satisfaction of phallic *jouissance*. It is evoked on the basis of castration, as an extra-linguistic *jouissance* that does not fail in the manner of phallic *jouissance*. In delineating femininity in *Guiding Remarks* in terms of differential aspects of feminine desire and an unrepresentable *jouissance* that is drive-related and oriented to a point beyond the Name-of-the-Father, Lacan lays the groundwork for his assertion later in *Encore* that there is no such thing as Woman (S20, 1972–1973: 72). In specifying a woman's Other relation as a structural position, Lacan goes further than in *Guiding Remarks* in unhooking femininity from anatomy, and indicates that the relation to S(Ⱥ) is possible regardless of anatomical distinction and genderisation. While other structural factors may impede access to the Other relation and limit access to the cut of castration and its 'beyond,' it is not the exclusive domain of women, even if, as indicated in *Guiding Remarks*, women are disposed in the symbolisation of their anatomical distinction to a relation with the first Other that does not suffer the same force of repression as it does for a man, in that, as Lacan puts it, it falls "under the sign of an organic minus-value" (614, 5).

Notes

1 Helpful here is Vanier's observation that although modern science is said to arise with Galileo, for Lacan the birth of the modern subject is linked to Descartes. The primary operation of the Cartesian method is doubt, and the mind must doubt in order to find certainty which is "announced in the *cogito*" and is expressed in "I think therefore I am." Thus the subject is produced by doubt which Descartes links to a thinking being and conscience (Vanier, 2000: 38–39).

2 Freud writes in 'Female Sexuality': "We believe we are justified in assuming that for many years the vagina is virtually non-existent and possibly does not produce sensations until puberty" (1931/2001: 228). This is patently not the case. Young girls are aware of vaginal sensations and occasionally experience a menstrual period during infancy.

3 In his 1949 paper on the mirror-stage, which is a re-writing of Freud's theory of narcissism through the structuring dynamics of projection and misrecognition via the field of the imaginary, Lacan demonstrates that the body is a psychically invested projection, an idealising fiction of the body as both a totality and locus of control. Ultimately, the emphasis on the body-imaginary is unsatisfactory, one-sided and fated to call into being elaborations along imaginarised lines of distinction, an opposition between 'haves and 'have-nots' which inevitably leads to a greater imputation of power to the 'haves' as those that have are better off than those that do not have.

4 Likely references of Lacan here are Jones 'The Early Development of Female Sexuality' (1927/1999: 135–136) where he asserts the importance of 'aphanisis' for both sexes and Klein in 'Early Stages of the Oedipus Conflict' (1927/1986: 147–148) where she asserts the importance for both sexes of the role of anatomical difference and the 'femininity phase' as common to both sexes.

5 What is essentially frustrated is that the child feels itself dispossessed of something it demands from the mother, this being love, meaning that every interpellation, every call aims at a beyond, at the love of the mother and the object that substitutes for the satisfaction of the child's needs (S4, 1956–1957: 137–138). The object in this sense is symbolic and dialectical because it invokes the Other of speech via the call and it is thus a speech effect of the relation to the big Other. So while the object impinges on the earliest age of life, it is not a mythic phallic property of the interior of the mother's body as Klein would have it, but in being incomplete evokes a presence–absence quality that includes the mother's comings and goings.

6 Freud links feminine defloration and frigidity on the side of woman to the wish to avoid the awakening of aggressive trends in the marital field. Karen Horney, by contrast, asserts that this is not about man's secret dread of woman or even castration-anxiety but it is "a reaction to the menace to [a man's] self-respect" (1932/1999: 243, 248). While Horney is right to dispute Freud's idea that the vagina remains 'undiscovered,' her emphasis on the man's side in her analysis of feminine defloration reduces the field of femininity to a masochistic passivity equivalent to a woman performing, as she puts it, "her part by merely being, without any doing" (250).

7 Castration anxiety in men is often revealed in their desire for approval, in their sense of inadequacy in the face of life decisions and satisfying their fathers' ideals and expectations. The attempt to live up to such ideals demonstrates that approval from fathers is conditional upon achievement, as if that approval could somehow make up for the *jouissance* that has been sacrificed. Yet no achievement can meet the expectation of the Other and it is an impossible task.

In the case of women, Freud postulated that their resentment of the Other, arising from their sense of deprivation is found in their indictment of their mothers for having deprived them of all manner of things, including the penis but also of failing to give them enough milk, enough love and for introducing a new sibling (Freud, 1931/2001: 231–235).

The only way out of this never-ending cycle is for a man to change his stance in relation to his demand for approval and for a woman to rescind blaming her mother as cause of her lack in relation to the Other.

8 As Freud notes in 'The Splitting of the Ego in the Mechanism of Defence,' an exemplary example of this is found in the story of Kronos from Greek mythology. He was the leader and youngest of the Titans and the father of Zeus. When he learned he was destined to be overthrown by his son, he devoured his sons as soon as they were born (Freud, 1938/2001: 275–287).

9 Morel (2002: 84–85) helpfully delineates three modalities of feminine frigidity. *The adulterous woman* in love is faithful to her companion but attains *jouissance* in liaisons with men she desires but does not love. *The collector of men* is a woman who is desirous and pursues *jouissance* with men but does not love them. *The disgusted woman* overestimates love but neither desires nor experiences *jouissance*. This is often found in hysteria when the penis is refused out of disgust.

10 Castration's structuring function culminates in the encapsulation of drive-related *jouissance* and narcissistic self-love within new libidinal ties cathected by the processes of sublimation and the substitution of creative, artistic and work-related aims for sexual activity.

11 Freud (1908/2001: 209–226) introduces this idea in 'On The Sexual Theories of Children' where he shows that the sexual theories of children, phallic, cloacal and sadistic are the responses of the emerging subject marked by libidinal development to the insoluble mysteries of origin and sexual difference.
12 These women were frequently ridiculed in satirical drama and poetry, for example in two Moliere plays, *Les Precieuses ridicules* and *Les femmes savantes*. See Faderman, 1997: 87–90.
13 The Central Statistics Office of Ireland indicates that marriage rates in Ireland, in spite of high levels of emigration, have been at their highest levels every year from 2007–2016.
14 The foundation of the subject by the *petit object a*, which precedes gender, privileges the subject's relation with the *petit object a*. Lacan states that "this object ought to be conceived by us as the cause of desire ... and the object is *behind* desire" (S10, 1962–1963, Session 16 January 1963).

Bibliography

Chiesa, L. (2007) *Subjectivity and Otherness: A Philosophical Reading of Lacan*, London: MIT Press.

Deutsch, H. (1930/1999) 'The Significance of Masochism in the Mental Life of Women,' in R. Grigg, D. Hecq and C. Smith (Eds.), *Female Sexuality: The Early Psychoanalytic Controversies*, London: Rebus Press, pp. 183–194.

Deutsch, H. (1932/1999) 'On Female Homosexuality,' in R. Grigg, D. Hecq and C. Smith (Eds.), *Female Sexuality: The Early Psychoanalytic Controversies*, London: Rebus Press, pp. 220–240.

Faderman, L. (1997) *Surpassing the Love of Men*, London: The Women's Press.

Freud, S. (1895/2001) 'Project for a Scientific Psychology,' in J. Strachey (Ed.), *The Standard Edition of the Complete Psychological Works of Sigmund Freud*, Vol. 1, London: Vintage, pp. 281–397.

Freud, S. (1905/2001) 'Three Essays on the Theory of Sexuality,' in J. Strachey (Ed.), *The Standard Edition of the Complete Psychological Works of Sigmund Freud*, Vol. 7, London: Vintage, pp. 130–245.

Freud, S. (1908/2001) 'On The Sexual Theories of Children,' in J. Strachey (Ed.), *The Standard Edition of the Complete Psychological Works of Sigmund Freud*, Vol. 9, London: Vintage, pp. 209–226.

Freud, S. (1909/2001) 'Analysis of a Phobia of a Five-Year-Old Boy,' in J. Strachey (Ed.), *The Standard Edition of the Complete Psychological Works of Sigmund Freud*, Vol. 10, London: Vintage, pp. 5–149.

Freud, S. (1920/2001) 'Psychogenesis of a Case of Homosexuality in a Woman,' in J. Strachey (Ed.), *The Standard Edition of the Complete Psychological Works of Sigmund Freud*, Vol. 18, London: Vintage, pp. 147–172.

Freud, S. (1925/2001) 'The Infantile Genital Organisation,' in J. Strachey (Ed.), *The Standard Edition of the Complete Psychological Works of Sigmund Freud*, Vol. 19, London: Vintage, pp. 141–145.

Freud, S. (1931/2001) 'Female Sexuality,' in J. Strachey (Ed.), *The Standard Edition of the Complete Psychological Works of Sigmund Freud*, Vol. 21, London: Vintage, pp. 225–243.

Freud, S. (1933/2001) 'Femininity,' in J. Strachey (Ed.), *The Standard Edition of the Complete Psychological Works of Sigmund Freud*, Vol. 22, London: Vintage, pp. 112–135.

Freud, S. (1938/2001) 'Splitting of the Ego in the Process of Defence,' in J. Strachey (Ed.), *The Standard Edition of the Complete Psychological Works of Sigmund Freud*, Vol. 23, London: Vintage, pp. 275–278.

Horney, K. (1932/1999) 'The Dread of Women: Observations on a Specific Difference in the Dread Felt by Men and Women Respectively for the Opposite Sex,' in R. Grigg, D. Hecq and C. Smith (Eds.), *Female Sexuality: The Early Psychoanalytic Controversies*, London: Rebus Press, pp. 241–252.

Jones, E. (1927/1999) 'The Early Development of Female Sexuality,' in R. Grigg, D. Hecq and C. Smith (Eds.), *Female Sexuality: The Early Psychoanalytic Controversies*, London: Rebus Press, pp. 133–145.

Jones, E. (1935/1999) 'Early Female Sexuality,' in R. Grigg, D. Hecq and C. Smith (Eds.), *Female Sexuality: The Early Psychoanalytic Controversies*, London: Rebus Press, pp. 276–285.

Klein, M. (1935/1986) 'A Contribution to the Psychogenesis of Manic-Depressive States,' in J. Mitchell (Ed.), *The Selected Melanie Klein*, London: Penguin Books.

Lacan, J. (1975/1998) *Book XX: Encore, On Femininity, Love and the Limits of Knowledge* (1972–1973), trans. B. Fink, ed. J.-A. Miller, London: W. W. Norton & Company.

Lacan, J. (1981/1993) *The Seminar. Book III: The Psychoses* (1955–1956), trans. R. Grigg, London: W. W. Norton.

Lacan, J. (1994) *Le Séminaire. Livre IV: La relation d'objet* (1956–1957), texte établi par J.-A. Miller, Paris: Éditions du Seuil.

Lacan, J. (1998) *Le Séminaire. Livre V: Les formations de l'inconscient* (1957–1958), texte établi par J.-A. Miller, Paris: Éditions du Seuil.

Lacan, J. (2004/2014) *The Seminar. Book X: Anxiety* (1962–1963), trans. A. R. Price, ed. J.-A. Miller, Cambridge: Polity.

Lacan, J. (2011) *Le Séminaire. Livre XIX: … ou pire* (1971–1972), texte établi par J.-A. Miller, Paris: Éditions du Seuil.

Leader, D. (1996) *Why Do Women Write More Letters Than They Post?* London: Faber and Faber.

Mitchell, J. and Rose, J. (1982) 'Guiding Remarks to a Congress on Feminine Sexuality,' in *Feminine Sexuality*, London: Palgrave Macmillan, pp. 86–98.

Morel, G. (2002) 'Feminine Conditions of Jouissance,' in S. Barnard and B. Finks (Eds.), *Reading Seminar XX, Lacan's Major Work on Love, Knowledge, and Feminine Sexuality*, Albany, NY: State University of New York Press, pp. 77–92.

Muller, J. (1925/1999) 'A Contribution to the Problem of Libidinal Development of the Genital Phase in Girls,' in R. Grigg, D. Hecq and C. Smith (Eds.), *Female Sexuality: The Early Psychoanalytic Controversies*, London: Rebus Press, pp. 122–128.

Roudinesco, É. (1997) *Jacques Lacan*, New York: Columbia University Press.

Soler, C. (2002) 'What Does the Unconscious Know About Women,' in S. Barnard and B. Finks (Eds.), *Reading Seminar XX, Lacan's Major Work on Love, Knowledge, and Feminine Sexuality*, Albany, NY: State University of New York Press, pp. 99–108.

Soler, C. (2006) *What Lacan Said About Women*, New York: Other Press.

Vanier, A. (2000) *Lacan*, New York: Other Press.

5

THE YOUTH OF GIDE, OR THE LETTER AND DESIRE

Jean-Michel Rabaté

Context

Lacan had a fondness for the journal *Critique* that had been founded by Georges Bataille in 1946. In April 1958, it was still edited by the notorious French writer, whose first wife, born Sylvia Maklès, became Lacan's second wife, when '*The Youth of Gide, or the Letter and Desire*' was published in number 131. Lacan was to publish two articles in the celebrated journal, one on Gide and one on Sade. Each time, the template was similar: authors were asked (and still are today) to comment on one or several books, but were given the freedom to explore their own ideas at leisure. To deal with an author who interested him, Lacan chose to start from two books on Gide, Jean Delay's monumental biography, *The Youth of André Gide, (1869–1895)*[1], published in two volumes in 1956 and 1957 respectively, a voluminous study of the French writer's first years—it stops in 1895, but totals more than 1200 pages—and Jean Schlumberger's *Madeleine et André Gide*, a book that looks almost slender by comparison (it has only 250 pages), also published in 1956 by Gallimard.

Gide had received the Nobel prize in 1947 just before dying in 1951 at the advanced age of eighty-one; after his death, countless memoirs, collections of letters and critical books were published, most of them attempting to understand the conundrum exemplified less by the works than by the life of the French author. Although he had been one of the first visible French authors to come out as a gay man, and had reproached Marcel Proust for not being as sincere or outspoken as he was, it was known then that he had fathered a daughter. At the beginning of his life, he absolutely wanted to marry his first cousin despite his mother's and the family opposition, since this marriage appeared as almost incestuous. Although he had begun his career as a symbolist and an aesthete, this disciple and personal friend of Oscar Wilde as a young man turned into a fellow traveler of the Communist party in the thirties. In this role he courageously denounced French colonialism in Africa, bringing about less inhuman colonial policies, but then attacked publicly the perversion of Stalinism when he had toured Soviet Russia. When André Gide oversaw the publication of his *Selected Prose* for Gallimard in 1921, he chose the witty motto of 'Extremes move me' (*Les extrêmes me touchent*). The epigraph for this personal anthology, *Morceaux Choisis*, plays on Pascal's famous remark, *Les extrêmes se touchent*, ('Extremes meet'). In the manner of Walt Whitman, Gide's vaunted egotism was capable of absorbing all contradictions, even when they reached metaphysical endpoints in which, for Pascal, God could be seen lurking, both in the infinity of smallness and in the infinity of bigness. Touched as well by similar extremes, Lacan had read Gide closely for some time, as we can judge from a passage of '*The Instance of the Letter in the Unconscious*,' another paper from the *Écrits* from 1957 to which I will return.

When the committee of *Critique* looked for a reviewer capable of doing justice to Delay's monumental book, the name of Lacan was not slipped at random by Bataille. Lacan was known to him, of course, and he was seen as a younger colleague and disciple of Jean Delay, like Lacan, a well-known psychiatrist in Paris. Delay had the distinction of being a celebrated author, a world-renowned physician who had elaborated some of the first successful psychotropic medication for psychotic patients, and who had the great honor of being elected to the Académie Française in 1959. He had been an intimate friend of Gide himself who granted him open access to his private archives. In his field of specialization, Delay was not opposed to psychoanalysis and he had invited Lacan to speak at his service on several occasions—the most important lecture being *Freud in the Century*, Lacan's presentation on the role of the founder of psychoanalysis to Delay's students in psychiatry, to be found as section XIX of *Seminar III* on *Psychoses*. A rapid look at Lacan's beautiful presentation will allow one to verify that he was not at all hostile to biography: he has a long section on Freud's name, his family, his background, his career, etc.

Jean Schlumberger has been even closer to Gide than Delay—they had founded the *Nouvelle Revue Française* together in 1906, and had exchanged letters, subsequently published, since 1901. Schlumberger never obtained great notoriety or distinction for his many essays, novels and plays, but he had the stature of a visible man of letters. His biographical study of the couple made by Madeleine and André Gide was to lead Lacan to his main questions even though he reacted negatively against its rather censorious tone, finding Schlumberger's wish to bring all the truth to an obscure relationship at any cost somewhat naïve. Here is a typical aside: "Jean Schlumberger reproaches Gide for having obscured his wife's face with the blackness of the shadows in which he moved toward her. Does he think he can dissipate these shadows with his fair-skinned memories?" (639, 2). Like Gide, Schlumberger was a Protestant coming from a rich and rigid provincial family, and they may have had too much in common. At least, Schlumberger attempted to save the "patrician virtues" (639, 4) embodied by their bourgeois class, whereas Gide had rejected these values much earlier in his life. Obviously, Lacan preferred Delay's subtle and textual psychobiography even if it covered only the first decades of Gide's life.

Since Delay was a gifted novelist even though he was best known for books on memory, psychological testing, and various issues of contemporary psychiatry, Lacan felt the need to foreground his literary credentials, which is why his essay is preceded by two rather forbidding epigraphs. The first one is in Greek and not translated. It comes from Euripides' *Medea.* Lacan chose a well-known passage from the play. It is often quoted since it seems to present Euripides' defense of his role as a poet in a political context defined by conformity and doxa. Here is a rather literal translation:

> If you introduce new, intelligent ideas to fools,
> you will be thought frivolous, not intelligent.
> If the citizens think you surpass those they deem smart,
> you will appear like a thorn in the city's flesh.[2]

It is Medea who replies bitterly to Creon, adding that this has been her fate. This alludes clearly to Lacan's sense that people could not understand him, and saw him either as a charlatan or a buffoon. The reference to tragedy is telling in this context: Lacan can be seen grappling with an ethics of psychoanalysis that he defines as fundamentally tragic. He will focus on one 'tragedy' in Gide's life, the burning of his correspondence with his wife by his wife. One might say that it was the only tragedy of note in Gide's long, successful and rather happy career.

The second epigraph is taken from a rather invisible passage in Gide's works—it comes from the endnote added to *La Tentative amoureuse*, a short novel subtitled "… or a Treatise of the vanity of desire." It is a novel about desire and love-making between a man and a woman. This is a melancholy text that Gide wrote in 1893 to sort out his indecision facing his own desire, caught up as he was between his sexuality (his attraction to young men) and his intense love for his cousin, Madeleine. The passage asserts that a good novel will describe a single line defining the trajectory of a soul untied with a body, but in order to do so, it sketches an original theory of desire. A purified desire will give access to truth, and truth can be heard speaking even in obscure and knotted metaphors; Gide's knot seems to announce the formulations of the later Lacan. I quote the original context: "*L'unité –autant dire la pureté du désir, fait la rectitude de la ligne. (…) Et, métaphores ou non, ce que je dis ici est parfaitement vrai*" (Gide, 2009: 256). One could translate this as: "The unity, let us say the purity of desire is what makes the line be straight. (…) And, whether I use metaphors or not, what I say here is perfectly true." Gide articulates key principles of Lacanian metapsychology: desire underpins an ontology of lines, patterns and structures defining the subject as desiring subject; the writer, poet or psychoanalyst who attempts to set down these insights may or may not speak in metaphors, since truth takes the form of fiction to express itself.

If Gide has often been mentioned in Lacan's texts and seminars, the years 1957–1959 saw the most systematic engagement with the work of the French novelist. One example of this comes at the end of '*The Instance of the Letter in the Unconscious*,' a text dated from May 1957, which concludes with an involved paragraph that has often baffled commentators. It is based on a passage of André Gide's main autobiographical text, *If it die*.... To wrap up a long and programmatic essay, Lacan attempts to pin down the links between the letter, being, and otherness. At the same time, he criticizes psychoanalysts who believe that they must become 'the others' of their analysands (that is, those who rely on subjective projection and deny the role of the Other.) It is in this context that he presents a section from Gide's autobiography as a blueprint for the way in which psychoanalysts should be attentive to the role of 'otherness' in their practice. In advance of his essay on the Youth of Gide, he is glossing one incident in Gide's youth:

> Which other was the young André Gide aiming at when he defied the landlady, in whose care his mother had placed him, to treat him as a responsible being by unlocking right in front of her—with a key that was fake only insofar as it opened all locks of the same kind—the lock that she herself considered to be the worthy signifier of her educational intentions? Was it she who would later intervene and to whom the child would laughingly say: 'Do you really think a lousy padlock can ensure my obedience?' But by simply remaining out of sight and waiting until that evening before lecturing the kid, after giving him a suitably cold reception upon his return home, it was not simply a female other whose angry face she showed him, but another André Gide, one who was no longer really sure, either then or even later when he thought back on it, what he had wanted to do—who had been changed right down to his very truth by the doubt cast on his good faith.
>
> (437, 4)

Gide narrates a moment of his adolescence, the stay he was forced to make in a private boarding house in Passy, where he was studying with a tutor in 1883. He had been expelled from several public and private schools because of the habit he had contracted of masturbating openly in public places. Having lost his father in 1880 when he was eleven, he experienced panic attacks that he called moments of '*Schaudern*,' unbearable fits of anxiety concerning the death of his loved ones. Besides, he had discovered that he was "not like the others" (Gide, 2001: 166). At this point, the thirteen-year-old, obliged to do boring homework, had taken refuge in the observation of pets. He had found mice that he tamed, but they were killed by the teacher. They were replaced by a couple of turtle doves who cooed happily all day and finally laid an egg. Mrs. Bertrand, the strong lady of the house, restricted

Gide's access to the birds, arguing that his passion for animals made him lose interest in his studies. In order to enforce this she put a padlock on the cage. The boy had noted that it was easy to buy a similar key, and he did this defiantly (Gide, 2001: 173). Now Gide arranged to be seen by the landlady as he opened the lock with the new key he had bought. Having opened the cage, he left the key in the lock and returned to his homework. He waited for a long time, finished a long and tedious Latin translation and only then was summoned by Mrs. Bertrand. This calculated delay was enough to annul his victory. Mrs. Bertrand pounced on him, preventing him from saying anything. She accused him of being dishonest and threatened him with jail. Finally, she appealed to the feelings of his mother, letting him imagine that his action would sadden her. Facing these contradictory reproaches, Gide forgot his motivation. His prank lost its revolutionary thrust and turned into a mere childish rebellion. Unable to justify himself, his desire vanished and he sank into silence. Then he lost interest in the birds, which made him work better. Sublimation and repression could for a while continue to work hand in hand.

In '*The Instance of the Letter in the Unconscious*,' Lacan presents this apparently minor incident. He prefers it to more explicit scenes as when Gide narrates his discovery of gay sexuality with young boys in Biskra. By focusing on a simple vignette like this, Lacan implies that what matters may not be contained in life-changing revelation but in everyday events. This explains why *The Youth of Gide* (627, 4–6) quotes with approval Gide writing to his mother that he had learned more about Goethe when he knew how he blew his nose than by reading his plays.

In the vignette about the birds and the key, we recognize the elements of a structure that will be repeated. There is the boy's curiosity for the riddle of procreation. The enigma of sexuality accounts for the observation of birds producing an egg, and it is barred by the teachers' repression. The mother stands out in her idealized role as the gaze of a symbolic power that remains blind, since she must never know anything of the defiant transgression.

We are told in no uncertain terms by Delay that when Gide's mother began suspecting her son's homosexuality, when she was alerted to what her son's sense of an 'exception' to the rule really meant, above all because of his friendship with the notorious Oscar Wilde, she was struck by a paralysis that was soon to bring about her demise.[3] Thus, before even embarking on a psychobiography of a famous writer who chose to be a homosexual, Lacan's point is more minimalist. He deploys a dialectics of desire as it underpins an othering mechanism. Truth is conveyed by the confession of a minor transgression because Gide's narrative takes time into account. Gide is talking about a calculated delay. His text enacts a delayed narrative when the adult writer speaks for the child in him. He speaks as the child he was when he had not been allowed to explain his motivations for a show of defiance. The confession retraces a progression from a moment of defiance, almost a victory, to failure because the landlady refused to play the part planned for her. She was supposed to scream at him immediately; instead, she let remorse accomplish its work. Gide's transgression 'fails'[4] and turns into discomfiture. Lacan captures the subjective alteration due to the time it takes to understand something. This calls up the notion of a 'logical time,' which may not be identical with the time it takes to understand. At the end of his narrative, Gide the boy who acted badly in his chronicle has become 'other' than he was at the beginning. His moral nature has shifted, and such an alteration derives from the temporality of an after-effect that is redoubled by the process of writing. After this experience, Gide the boy is 'other' because he has lost his initial desire. He abandons a 'perverse' impulse to rebel and contradict the law laid down by adults. However while he identifies with parental work ethics, he is about to plan decisive campaigns against the social link established by academic recognition and sexual repression. Here is the meaning recaptured by the two epigraphs chosen by Lacan for his essay in *Critique*: the writer who creates a truth has to fight against the *doxa* of common morality; in the end, the poet's metaphors (here, condensed in a self-defeating game with a lock) can state the truth, and it will shake the foundations of the *polis*.

Lacan was aware of the fact that Gide's life had been marked by the early disappearance of the father; his untimely death prevented him from laying down the law. Gide had to face his mother's desire with all its religious fanaticism and its heightened demands. She was a devout woman, whose hold on her son was to last, while she was to have a passionate friendship with an English woman after she became a widow. In *Seminar V*, Lacan's reading of Gide's 'perversion' indicates that perversion does not stem from his pederasty, that is from his longing for young boys, but from a desire to remain the little boy he once had been. Gide wants to be the 'desired child,' who had once been the sexual object of an aunt's attention and had run away, aghast. In order to ward off and preserve at the same time the horror of this feminine desire, he decided to marry his aunt's daughter, his own cousin. His desire remained stuck at a narcissistic stage, mostly choosing those exotic boys in Algeria (S5, 1957–1958: 257). Gide loves the cousin whom he was to marry because he could identify with her. His wish was to live securely but chastely with his wife and have sex with boys as he did even during his honeymoon spent in Algeria. Madeleine could observe her husband's libido. Because she was never the object of his desire, she understood the horror of it. She saw how lust distorted Gide's features during their wedding trip to Algiers. Gide, sitting in front of her in a train, caressed the arms of playfully seductive Arab boys through the window. "You looked like a criminal or a madman," she told him (Gide, 2001: 948). Lacan identifies a root of perversion in this structure, however perversion is not located in what popular *doxa* assumes, that is in same-sex desire, but in a certain rapport to the same or the other in a knot between writing, love and desire. Gide's love for his cousin was still-born, it felt like 'embalmed,' as he would say. Lacan goes on:

> This wife whom he does not desire becomes the object of a supreme love, and when this object with which he has filled up the hole of a love without desire comes to disappear, he cries out the miserable shout whose connection I have pointed out with the comical cry par excellence, that of the miser—*My casket! My dear casket!*
>
> (S5, 1957–1958: 260–61)

The 'hole of a love without desire' refers to the famous letters that will be destroyed, and to which we will soon return.

When he died, Gide's father had left as his main heritage a well-stacked library. This was a cultural treasure-trove that the young man was only allowed to enter when he turned sixteen. Once established in the library, Gide kept wondering whether the pact that he had made with himself very early, namely an effort to tell the truth, could be sustained. If such a commitment to truth led to a transgression of accepted norms, could it resist becoming perverse? Did Gide take a perverse pleasure in pushing the limits of sincerity and confessional authenticity? Gide attempted to deal with this issue by establishing a stark contrast between the two halves of *If it die*.... His memoir is divided into two sections; the first, which looks like a traditional *Künstlerroman*, leads to a meditative pause, during which Gide expatiates on the impossibility of actually telling the whole truth: "My intention has always been to say everything," he writes but adds:

> I am a being of dialogue; everything in me fights and contradicts itself. Memoirs are never more than half sincere, however great one's wish to tell the truth: everything is half more complicated that one says. It may even be that one approaches truth best in a novel.
>
> (2001: 267)

Such a narrative hinge was necessary before reaching the sexual aspect of the memoirs, and it is accompanied by a number of disclaimers as to the exact correlation of his memories, complemented by corrections of erroneous details later provided by a cousin (Gide, 2001: 328–329), a worry about exact factual reports that will rebound in Jean Schlumberger's book on Madeleine.

The second half of the memoir is much more daring and centers around the figure of Oscar Wilde, whereas the first part was dominated by positive tutelary figures: the poet Stéphane Mallarmé and the model of artistic devotion met in de la Nux, his devoted piano teacher. In the second part, we meet the perverse, outrageous and almost satanic (given Gide's belief in the devil highlighted in the first part) figures of Wilde and Lord Douglas—yet it was to them that Gide owed the revelation of his sexuality. What had remained hidden at the beginning comes to the fore in the intense sunlight of Algeria, a colonial locale less repressive than metropolitan France. There, little boys know exactly what is expected of them. The sharp glare of Africa banishes the shadows of bourgeois childhood, it dispels the puritanical gloom and the 'devils' hallucinated there, wipes away studious boredom, and the pseudo-artistic *chiaroscuro* of Parisian interiors. Like Nietzsche's blinding light of noon, the pitiless sun annihilates the ghosts of the religious past. Gide's true nature is revealed to him when he has sex with the young Mohammed, one of Lord Douglas's 'mignons' lent to Gide by Wilde for an unforgettable night of pleasure. The narrative becomes lyrical when evoking the transports and intense joy that come close to an extreme *jouissance.* Gide confides that he had five orgasms with his partner, and kept masturbating several times before he could regain his composure and return to his "normal self" (Gide, 2001: 310.)

The discovery of erotic ecstasy leads to sexual feats à la Flaubert when he enjoyed Kuchuk Hanem, the famous prostitute, an impressive number of times in an Egyptian brothel. Like Flaubert, Gide discovers pure pleasure, a pleasure that merges with *jouissance*: this sexual enjoyment is excessive, transgressive, and above all not tainted by love. Gide verifies then an insight he had only glimpsed before, that for him love and desire will never coincide or overlap. This becomes his truth. It is a new evidence, an almost blinding certainty, and it provides him with a basis for what he then calls his 'normalcy.' Before, there had been other attempts, as with the young female prostitute Meriem whom he shared with his friend Paul; but because Paul seemed to enjoy himself more with her, Gide had felt "foreclosed" (literally "*forclos*" in Gide, 2001: 284). Foreclosure refers to the subject's destitution when he can suppose pleasures that are more intense with others. Opposed to this, the absolute truth that Gide has reached in a climax of sexual *jouissance* capable of transgressing all limits gives him a secure foundation. This is Gide's *cogito*, a quasi-Cartesian concept or main lever, less a '*cogito ergo sum*' than a '*gaudeo ergo sum.*'

It is on the strength of a *jouissance*, which was actually masterminded by Oscar Wilde against Lord Douglas, that Gide assumes his sexual orientation, an orientation that he decides to call 'pederasty.' In confessing the truth about his homosexuality overtly, Gide rejects the fake femininity of some gay men he knows; above all, he disavows the myth of a 'race of inverts' that Marcel Proust presented in *Sodom and Gomorrah.* Gide felt that he had become a manly and healthy man, as if he had been reborn after a grave illness. The autobiographical narrative thus allowed Gide to become one with his previous fictional alter-ego in the novel *The Immoralist.* As Delay shows in a number of masterful analyses, Gide became an 'immoralist' only after he had written his autobiography, whereas his fictional character, Michel, whose wife's death forces him to 'confess' to his friends, is a half-hearted Nietzschean. Michel hasn't shaken off the specters of religion and morality. Curiously, the fictional wife's death anticipates the untimely death of Gide's wife, Madeleine, her real life model. However *If it die…* ends with a different drama: the death of Gide's beloved mother. In spite of the terrible loss, Gide exhibits a strange ambivalence. In addition to his chagrin and despair, what he experiences at the loss of a mother who was everything to him, is akin to absolute freedom in "an abyss of love, despair, and freedom" (Gide, 2001: 326). This was the freedom the young Gide had longed for—but this alone was not enough to trigger his decision to write an autobiography.

Gide's decision to write his autobiography was triggered by an even more painful event. It was the famous crisis of 1918 on which Lacan focuses, when Madeleine told him that she had burned all their letters. This she did after she learned that her husband, full of desire for a young man and of barely hidden contempt for her, was leaving her for a month and would go to England to spend a vacation with a male friend, Marc Allégret. Later, when she told him what she had done, Gide was inconsolable. This incident is the main focus of Lacan's essay, '*The Youth of Gide, or the Letter and Desire*', and one can say that it also constitutes the point of perspective of Delay's psychobiography, even though Delay stops twenty-three years before, in 1895.

Commentaries on the text

In the *Critique* essay, Lacan begins by paying homage to Delay's eminence as a psychiatrist and literary figure while remaining rather reserved facing Schlumberger's book whose explicit aim was to correct Gide's portrayal of Madeleine. Even though Lacan cannot agree with the intention of Delay's 'psycho-biography' he recognizes that by exploring in depth one particular subject, Delay has managed to get hold of the central core of the subject (624, 5). Lacan is alerted quite early by a textual lack that Delay mentions in the acknowledgments when he notes the curious fact that the entire correspondence between Gide and his wife is missing. Delay's attention to archives announces the rise of what would be called 'genetic criticism' in France, a critical school that has dominated the study of modern and contemporary literature since the 1990s and takes pre-publication materials such as drafts, letters and diary entries as it main object. Lacan agrees with Delay's promotion of these shorter writing or "stray papers (*petits papiers*)" (625, 6) to the status of literary symptom.

Lacan alludes to Delay's effort at psychological reconstitution, which would present a "marriage of psychology and the letter" (629, 4). Lacan gives to this the 'Blakean title' of a *Marriage of Heaven and Hell* before arguing that the letter will triumph and render pure psychology irrelevant. Delay himself was not ignorant of psychoanalysis, even if he refused to produce a work of "applied psychoanalysis" (629, 7). Praising Delay's honesty and rigor in the method he follows, Lacan concludes that the biographer was able to expose the very "structure of the subject" (630, 3) and thus be true to a method that psychoanalysis had outlined. Lacan praises Jean Delay's exhaustive and authorized biography while expressing reservations about Jean Schlumberger's project in *Madeleine and André Gide.*

Schlumberger aims at correcting Gide's portrayal of Madeleine, possibly because he was an old friend of both. Indeed, Gide and Schlumberger had founded the NRF press in 1911 with Gaston Gallimard. Like most biographical investigations, Schlumberger's memoir underlines discrepancies between Gide's autobiographical texts and what we know of historical reality. Lacan does not seem interested in this revisionist effort and prefers Delay's psychobiography because it remains faithful to Gide's project. Delay remains focused on Gide, and explores in depth one particular subject so as to reach the central core of humanity. Biographer and autobiographer agree that the point is to throw light on "*man's relationship to the letter*" (623, 3). If Delay could devote thirteen hundred pages to an examination of Gide's life between 1869 and 1895, it was in the hope of providing a psychological key to the contradictions of the French novelist. His aim was not to show discrepancies between the texts and the 'facts.' The truth of the work appears through the delusions and falsifications it records, a fact of which Gide himself was aware, so that "... the only thing that is of importance is a truth that is based on the fact that the message condenses in its unveiling. There is so little opposition between this *Dichtung* and *Wahrheit* in its nakedness that the fact of the poetic operation must make us notice, instead, the following feature which we forget in every truth: truth shows itself in a fictional structure" (625, 5). Indeed, Gide derided de Gouncourt's flatness and timidity because the French memorialist believed that he needed 'proof' for everything he wrote, "as if," Gide added ironically "proof by reality were necessary" (642, n.3.) Delay's rigorous reconstruction exposes the structure of the subject that psychoanalysis outlines. Gide had indeed been introduced to psychoanalysis even if he remained wary of Freud whom he would call an "idiot of genius" (Gide, 1951: 785).

Given Gide's reservations, there is something to learn from the fact that he chose Delay, a well-known psychiatrist, to be his own Eckermann. Lacan adds that the power granted to the therapist, whether a psychoanalyst or a psychiatrist, is akin to that granted to God in former times (627, 4). Yet "Gide knew how to do what it was appropriate to do with God and thus expected something else" (627, 6). Gide had left room for the unconscious in his writings quite early, as was attested by the introductory note he added to his witty satirical novel, *Paludes*, a book to which I will return at the end. It is a Virgilian pastoral that makes fun of the symbolist literary milieu that Gide knew so well and described at length in *If it die*... Here, Gide announces that his readers are free to make sense of an open text:

> Before explaining my book to others, I wait for others to explain it to me. (...) ... what interests me is what I have put there without knowing it, -- that part of Unconscious that I would like to call God's part. A book is always a collaboration, and whatever it is worth, the more the scribe's part is small, the more God's welcome will be great.
>
> (1920: 12)

Lacan includes in the discussion the fact that Gide had been initiated to psychoanalysis by a Polish psychoanalyst who had come from Vienna and was the first to introduce Freudian ideas to Paris (630, 6). She was a friend of Jacques Rivière, and when she came to Paris for the second time in 1921, Eugénie Sokolnicka, the first Freudian psychoanalyst to come to Paris, attracted huge interest among the circle of friends around Gide. Gide was among those who would gather to hear her expound Freudian theories, especially regarding the cure of children, which was one of her specialties. Gide was to use her in an oft-quoted chapter of *The Counterfeiters*, in which her role is not positive. Sokolnicka appears barely disguised as Mrs. Sophronicka, and attempts to understand the symptom of the doomed hero, Boris, but fails. Boris will end up committing suicide in front of his schoolmates. Like Delay, Lacan assumes that Gide projected himself in Boris, but then pushed psychoanalysis away, and rejected its interpretive methods as unsound or blinkered (630, 7). Lacan is also aware of the fact that Gide's mother had become ostensibly a lesbian after she had lost her husband—her passionate friendship with her governess, Anna Shackleton is duly noted (631, 6).

When Delay follows Gide throughout all his games with masks, Lacan tends to sum up this painstaking reconstruction. A revealing comment situates the interaction of jouissance and desire:

> When Gide declares to Robert de Bonnières that 'We must all represent,' and when in his ironic *Paludes* he speculates about being and appearing, those who, because they have a rented mask, persuade themselves that they have a face underneath it, think 'Literature!'—without suspecting that Gide is expressing here a problem that is so personal that it is the very problem of the person. // Freud's ego-ideal is painted on this complex mask, and it forms itself, along with the repression of one of the subject's desires, by the unconscious adoption of the very image of the Other who has the usufruct [*jouissance*] of this desire and both the right to enjoy it and the means with which to do so.
>
> (633, 8, 9, slightly modified)

Here, when Lacan quotes Delay's second volume he is in fact rehearsing the main thesis of his own dissertation on paranoia and the structure of human 'personality.' As he had explained about the case of one paranoid patient he called Aimée, a 'person' is above all a *persona*, that is the mask that one finds in Roman comedies or tragedies (633, 4). Becoming aware of his own masks and disguises, Gide was attempting to capture the point of juncture between desire and jouissance. He has painted on this mask the ego ideal he has found in his cousin, hence this passionate love for her. This love entailed a repression of desire. The unconscious Other has the legal ownership of Gide's desire and the actual means to enact it, but it is hidden by the painted face on the mask.

The decision to marry his cousin was a life-changing moment for Gide: if it was the exact reverse of Kierkegaard's decision to abandon his bride just before the marriage, for Gide and for Kierkegaard both, the decision was a radical gesture meant to change their lives for ever.

Madeleine then became the sublimated Woman, perhaps a wonderful companion and devoted collaborator, but also a very unhappy wife. Gide's ambivalence toward her was revealed in the journal published after the death of Madeleine, *Et nunc manet in te*. Gide's obstinate desire to marry a cousin who was like a sister for him was an attempt to make The Woman set a limit to his own homosexual inclinations. Gide, whose sensuality had bloomed early, as we have seen, and whose homosexuality was not closeted, decided to marry in an almost incestuous union a cousin whose sexual urges would remain unsatisfied: here was a type of "mystical love" based upon sexual renunciation, and one that divorced pure love from sexual satisfaction with boys (635, 4). The unconsummated marriage exacted its toll with a Madeleine who was kept in the dark as to her husband's sexuality. *Et nunc manet in te* unflinchingly documents how drained and aged his wife Madeleine soon became; in public, they were often taken for a mother and her son.

However, in 1918, Madeleine acted decisively when she burned her only treasure, which was the huge collection of letters that Gide had written to her every day (there were often several letters a day) since they had known each other, that is for more than thirty years. Gide's reaction to this loss was excessive: he cried for one week and felt as if he had lost a "child" (Gide, 2001: 961). Lacan's reaction to this grievance is ironical, even sarcastic. Moreover, turning this time more to Schlumberger's book for his material, he notes with approval that Madeleine was not only "refined, cultured, and gifted" (639, 7) but also that she had an "icy determination" (639, 9). Her radical gesture, burning the letters that embodied love in a series of signifiers, those cherished letters, proves that she was able, at least for once, to resist the role prepared for her by her husband, for whom she had to be the pious, ethereal and asexual Alissa. Here was a true 'gesture' from this desperate woman, and Lacan fully approves of it:

> To what extent she managed to become what Gide made her into remains impenetrable, but the sole act in which she clearly showed that she was separate from it was the act of a woman, a true woman, in her uncompromising nature as a woman (*d'une femme, d'une vraie femme, dans son entièreté de femme*).
>
> (640, 1)

By a strange inversion, her nihilistic act made a true woman of her while exposing Gide's femininity, a femininity that he had denied (he explains everywhere that his sexual orientation was "active"). Gide felt as if he had lost a child. "I am suffering as if she had killed our child" (Gide, 2001: 961). For

Lacan, this attitude evokes the wail of a "female primate struck in the stomach" (640, 4).

Indeed, Madeleine had burned a trove of letters, to which both had access, and they filled large drawers. According to her account, she had to 'do something' that would be irrevocable after this betrayal in order not to become mad. After a mourning period, Gide took some distance, and he could comment more ironically on his infatuation with his own letters. Following his insight from *Seminar V* (S5, 1957–1958: 261), Lacan again compares Gide's cry with that of Harpagon, Molière's famous miser. Harpagon cries out for the treasure that he thinks has been stolen: "My casket!" whereas he should be concerned for his daughter's fate (S5, 1957–1958: 261). Here, unwittingly, Gide becomes a character of comedy, even if this comedy had come very close to tragedy. His truth will continue being written, but in letters deprived of this privileged and beloved addressee—letters for all, that is to say, literature.

Just as Harpagon bemoans the disappearance of a casket whereas he should investigate his daughter's loss, Gide could only understand what had happened to the strange couple they formed after Madeleine's death. The letters have been left in the hole into which desire vanished. This was how Gide turned into a 'man of letters,' someone who could universalize a 'truth' equally valid for all readers. Lacan quotes the last page of *Et nunc manet in te*, admitting to a felicitous misreading. In 1939, Gide had written in his journal:

> Before leaving Paris, I was able to revise the proofs of my *Diary*. Rereading it, it appears to me that the systematic excision (until my mourning at least) of all the passages concerning Madeleine have in a way *blinded* the text. The few allusions to the secret drama of my life thus become incomprehensible because of the absence of what could throw light on them. Incomprehensible or inadmissible, the image of my mutilated self I give there, offering only, in the burning place of the heart, a hole.
>
> (2001: 977)

Lacan thought that Gide referred to the burnt correspondence, then realized his mistake. He concluded that he had been right to misread, since the text points to the same structural function. Here is the point where Gide's famous irony, so visible in many novels, finds a limit, the limit of the letter as such. Lacan goes on:

> The letters in which he placed his soul had … no carbon copy (*double*). When their fetishistic nature appeared it gave rise to the kind of laughter that greets subjectivity caught off guard. // It all ends with comedy, but who will put a stop to the laughter?
>
> (641, 8, 9)

Lacan is always on the alert for signs of Gide's famous irony, seemingly wondering who is the laughing stock here: "Is it the Gide who contents himself in his final days with writing down on paper silly stories, childhood memories, and lucky deeds all mixed together, which take on a strange glow in his *Ainsi soit-il?*" (641, 10). At the end of the double review, Lacan pinpoints a last text that critics have all but bypassed. *Ainsi soit-il?* is a curious medley of memories and silly jokes narrated with obvious glee by Gide who was then eighty-one. One of these offers a wry comment on the vignette I had started with, the story of the two turtle doves. It is presented as an 'American joke' by Gide. In fact, it is a simple cartoon. A hen looking like a nurse opens the door of the waiting room in a maternity hospital; the rooster, waiting anxiously, smoking nervously, wings crossed behind him à la Napoléon, paces up and down the room littered with cigarette stubs; the nurse calls out: 'It's an egg!' Gide explains that this makes him laugh each time. He adds mischievously "Too bad for you if you don't see the connection" (Gide, 2001: 1016). This belated joke, discussing among other things the comic annulment of sexual difference, is obviously the *Witz* that Gide was waiting for when he was thirteen and obsessed about doves' eggs.

In this last diary written by Gide one year before his death, we have a testament of some sort. Even if the text has been heavily edited by Jean Schlumberger, the tone remains light, witty, and juvenile. In this last autobiographical sum, which had been dedicated to his daughter Catherine Lambert, Gide sounds younger and sprightlier than in his early and rather pompous *Notebooks of André Walter.* Lacan reads these vignettes with great attention, relishing their non-sequiturs and poetic absurdities. He alludes to one of these, albeit rather cryptically:

> 'Are you almost done, Signora Velcha?' – where did this incantation come from which was repeated by his cousins, little girls like any others, this incantation that was irrevocable for them if they risked saying it, and that they revealed to him once in the attic retreat where it scanded their dance? From the same fateful trio of female magicians who reappeared in his destiny.
>
> (641, 11; 642, 1)

Here, Lacan summarizes a strange ritual that had been mentioned by Delay in his first volume, p. 184 of the French edition. It was a game played by the three cousins (including Madeleine), and one day Gide was drawn into it forcefully, which made him grow ecstatic. The game was an elaborate dance; the participants would go round and round in a procession, until at a given signal two would face each other, one would then ask: "Are you almost done, Signora Velcha?" after which they would resume the procession (Gide, 2001: 1028). The fact that one of the young women who had invented the game was his future wife, here with her two sisters who were competing for

André's attention, has some importance. However the magic did not work in the end, and the foreclosure of the little boy from a purely feminine ritual could not be overcome. Lacan adds the ominous question: "And the hand that transcribed that incantation, was it still his, when he already at times believed he was dead?" (642, 2).

To conclude his own essay, Lacan connects the psychobiography of Gide with Delay's announced book on Nietzsche. However, this book was never published. Delay had shown clearly that Gide was in great debt to Nietzsche. Gide's amazing facility as a writer did not prevent him from being a philosopher too. In the end, Lacan answers his own question with another reference to Nietzsche:

> This movement will only stop when it reaches the appointed place of which you are already aware, since you are on your way to it, when it reaches the question on the face offered by the Word beyond Comedy, at the moment at which comedy turns, of its own accord, into farce: How can we know which of the jugglers holds the real Punchinello?
>
> (642, 4)

Here, Death enters under the guise of the 'absolute master,' and this sends Gide back to his cousin's place. A footnote puts us on the track: Lacan alludes to Nietzsche's cry of: *Ecco, ecco, il vero Pulchinella!* That he cried out when a priest showed him a crucifix in Turin. Christ turns into the 'true Punch,' and thus parody will not spare the letter of desire. This is implied by Nietzsche (1976: 687) in his last letters, after the collapse in Turin, when he writes that he goes round in the streets, taps people on the shoulder and asks them: "Are we happy? I am god, it is I who made this caricature."[5]

Conclusion

Lacan's essay for *Critique* concludes in a tone reminiscent of Georges Bataille. Nietzschean parody dominates all the rest, even the ontology of desire that underpins the letter, as we have seen in the first example of Gide's adolescent transgression. We may remember that Madeleine had to do something radical after André had left with his lover, otherwise she would have gone mad like Nietzsche. The personal tragedy caused by the simple fact that there were no copies of the letters encouraged Gide to write more frankly, with less narcissism, while publishing autobiographical texts that had hitherto remained private (or for a close circle of friends). Gide attempted then to portray his conflicted libido in the colder light of analysis, and he also moved away from his lyrical transference to an idealized feminine addressee. If Gide's 'perversion' was to recreate the little boy he had been, to be once more the object of his aunt's sexual attentions, this auto-erotic graphomania aimed at perpetuating a family drama, at rebuilding endlessly a private theater of unlimited adoration, could only be put to an end by the radical gesture of his wife when she burned the letters. Before, Gide was 'his majesty the baby' strutting on a quasi-incestuous stage; there, he was the hero no matter what. The mirroring process keeping him desiring and desired, was buttressed on a correspondence that was the loving heart of his work.

The correspondence with his wife has been a work of love, transference and imaginary projection. Gide truly loved the pure Madeleine, the Alissa of the novel *Straight is the gate.* This love followed the Lacanian formula: Gide gave to Madeleine what he did not have, namely sexual desire, and desire was what Madeleine did not want, preferring to remain pure in an unconsummated incestuous union that would be sublimated. The destruction of the correspondence did create a 'hole' in Gide's heart whose contours would be identical with that of the letter as such. After Madeleine's death, the 'letters' would be metamorphosed into literature. Gide had became a 'man of letters,' his particular truth turned into a universal truth and it could be shared by the general reader.

This insight was developed in Lacan's next seminar, *Seminar VI, Desire and its interpretation.* One year later, Lacan returned to Gide in the conclusion of a seminar wholly devoted to desire. Going back once more to Delay's excellent psychobiography, Lacan deployed the concept of sublimation when commenting on another childhood vignette of Gide's. It is another passage of *If It Die…*, when Gide mentions the summer vacations he took in the family house in Uzès. There, his father had lost a marble that he had let fall into a hole made in an old oak door. The child tried to push and touch the marble but it had gone too far to be lifted up. Then he kept thinking about it during the subsequent year he spent in Paris, letting the fingernail of a little finger grow all that time. Then one year later, he was successful: with his long and sharp nail, he was able to catch the marble at last. But this led to another disappointment. What he held was just another dull and banal marble, similar to all the others, devoid of mystery or interest (Gide, 2001: 114). The object of desire, first lost then found, had to fall again. Here is a metaphor of the paternal phallus, an imaginary phallus this time.

Lacan comments on this passage by adding that Gide allegorizes the function of the object that has been "pushed back into a magnificent *Sublimierung*" (S6, 1958–1959: 551). It will only be with the following year's seminar on ethics that Lacan will disentangle himself from the Freudian dialectics of sublimation. He will find in Freud's *Project* the term of *das Ding*, which will become the *Thing.* With this new concept, Lacan will assert that sublimation is, in fact, a way of raising the object to the dignity of the Thing. In this vertical propulsion, the letter will once more come close to a hole, but it will be the hole left open by *jouissance*. The desire and the literary symptom to which Gide testifies so forcibly will be replaced by Joyce the 'sinthome' of literature.

Joyce and Gide would be linked by Lacan once more, in April 1975. Just then, as Lacan was immersing himself in critical approaches to Joyce because of the forthcoming invitation to open the June 1975 international James Joyce Symposium in Paris, he alluded to Gide's novel, *Paludes*—that I have already quoted—in his Seminar:

> It is worth giving all its due to the proverb translated and glossed by André Gide in *Paludes* -- *Numero deus impare gaudet*, which he translates as 'Number two is happy being odd' (*'Le numéro deux se réjouit d'être impair'*). As I have said for some time, this is quite right, since nothing would realize the two if there was not the odd, the odd that begins with three -- which is not obvious immediately and makes the Borromean knot necessary.
>
> (S22, 1973–1974: 49)[6]

To understand this schoolboy's joke, one needs to imagine the usual mistranslation of the second half of a well-known line in Virgil's Eclogue 8: "… numero deus impare gaudet" (meaning: "uneven numbers please god," or more literally: "god rejoices at uneven numbers") into French. By a French over-literalization, the mistranslation generates a Lacanian paradox: number two becomes an odd number and rejoices at being so odd.

In Virgil's Eclogue, as replayed in Gide's *Paludes*, we meet two shepherds who rival each in their songs while trying to outdo Orpheus. The power of poems or charms is compared to Circe's craft when she used to 'spellbind the shipmates of Odysseus':

> (*Draw Daphnis back from town, my spells, draw Daphnis home.*)
> First with these three triple threads in separate colours three
> I bind you, then about this altar thrice I bear
> Your puppet self; uneven numbers please the god (numero deus impare gaudet.).
>
> (Virgil, 1980: 90, 91)

Gide's novel suggests that freedom derives from odd numbers, which alludes to sexual "oddity," (Gide, 1920: 70), while introducing the theme of God's enjoyment, or more precisely, God's *jouissance*, or the *jouissance* of the Other. This maps a domain that Lacan explored later with Joyce and Duras, the variegated field of knots, triple strings bound together in different colors, and the notion of the letter of a hole providing a limit of a rim to *jouissance*. The combination of Gide and Joyce announces the investment in the 'Borromean planet' that dominated in Lacan's last years. The *jouissance* of God underpins the practice of the letter in true literature. Showing that '*Numero deus impare gaudet*' can be mistranslated as '*Le numéro deux se réjouit d'être impair*,' Gide notes that 'l'impair' entails a promise of happiness or freedom, while Lacan sees a promise if not of happiness (*bonheur*), at least of '*bon noeud*' (a good knot). Such a good knot will confirm that we can begin to perceive an even number as a pair from the point of view of its oddness or imparity, which sends us back to Poe's speculations on oddness and evenness in the *Purloined Letter*. Thus we need to count to three in order to understand the letter: here, at least, we have Delay, Schlumberger and Gide. But it was Gide who first sent Lacan on the right track by linking the letter and the hole in the heart branded by a terrible truth.

Notes

1 A good abridged version has been provided by June Guicharnaud, see Delay (1963).
2 Euripides, *Medea*, lines 298–302, in Easterling and Knox, 1985, p. 317, trans. modified.
3 "Between Wilde's conviction on May 25 and the attack that paralyzed André Gide's mother at the end of May, the chronological coincidence is indeed disturbing" (Delay, 1963: 441).
4 "*Comme c'était manqué!*" ("What a misfire!") the youth exclaims (Gide, 2001: 174).
5 Nietzsche wrote in Italian: *Siamo contenti? Son dio ho fatto questa caricatura.* I have modified Kaufmann's translation.
6 See Lacan (1975/1976).

References

Delay, J. (1963). *The Youth of André Gide.* Chicago, IL: University of Chicago Press.
Easterling, P. and Knox, B. (1985). *The Cambridge History of Classical Literature, I, Greek Literature.* Cambridge: Cambridge University Press.
Gide, A. (1920). *Paludes.* Paris: Gallimard, Pléiade.
Gide, A. (1951). *Journal 1889–1939.* Paris: Gallimard, Pléiade.
Gide, A. (2001). '*Si le grain ne meurt*,' in *Souvenirs et Voyages*, edited by Pierre Masson, Daniel Durosay and Martine Sagaert. Paris: Gallimard, Pléiade.
Gide, A. (2009). *Oeuvres, Romans et Récits, I.* Paris: Gallimard Pléiade.
Lacan, J. (1975/1976). 'R.S.I. Séminaire 1974–75,' edited by J.-A. Miller, *Ornicar?*, 5.
Nietzsche, F. (1976). *The Portable Nietzsche*, edited and translated by Walter Kaufmann. New York: Penguin.
Virgil (1980). *The Eclogues*, translated by Guy Lee. New York: Penguin Classics.

6

KANT WITH SADE

Dany Nobus

Context

Of the twenty-eight substantial papers and six shorter contributions that make up Jacques Lacan's *Écrits*, the piece entitled '*Kant avec Sade*' ('*Kant with Sade*') is generally regarded as one of the most difficult essays in the collection. The qualification of 'difficult' would probably not be very significant in this context, if the other texts in *Écrits* were an easy read, but since the others are already widely considered to be distinctly cryptic the word 'difficult' could only be synonymous here with 'inaccessible' or 'impenetrable'. Remarkably, this qualification would not be too far removed from how Lacan himself put it to an Italian journalist in October 1974: as to '*Kant with Sade*', "I am incomprehensible" (Lacan, 1975/2013: 83).

The title '*Kant avec Sade*' is effectively a double metonymy. Lacan is not at all interested in comparing and contrasting the (rather uneventful) life of Immanuel Kant, the famous academic philosopher of Königsberg, with the (rather tumultuous) life of D.A.F. de Sade, the infamous French Marquis who spent twenty-seven years of his life behind bars. When, starting from section eight in the text (656), he intermittently refers to key events in Sade's life, it is primarily to demonstrate the limits of his 'art', insofar as to Lacan one should not assume that the licentious content of Sade's novels is a reliable indicator of the author's morals, his politics and his lifestyle, much less that the prevailing sexual tendencies in Sade's work are but a fictional extension of his own mental economy—the 'sadists' in the novels having been created by a man who is himself an inveterate 'sadist'. One of the crucial lines of Lacan's argument in '*Kant with Sade*' is precisely that the contents of Sade's libertine novels, which he also designates as "the Sadean fantasy" (653, 9), that is, the fantasy Sade articulated as a literary text within the space of his creative imagination, cannot be mapped directly onto the author's life. More specifically, the fact that it is the 'sadistic' fantasy of Sade's libertine heroes that tends to dominate within the Sadean fantasy—whose full spectrum also includes the more 'masochistic' side of the victims, as epitomized by the perennially virtuous Justine—did not, for Lacan, demonstrate that this is also the type of 'practical reason' which would have presided over his daily routines, outside the fictional space of the literary narrative. Although Sade's incessant articulation of the libertines' 'sadistic' fantasy of absolute destruction inevitably played a crucial part in the author's own *Weltanschauung*, for Lacan the latter is much more constructed around Sade's relationship to his own act of writing, and to the specific function he wanted to accord to his libertine novels, as exclusive 'instruments' of fantasy, than to the personal realization of the cruel and barbaric fantasy of his fictional heroes.

Much like 'Kant' in the title of the paper refers to Kant's books and ideas rather than to the man, the 'Sade' in '*Kant with Sade*' is thus meant to be understood primarily as Sade's works, and the views expressed within them by a host of fictional characters. As a matter of fact, the focus of Lacan's paper is even tighter, because rather than aiming to combine all of Kant's writings with the whole of Sade's literary output, which also includes much more mainstream short stories, novels, essays and plays, it essentially restricts itself—and this is the second metonymy—to a discussion of the links between a mere two texts: Kant's *Kritik der Praktischen Vernunft* (Kant, 1788/1997) and Sade's *La philosophie dans le boudoir* (Sade, 1795/2006). And because Lacan's text was originally intended as a preface to the latter volume, it should not come as a surprise that the emphasis is firmly placed on this one particular book—Kant's treatise being placed in a secondary, supporting role.

In the fourth paragraph of '*Kant with Sade*', Lacan mentions that, to the best of his knowledge, this link between Kant and Sade had "never been pointed out as such" (645, 4), thus emphasizing the originality of his direction of inquiry. Either Lacan's literature study had been too superficial, or he had conveniently decided to 'forget' some of his source materials, but the connection between Kant and Sade—their works and ideas, rather than their personalities, of course—had definitely been made before, and moreover along the same lines, notably in 'Excursus II' of Adorno and Horkheimer's *Dialektik der Aufklärung* (*Dialectic of Enlightenment*), which was first published in 1944 (Adorno and Horkheimer, 1944/1997). In this remarkable text, the principal proponents of the Frankfurt School drew a parallel between Kant's *Kritik der praktischen Vernunft* and Sade's *Juliette ou les prospérités du vice* (Sade, 1797/1968), in order to show that Sade's libertine heroes sound uncannily like Kant when they profess their moral maxims, with the proviso that they represent the dialectical underside of Kant's system. Much like Kant, Juliette and her acolytes reject any consideration of extrinsic, socially sanctioned moral values when advancing their doctrine. They believe unreservedly in the power of reason, provided it is stripped of its emotional dimensions (what Kant designated as the 'pathological'), so that it becomes a formal, rigorous, 'apathetic' faculty. But Adorno and Horkheimer also argued that Sade's heroes are Kantian philosophers who are actually purer than Kant himself, if only because they do not believe that autonomous, dispassionate, scientific reason will automatically engender moral benevolence and contribute to the establishment of a harmonious world order. According to Adorno and Horkheimer, Sade's libertines are far more rational than the philosopher of Königsberg, insofar as the latter's conviction that the simple 'fact' of pure reason would spontaneously generate a practical, moral law of mutual respect constitutes in itself a point of irrationality. These propositions are not at all dissimilar to what Lacan posits in '*Kant with Sade*', yet I cannot prove that he was familiar with Adorno and Horkheimer's work, much less that he relied on it when developing his own theses.

Given the cultural prominence of Sartre and de Beauvoir in France during the 1950s, I would definitely be surprised if Lacan had not read de Beauvoir's seminal essay '*Faut-il brûler Sade?*', which was originally published in '*Les temps modernes*' (de Beauvoir, 1950–1951/1990). In this particular text, de Beauvoir averred, almost in passing and without any further elaboration: "With a severity similar to Kant's, and which has its source in the same puritan tradition, Sade conceives the free act only as an act free of feeling" (de Beauvoir, 1950–1951/1990: 55). Lacan never refers to de Beauvoir's work on Sade, but the two had met during the 1940s at a private performance of a play by Picasso, and continued to be on friendly terms (Roudinesco, 1993/1997: 168–169). De Beauvoir's coupling of Kant and Sade was not nearly as tight as Horkheimer and Adorno's intricate intellectual braid of Kant, Sade and the Holocaust, but at least it demonstrates again that Lacan is clearly mistaken when he claims that the link between Kant and Sade had never before been made.

It should also be noted, here, that when Lacan associated Kant with Sade for the first time on 23 December 1959 (Lacan, S7, 1959–1960: 78), French Sade-scholarship was already highly advanced, by virtue of a series of influential studies by Maurice Heine (1950), Jean Paulhan (1945), Pierre Klossowski (1947), Maurice Blanchot (1949/1986) and Georges Bataille (1957a, 1957b), and the painstaking biographical work by Gilbert Lely (1952, 1957). It is highly likely that Lacan was introduced to Sade's works by Bataille, but even without this direct line of influence, he would have been immersed in a post-War cultural and intellectual atmosphere that took Sade very seriously, perhaps for the first time in French history (Marty, 2011). Furthermore, one year before Lacan started writing '*Kant with Sade*', Michel Foucault published *Folie et déraison*, his massive thesis for the French State Doctorate, in which Sade featured prominently as a major figure of contestation in the history of French institutional psychiatry (Foucault, 1961). Although he was not in the habit of acknowledging all his sources, Lacan was clearly inspired by all these works when he wrote up '*Kant with Sade*', and in what follows I will endeavour to show that the contributions of Blanchot, Klossowski and Bataille in particular, constitute an important intellectual backdrop for Lacan's arguments.

Finally, I should mention that on 11 April 1961, Adolf Eichmann, one of the most highly ranked Nazi officials, was put on trial in Jerusalem, charged with the mass deportation and large-scale extermination of millions of Jewish people. At one point during the trial, Judge Raveh questioned Eichmann about a remark he had made previously under police interrogation, in which he had emphasized that he had only ever lived his life in accordance with the Kantian definition of duty. In response to the judge's question, Eichmann surprised everyone by reciting, almost *verbatim*, Kant's definition of the categorical imperative: "I [Adolf Eichmann] meant by my remark about Kant that the principle of my will must always be such that it can become the principle of general laws" (Arendt, 1963/2006: 136). Following this statement, Eichmann declared that he was familiar with Kant's *Kritik der praktischen Vernunft*, but that he had stopped complying with its precepts from the moment he was charged with the duty to implement the so-called Final Solution. In her reading of this extraordinary moment, Hannah Arendt argued that Eichmann never really relinquished his Kantian sense of duty at all, but that he simply

> distorted it to read: Act as if the principle of your actions were the same as that of the legislator or of the law of the land—or … 'Act in such a way that the Führer, if he knew your action, would approve it'.
> (1963/2006: 136)

Arendt did not go so far as to say that Eichmann had interpreted Kant in a Sadean fashion, but in her report Eichmann definitely appeared as a diligent, albeit twisted Kantian and, by extension, as a cold and callous, yet rational mass-murderer who incarnated the destructive obverse of Kant's categorical imperative—the kind of figure Adorno and Horkheimer may have had in mind when, in response to the atrocities of World War II, they exposed the Sadean dangers of Kant's moral philosophy, and of the Enlightenment values in general. Arendt reported on the case for *The New Yorker* in February and March 1963, but in France, too, the newspapers devoted numerous pages to the events in Jerusalem. Lacan had already linked Kant and Sade sixteen months before the trial started, but Eichmann's declared Kantianism may have emboldened him in his views, and may have given him a renewed strength of purpose when he began composing '*Kant with Sade*' during the Spring and Summer of 1962.

In what follows, the reader will find a step-by-step commentary on '*Kant with Sade*', in which I shall articulate the central lines of Lacan's argument, and situate his ideas within their broader intellectual context. I have structured the commentary in accordance with Lacan's own textual divisions in '*Kant with Sade*', so that each section of my text corresponds to a specific division of the essay. However, because the twelfth part of '*Kant with Sade*' (663) is just one sentence, and serves as an introduction to the following division of the paper, I will take the twelfth and thirteenth parts as one. I have also felt it necessary to alert the reader on occasion to those passages in '*Kant with Sade*' where Lacan's own explanations and elaborations are rather contentious and problematic, because otherwise my text would have been in quite a few places no more than a paraphrase of Lacan's. At the same time, I do not wish to claim, of course, that my critical analysis of '*Kant with Sade*' is the only possible interpretation of the text, let alone that it is the most accurate exegesis of what remains an exceptionally demanding *écrit*.[1]

Commentaries on the text

Section 1

In 1904, the German sexologist Iwan Bloch published, under the pseudonym of Dr Eugène Dühren, the first edition of Marquis de Sade's mammoth *Les cent vingt journées de Sodome* (*The Hundred-and-twenty Days of Sodom*), the manuscript of which had been deemed lost after Sade's transfer from his prison cell in the Bastille to the asylum of Charenton on 4 July 1789, shortly after the outbreak of the French revolution (Sade, 1904; Pauvert and Beuchot, 1999: 101). Both in his preface and in his extended 'scientific annotations' to the book, Dühren repeatedly emphasized the striking similarity between Sade's fictional heroes and the clinical cases described by Richard von Krafft-Ebing, the most famous sexologist at the time, in his celebrated (and constantly updated) *Psychopathia Sexualis* (Sade, 1904: 3, 534—notes 70/71, 535—note 90; Krafft-Ebing, 1901). Twenty-five years later, a Lyonese medical doctor by the name of Salvator Sarfati devoted the first doctoral thesis to Sade, in which he endorsed Dühren's view by saying that Sade's writings were "illustrated monuments of sexual psychopathology which had contributed to science, before Krafft-Ebing did, the full range of perversions" (Sarfati, 1930: 1). Yet Sarfati also extended their 'scientific' value by identifying in them the seeds of a doctrine "that would be developed, one-hundred-and-twenty-five years later, by the Vienna School" (Sarfati, 1930: 117)—to be read as: 'by Freud'. This is the point that was picked up by the French medical doctor, journalist and Sade-connoisseur Maurice Heine in a review of Sarfati's work (Heine, 1932/1950: 107–108), and it emboldened him to promote the hybrid paradigm of 'freudo-sadism', which was received with great enthusiasm by the French surrealists. In his influential *Anthology of Black Humour*, the founder of the surrealist movement André Breton accordingly wrote: "[P]sychologically speaking, it [Sade's writing] can be considered the most authentic precursor of Freud's work" (Breton, 1939/2009: 46).

After World War II, the idea that Sade's libertine novels foreshadowed Freudian psychoanalysis reappeared in Jean Paulhan's '*Le Marquis de Sade et sa complice ou les revanches de la pudeur*' (Paulhan, 1945). In the fifth section of this essay, Paulhan opined: "Krafft-Ebing was to consecrate the categories and distinctions the Divine Marquis traced. Later, a Freud was to adopt Sade's very method and principle" (Paulhan, 1945/1990: 18). In his deposition at the court case against the French publisher Jean-Jacques Pauvert on 15 December 1956, Paulhan reiterated the intellectual synergies between Sade and Freud on three separate occasions (Garçon, 1963: 48–50), but by that time other key figures within the new wave of French Sade-scholarship had also ascertained Sade's proto-freudianism. For example, in his seminal 1949 article '*La raison de Sade*', Blanchot had identified a number of themes in Sade's work that could be easily interpreted as anticipating Freud (Blanchot, 1949/2004: 39), whereas in 1957 Sade's biographer Gilbert Lely rekindled Heine's 'insight', quoting the same passage from Sade's *Justine ou les malheurs de la vertu* as Blanchot had used, in support of the thesis that in 1791 the Marquis was already professing some of the ideas that would later become cornerstones of the Freudian edifice (Lely, 1957: 333, 555, footnote 1). And in 'Must We Burn Sade?', Simone de Beauvoir wrote that in *Philosophy in the Boudoir*, Sade had clearly anticipated Freud's 'pan-sexuality' (de Beauvoir, 1950–1951/1990: 38).

In the opening paragraph of '*Kant with Sade*', Lacan (645, 1) designates this portrayal of Sade as a precursor of Freud as "a stupidity" (*une sottise*). Although he does not clarify his reasons nor his precise target, one plausible explanation could be that for Lacan the analogies that had been drawn between Sade and Freud (and Krafft-Ebing) should not be taken seriously, since they had primarily served the purpose of rendering Sade more palatable, and the publication of his work more justifiable. Instead of seeing Sade as presaging Freud, Lacan aligns the Sadean boudoir with the famous locations where the ancient philosophers had debated the meaning of life, and where eager young citizens had received instruction into the ethical principles underpinning the establishment of a sustainable social system (645, 2). Rather than calling him a precursor of Freud, Lacan suggests that Sade should thus be recognized as a (moral) philosopher, and that his works should be situated within the history of ethics. If there is a link at all between Sade and Freud, it has nothing to do, then, with the former anticipating the latter, but merely with the latter being able to formulate his fundamental 'scientific' concept of the 'pleasure principle' and especially its ostensible contradictions—the fact that one can experience pleasure in one's own and someone else's pain—because Sade had somehow prepared the *ethical* ground for it (645, 3). Indeed, Sade's libertine heroes relentlessly insist on the 'natural fact' that human beings are driven by but one 'moral' principle, notably that of the selfish pursuit of pleasure, whereas Freud argued that unconscious mental processes are governed by the sole aim of obtaining pleasure and avoiding pain (Freud, 1911/1958: 219). In addition, for Sade's libertines, there should be no limit to a human being's compliance with this natural 'moral' principle; even when someone only derives pleasure from inflicting pain, torturing and killing others, or from his or her own suffering, the acts are legitimate on account of their being authentic and truthful. For Freud too, the pleasure principle by no means excludes the existence of a primary (erotogenic) masochism, which is tantamount to human beings finding 'pleasure in pain', and which may be reinforced by outward-facing destructive impulses being re-directed towards the ego (Freud, 1920/1955: 54–55; 1924/1961: 161–170). Hence, if Freud came up with his own psychoanalytic 'pleasure principle'—without running the risk of being misunderstood as defending Rousseau's belief in the virtuous, uncorrupted state of human nature—it is, according to Lacan, because Sade had somehow cleared the ethical path for it, roughly one hundred years before Freud, and because throughout the nineteenth century the theme of 'delight in evil' (*bonheur dans le mal*) had gradually gained momentum (645, 3).[2]

For Lacan, Sade had thus been the first to formulate, through the mouth of his libertines, a concrete ethical system that does not take its bearings from common principles of moral goodness, and that does not aim to secure a set of socially sanctioned values about mutual support, benevolence, courtesy and respect. For this in itself to become possible, Lacan asserts, Kant's *Critique of Practical Reason* (Kant, 1788/1997) had been the necessary turning point, if only because Kant had set out to propose a theory of morality which does not rely on conventional distinctions between good and bad, which regards emotional factors of sympathy and compassion as 'pathological', which deems the anticipated consequences of one's actions to be irrelevant with regard to human beings proceeding to fulfil their moral duty, and which constructs the moral law as simultaneously subjective and universal (645, 4). Yet instead of seeing Sade as an extension of Kant, Lacan posits that Sade's work—here, *Philosophy in the Boudoir* (Sade, 1795/2006)—in a sense completed Kant's *Critique of Practical Reason*, and even revealed its truth (646, 1). This is indeed one of the most important theses of '*Kant with Sade*': in *Philosophy in the Boudoir* Sade presented the disturbing truth of Kant's *Critique of Practical Reason*, a truth which Kant himself had failed to recognize and disclose.

At the end of this section (646, 2), and in order to show how Kant's work is already highly subversive in and of itself, Lacan summarizes two of Kant's 'postulates (presuppositions) of pure practical reason' (Kant, 1788/1997: 102–111). The first postulate is that of the immortality of the soul (*Unsterblichkeit der Seele*). For Kant, the ultimate object(ive) of the moral law is the realization of the 'highest good' (*Bewirkung des höchsten Guts*), which is the moment when supreme virtuousness and supreme happiness coincide. For this highest good to be achieved, a rational being's will would need to be in 'complete conformity' (*völlige Angemessenheit*) with the moral law, that is to say, a rational being would need to attain a state of 'holiness' (*Heiligkeit*). Since no rational being will ever be capable of holiness during his or her earthly existence, and because the moral law should neither be adjusted nor imposed unrealistically, Kant argued that the immortality of the soul needs to be postulated in order to understand why a rational being would never give up trying to comply with the moral law.

Kant's second postulate of practical reason is the existence of God, who is designated as a 'supreme intelligence' and the 'supreme cause of nature', and whose existence needs to be presupposed in order to render the highest good altogether possible (conceivable, thinkable and achievable). In the absence of God, the ultimate object(ive) of the moral law cannot be guaranteed, which will inevitably affect a rational being's will to promote the realization of the highest good. In other words, the existence of God needs to be postulated, because the object(ive) of the moral law needs to appear as a consistent, intelligible and feasible achievement to the rational being whose duty it is to comply with the law. In the last paragraph of Section 1 of '*Kant with Sade*', Lacan does not refer to Kant's God, but simply highlights the *Critique*'s "need for a [divine] will to which the object that the law concerns [i.e., the highest good] is intelligible" (646, 2). Lacan does not say anything, here, about Kant's third postulate—that of a rational being's freedom from the sensible world (Kant, 1788/1997:110)—but he points out how in the *Critique* Kant had gone so far as to completely eradicate the function of 'usefulness' or 'utility' (*das Nützliche*) as a possible good in itself (Kant, 1788/1997: 51), a function which he had still included, albeit only as a 'setting' (*Einfassung*) of the will, in his first treatise on moral theory, the 1785 *Groundwork of the Metaphysics of Morals* (Kant, 1785/2012: 10). Following all of this, Lacan cannot resist telling his readers (and apparently he shared his elation with everyone else in his environment) how, in studying Kant's work, he had experienced 'incredible exaltation' (646, 2) (Miller, 2003: 27).

Section 2

In the first four paragraphs (646, 3–6) of this section, Lacan outlines Kant's account of the 'concept of an object of pure practical reason' from the second chapter of the first book of the *Critique of Practical Reason* (Kant, 1788/1997: 50–58). In this part of his work, Kant underscored that the German language is at an advantage compared to languages whose vocabulary is strongly indebted to Latin, because German has two words to express 'good' and another two words for 'bad'. In German, 'good' can be rendered as '*das Wohl*' or as '*das Gute*', whereas for 'bad' one can use '*das Übel*' or '*das Böse*'. '*Wohl*' and '*Übel*' generally capture how an individual feels ('good' or 'bad') in response to a certain object, event or situation. In Kant's own terms, the words refer to "our sensibility and to the feeling of pleasure or displeasure it [the object] causes" (Kant, 1788/1997: 52). The upshot is that the lexical ambiguity of the English sentence 'I'm feeling good about doing (a) good (deed)', and its French equivalent '*On est bien dans le bien*', disappears in German, where a literal translation of the sentence would read: '*Man fühlt sich wohl im Guten*' (646, 3). Yet because '*das Wohl*' is associated with a personal sensation of pleasure, that is to say with the subjective experience of *feeling* good, it does not by definition accord with what a reasonable human being would conceive as a 'good' thing to do. It is quite possible for someone to *feel* bad about doing a good thing and *mutatis mutandis* for someone to *feel* good about doing something bad. For a dedicated Enlightenment philosopher like

Kant, it would have been difficult to imagine the latter possibility and so he did not really consider it, but as Lacan points out in the opening paragraphs of '*Kant with Sade*' (645, 3) the idea of 'delight in evil' ('*bonheur dans le mal*') had gradually infiltrated the Western cultural imagination during the nineteenth century.

Purely on the basis of Kant's definition of '*das Wohl*', a term which can be rendered in English as 'well-being' or 'feeling good', and without needing to subscribe to Freudian psychoanalysis, it already becomes apparent, then, that the rules governing the pursuit and maintenance of subjective well-being can be designated as a 'pleasure principle' (646, 4). Yet according to Kant, this type of regulatory system could never constitute the foundation for a moral law, because good (pleasure) and bad (displeasure) are merely a subject's affective responses to an arbitrary and capricious empirical object. The experience of well-being is taken up in a chain of transient and unpredictable phenomena, whereby 'good' and 'bad' are but momentary effects of a set of specific circumstances whose precise nature and impact cannot be accurately foreseen. Moreover, apart from the fact that the link between the subjective experience of well-being and the empirical object is fragile—for no phenomenon, as Lacan put it, "can lay claim to a constant relationship to pleasure" (646, 4)—the sensation that results would be all too idiosyncratic and short-lived for it to become the foundation for a moral law that is universal, and would therefore be applicable to everyone.

By way of radical alternative, Kant proposed the establishment of a moral law which completely bypasses all considerations of 'goodness' that take their bearings from a certain relationship between the subject and the object. Whether something is 'good' or 'bad' should not depend on what an object elicits in the subject (pleasure or displeasure), but on the extent to which the subject's will acts in accordance with an *a priori* law. If there is an object of the moral law, it can only involve, in Kant's perspective, the convergence of a rational human being's will with the formulation of this very law, and not—as in traditional conceptions of morality—a certain set of precepts as to which empirical objects (events and situations) are agreeable and which are not. Beyond '*das Wohl*', Kant thus continued to recognize '*das Gute*' as the object of the moral law, but this is very much a 'concept' of an object rather than an object *per se*, partly because it has no connection with any empirical object whatsoever, and partly because (as I explained above, in the context of Kant's postulate of the immortality of the soul) the object cannot actually be attained by any rational human being during his or her earthly existence (646, 5).

Following Kant, when the will frees itself from the lures of all empirical sensibilities—which he did not hesitate to call 'pathological' (Kant, 1788/1997: 17)—it will hear the 'voice of reason' (*die Stimme der Vernunft*) (Kant, 1788/1997: 32). This voice will distinctly articulate the moral law as a categorical imperative: "So act that the maxim of your will could always hold at the same time as a principle in a giving of universal law" (Kant, 1788/1997: 28)

(646, 6). Although Kant's moral law appears to the rational human being as a command (imperative), it is radically different from the Biblical 'ten commandments', for instance, because it is devoid of contents, stripped of every reference to specific objects, and reduced to a pure form. As Kant described it, the moral law is categorical (as opposed to hypothetical), universal (applicable to all rational beings) and unconditional (unaffected by any condition that would be imposed upon it by an empirical object, event or situation).

Of course, the question is why a rational human being would decide to follow this moral law or, more concretely, what incentives (*Triebfeder*) a will would require for it to comply with the categorical imperative. This is the issue Kant addressed in the third chapter of the first book of the *Critique of Practical Reason* (Kant, 1788/1997: 62–89), and Lacan summarizes some key points of it in the fifth paragraph of Section 2 of '*Kant with Sade*' (647, 1). In essence, Kant argued that the moral law should determine a subject's will directly, in an unmediated fashion, and not owing to the "cooperation of sensible impulses"—amongst which he did not hesitate to include 'regard for oneself' (*Selbstsucht, solipsismus*), which is in itself made up of 'self-regard', 'benevolence toward oneself' (both also known as self-love) and 'satisfaction with oneself' (*Arrogantia*, self-conceit) (Kant, 1788/1997: 63). Needless to say, when the moral law infringes upon self-love and strikes down self-conceit, this will be experienced by the rational human being as painful. Yet since the moral law remains something positive in itself, it will actually become weightier (more powerful, important and influential) when 'regard for oneself' is removed, because the latter acts as a counterweight to the subject's direct observance of the moral law (and the highest good that can be expected of it). And so Lacan states that in Kant's moral philosophy, the Good (which coincides with the moral law directly determining the subject's will) is some kind of 'anti-weight', which derives its force from the reduction (subtraction) of the weight of *Selbstsucht* (647, 1).

In the remaining paragraphs of Section 2, Lacan formulates two criticisms of Kant's theory. First, he alerts the reader to an ostensible paradox (647, 2): when Kant insisted on the necessity for all empirical objects (and subjective sensibilities) to be excluded as possible grounds for morality, there seemed to appear a new, incontrovertible object, notably the object of the moral law itself, which is heard by the subject as "something that is already signifying", a "voice in conscience" (647, 2). Lacan intimates, here, that Kant's persistent attempt at securing a strictly rational, exclusively formal and distinctly non-empiricist foundation for morality runs aground on the manifestation of the categorical imperative as a new empirical object in its own right—the meaningful sound of the voice of reason.

Lacan's second critical comment concerns the status of the moral law as a categorical imperative. Drawing on Kant's distinction between analytic and synthetic propositions in his *Critique of Pure Reason* (Kant, 1781/1998), Lacan posits that the logic of the categorical imperative requires that it can only be applied with certainty to analytic maxims, and not to synthetic ones. The requirement that the maxim of a rational human being's will should incorporate the principle of a universal law is, for Lacan, only something that can be accepted with positive conviction, if and only if it concerns a proposition whose predicate is already encapsulated within its subject concept, as in 'All triangles have three sides' or—with an example Lacan took from the *Critique of Practical Reason* (Kant, 1788/1997: 25)—as in 'All deposits have a worthy depository' (647, 5). Analytic (or expliative) maxims are by definition universal, because their predicate (three sides, a worthy depositary) does not add anything that is not already included in the concept of the subject (the triangle, the deposit), and so their universality does not need to be demonstrated. In synthetic (or ampliative) propositions, the predicate is not identical with the subject, and so the relationship between the two is not self-evident. Some form of argument, proof or demonstration is required before these propositions can be regarded as universally valid, and even then there may still be an element of doubt as to their validity.

Lacan (647, 6) illustrates this point with a famous sentence from Alfred Jarry's comic play *Ubu Rex*, in which the central character of Pa Ubu exclaims (and these are the final lines of the play): "Beautiful though it [Germany] may be, it's not a patch on Poland. Ah gentlemen, there'll always be a Poland. Otherwise there wouldn't be any Poles!" (Jarry, 1896/1968: 73). In Lacan's Kantian adaptation, the line reads: "Long live Poland, for if there were no Poland, there would be no Poles" (647, 6). What makes the sentence amusing, is that it presents a synthetic proposition ("All Poles are inhabitants of Poland") as if it were an analytic judgement. Lacan indicates that while the 'analytic explanation' of Poles' existence being dependent upon Poland "is [seemingly] irrefutable", because the predicate Poland is clearly included in the subject concept (Pole), it is of course perfectly possible for Poles to maintain themselves in the absence of their homeland (647, 7). Hence, although Pa Ubu formulated his salutation in analytic terms (with the object 'Poland' being included within, and as identical to the subject of the 'Poles'), in actual fact the relationship between the object and the subject is synthetic and needs to be demonstrated. And so Lacan asserts that, in having to rely on analytic propositions for the implementation of his categorical imperative, Kant once again showed himself to be incapable of attaching the moral law to an (empirical, phenomenal) object that is *not* already included in the concept of its subject *qua* maxim of the will (647, 8).

At the end of section 2 of '*Kant with Sade*', Lacan concludes that throughout the *Critique of Practical Reason* the object thus keeps slipping away (647, 9), although it leaves behind traces at each and every point of its involvement with the moral law. With the Kantian object refusing to be caught, but with it being felt 'behind the scenes' and it being detected in small remnants of its imposing presence—like the handkerchief the lady leaves to her knight before he is going into battle in the medieval accounts of courtly love—Lacan ends this section by declaring that Kant's work has certain erotic qualities, innocent no doubt, but distinguishable all the same, which he promises to evince by clarifying the nature of the endlessly receding object in question (647, 9).

Section 3

Sade's *Philosophy in the Boudoir* is essentially a play about the sexual and moral education of a delightful fifteen-year-old girl called Eugénie de Mistival, by a trio of unbridled libertines (Madame de Saint-Ange, her brother the Chevalier de Mirvel, and the philosopher-villain Dolmancé) and two 'extras'. The narrative structure unfolds as a series of seven dialogues in dramatic form, replete with stage directions. Lacan calls it a 'pamphlet' (648, 3), no doubt because it was printed in a limited edition, without the name of a publisher, and as a posthumous work of the anonymous 'author of *Justine*'. Rather than summarizing the text, he immediately draws attention to a strange peculiarity of its composition. In the middle of the fifth dialogue, Eugénie asks "whether a government truly needs a set of morals, whether they can really influence the essence of a nation" (Sade, 1795/2006: 103), to which Dolmancé responds that it so happens he has just bought a pamphlet entitled *Frenchmen, Some More Effort if you Wish to Become Republicans*, which will answer all of Eugénie's questions. Casting her eye over the document, Madame de Saint-Ange instructs her brother to read it aloud, and what follows is the full forty-five page text of the pamphlet, which takes up almost a quarter of the entire book. Lacan refers to it as a "pamphlet within the pamphlet" (648, 3) and as a 'factum', drawing attention to how it is commonly regarded as a 'mystification', but emphasizing that it deserves to be recognized for its "closer relationship to the real", similar to how Freud had interpreted the 'dream within the dream' (648, 4). Again, instead of summarizing its contents, Lacan restricts himself to pointing out that the gist of this 'factum' may be captured in a moral maxim, whose projected universality follows the key principle of the Kantian categorical imperative (648, 5).

In Lacan's version, the Sadean maxim sounds as follows: "'I have the right to enjoy your body', anyone can say to me, 'and I will exercise this right without any limit to the capriciousness of the exactions I may wish to satiate with your body'" (648, 6). Although the maxim appears in quotation marks in '*Kant with Sade*', Lacan does not lift it as such from *Philosophy in the Boudoir* nor, for that matter, from any other work by Sade. Lacan concedes that "any reasonable being" is likely to recognize the black humour in this sentence, and so we need to assume that, in formulating the Sadean maxim in this particular way, he also wanted to preserve something of Sade's satirical intent (648, 8). However, the maxim's humour, which would stem from the sheer absurdity of a society embedding this principle within its legal structures as an essential human right, should not detract from its seriousness, partly because (as Freud would have it) humour is in itself "a contribution made to the comic through the agency of the super-ego" (and thus of moral conscience) (Freud, 1927/1964: 165), partly because (in a strict Kantian sense) reasonable interpretations should not be confused with basic rationality and prospective universality, which are intrinsic formal aspects of pure practical reason (648, 9). Later on in the text (649, 7–9), Lacan maintains that the preposterousness of a social order endorsing this maxim has no bearing whatsoever on the value of its edict (its *kerygma*) as a universal and unconditional, categorical imperative. The Sadean maxim qualifies, because like Kant's moral law it is based on a "radical rejection of the pathological", and it does not take account of anything else but the rational, formal aspects of its exposition (649, 9). Lacan then proceeds to unpack the fundamental principle of non-reciprocity which underpins this Sadean maxim of the right to *jouissance*, and which he not only recognizes in the Sadean subjective structures, but in all developmental processes, insofar as they concern a relationship between the subject and the signifier (the symbolic order, the Other). In the Sadean universe, non-reciprocity is the non-negotiable foundation for each and every type of sexual configuration and, by extension, for all patterns of human interaction. Hence, in Lacan's formulation of the Sadean maxim, there is meant to be an absolute subjective disparity between the victim and the aggressor. At no given point will there be a shared, mutual experience of *jouissance*, although this does not by definition exclude the possibility of roles being redistributed, the victim becoming a tormentor at a later stage (and *vice versa*), which is what Lacan calls "my turn next time" ("*la charge de revanche*") (649, 7).

In order to understand the following parts of Lacan's text (650, 1–8), it is essential to analyze the syntactical structure of the Sadean maxim. The first thing to note is that the first person singular 'I', with which the sentence opens, does not coincide with the grammatical subject of the statement, which is situated at the level of the objective personal pronoun 'me'. The enunciating subject of the full sentence is the one who is being subjected (as a victim) to the law of *jouissance* of "I have the right to enjoy your body…", which is in itself enunciated by an abstract, anonymous Other ("*anyone* can say [it] to me") (648, 6).[3] Lacan (649, 10) points out that, by ostensible contrast with Kant's moral imperative, it transpires that in the Sadean maxim the law primarily imposes itself upon the Other, rather than upon ourselves, for after all it is from the Other that I (as passive target) hear the law being enunciated. The Other proclaims to have the 'right to enjoy', whereas I am no more than the body who is about to be enjoyed 'without any limit' by this Other. Yet Lacan declares that the difference between the Sadean maxim and the Kantian categorical imperative is only apparent, only occurring "at first blush" ("*de prime abord*") (650, 1), because in Kant's system too it is from the place of the Other that we are being called for by the command of the moral imperative. As I explained above, Kant believed that once a rational human being has relinquished all 'pathological' considerations for empirical objects, he or she will hear the moral law being articulated by the voice of reason. Kant assumed that rational human beings and the voice of reason are part and parcel of the same self-reflexive process, whereas for Lacan this is a false assumption, because the subject is effectively split (divided), here, between a position from where the moral law is enunciated (sent out), and a position to which the moral law is being applied (where it is received) (650, 2). Relying on the Sadean maxim, which he defines as "more honest than Kant's appeal to the voice within" (650, 4), Lacan thus also criticizes Kant for failing to acknowledge the fundamental 'bipolarity' in the way the moral law is being conveyed, that is, for covering up the subjective splitting that occurs as soon as the moral law is enunciated.

Emphasizing the disparity between the enunciating subject and the subject of the statement, Lacan also asserts that in the Sadean maxim the enunciating subject is being detached ("*s'y détache*") from the actual enunciation of the law (650, 5). Again, as with Pa Ubu's (slightly modified) "Long live Poland", one may deservedly wonder in whose name Sade's representatives of the moral law are speaking (650, 5). In the second part of *Frenchmen, Some More Effort if you Wish to Become Republicans*, the anonymous author of the revolutionary pamphlet drew on the first article of the 'Declaration of the Rights of Man and of the Citizen'—which had been adopted in August 1789 and which still counts as one of the most important documents in the history of human rights—not to nuance but to *justify* his law of *jouissance*. Here, the author of the pamphlet spoke in the name of human Nature, which (unlike Rousseau) he defined as brutal, selfish, cruel and merciless (650, 6). Hence, although the pamphleteer articulated the law of the right to *jouissance*, he was only reiterating a moral dictate emanating from the radically free Other of human Nature (650, 7).

Lacan adds to this that the detachment of the enunciating subject does not make the moral law less effective, both in its function as a command and in its determining effect on the subject of the statement (the 'target-subject', on whom the law is being imposed and which thus becomes victimized). In the first instance, Lacan claims, the Sadean discourse of the right to *jouissance*, despite its coming from the Other, is as commanding as the Kantian "So act that ...", the latter stemming from the depths of the 'voice of reason' (650, 7). Second, the law of limitless *jouissance* establishes a fundamental polarity between the Other (who articulates it, although in the name of Nature) and the 'target-subject', who is being enjoyed, and who shall bear the cross of the whole experience. As Lacan puts it, the right to *jouissance* "drills [a hole] in the Other's locus" (650, 8), because it cannot operate without the existence of someone who sacrifices, or is being forced to sacrifice, his or her own *jouissance* for the sake of the Other—a subject in the literal sense of the term.

Section 4

Throughout the *Critique of Practical Reason*, Kant hardly paid any attention to the experience of pain, save as a by-product of the will's virtuous compliance with the moral law, or as something that merely belongs to the empirical world of sensible experience and which, as such, should have no bearing on pure practical reason. Although he was critical of the Stoics' unwavering belief in a human being's moral capacity to attain virtue and the highest good during the time of his earthly existence (Kant, 1788/1997: 106), Kant also felt that the Stoics' radical contempt for pain was entirely justified, because pain does not "in the least diminish the worth of his [the sufferer's] person but only the worth of his condition" (Kant, 1788/1997: 53).

Gauging the status of contempt within the Sadean experience, Lacan invokes the oft-recounted anecdote of how Epictetus ended up with a crippled leg, which had first appeared in Book 7 of Origen's *Contra Celsum* as something the philosopher Celsus had mentioned in (the now lost text of) *The True Word* (*Αληθής Λόγος*): "When his master was twisting his leg," [Epictetus] said, smiling and unmoved "You will break my leg!" and when it was broken, he added "Did I not tell you that you would break it?" (Origen, 248/2013: 622). Were the target-subjects (the victims) in the Sadean experience to respond in this way, with radical contempt for their predicament, the libertines' *jouissance* would fall flat and turn into disgust (651, 1). As I explained above, under no circumstance should the victims experience *jouissance* themselves. However, as Dolmancé put it to Eugénie, it is much better for them not to be indifferent (or act contemptuously) either, and for them to experience a certain degree of pain, be it in the form of humiliation, personal disgrace, or an assault on their modesty [*pudeur*] (651, 2) (Sade, 1795/2006: 93). Lacan states that in the Sadean maxim, pain "projects its promise of ignominy" (650, 9), because as soon as the law is enunciated, through the mouth of the Other, the target-subject is likely to experience a sense of personal disgrace, dishonor and humiliation.

Lacan posits that, compared to Kant's pure practical reason, the Sadean 'moral' experience is modified, because it revolves entirely around *jouissance* (651, 2). On the side of the libertine aggressor, the will to *jouissance* is as absolute as the victim's will to resist should be. Because of this, the latter's suffering will always be the former's delight, and the latter's agonizing disgrace will always be the former's cherished immodesty. If the libertines experience pain, it is never as a passive empathic reaction to the victim's pain, but only ever as an intentional means to an end, proficient as they are in transforming pain into pleasure. Lacan claims that the libertines' will to *jouissance* appropriates and monopolizes the victims' will, insofar as it has already traversed it—insofar as it has already nestled itself at the point of the victims' modesty. In a sense, the same is true for the libertine aggressors themselves. The libertines can profess the law of the right to *jouissance* without suffering from it, because they are already positively affected by it on account of their 'immodest' disposition or, as Sade would have it, on account of the 'singularity of their organs'. That is why Eugénie is never a genuine Sadean victim, but always already a libertine, albeit a rather inexperienced one who requires some additional instruction.

In another cryptic sentence, Lacan writes that in the Sadean experience "modesty is an amboceptor with respect to the circumstances of being [*ambo-ceptive des conjonctures de l'être*]" (651, 3). What he seems to have had in mind, here, is the observation that whenever two or more complementary beings come together (are being conjoined) in the Sadean 'relationship' between the tormentor and the victim, modesty (sexual timidity and decency) is a liminal function, because it operates *between* the two poles of the interaction—the libertine's immodesty being in itself an assault (violation) on the modesty of the target-subject. The libertine would not be able to pontificate about the necessity of immodesty, were it not for the fact that he assumes the existence of modesty on the side of the target-subject. Were everyone to be immodest, and the moral law of the right to *jouissance* were effectively a universal rule, the libertine would no longer have a need to issue his edicts, and would paradoxically lose much of his *jouissance*.

For the Sadean libertine, *jouissance* is thus extremely precarious, because it is largely conditioned by the existence of a target-subject whose body can be enjoyed, without this subject itself being given the right to enjoy, or without it being allowed to react with the dismissive power of stoic contempt. The target-subject preferably needs to experience pain, whose verbal manifestation often appears as an echo of the libertine's own expressions of *jouissance* (651, 4). Yet the victim's pain needs to be maintained at a certain level so that the victim does not lose consciousness, which is often difficult to avoid on account of the horrible tortures to which it is being subjected.

At this point, Lacan introduces a third term into his analysis of the Sadean dynamic between the libertines and their victims (651, 5). After the Other and the subject, he now presents the object. As I detailed above in my discussion of Section 1 of '*Kant with Sade*', in Kant's philosophy the object of the moral law is endlessly receding. Having dismissed all considerations for an empirical object as purely 'pathological', Kant's only remaining object(ive) of the moral law was that of the rational will's perfect compliance with its edict, which would effectively result in the realization of the highest good, as the ultimate convergence of virtue and happiness. However, this object is in itself unattainable, at least during the time of a rational being's earthly existence. Hence, the object appeared here as a typical figuration of the 'thing-in-itself' (*das Ding an Sich*)—a noumenon which can be thought, but which cannot be experienced and known (Kant, 1788/1997: 47–49).

In the Sadean scenario, Lacan (651, 5) claims, the object of the moral law loses its Kantian inaccessibility, because it is materialized in the figure of the libertine tormentor, whom he designates as the incarnated 'tormenting agency', an object endowed with being-in-the-world (*Dasein*, in the Heideggerian sense of 'conscious human presence'). In the next section of '*Kant with Sade*', Lacan will explore this function of 'presence' in greater depth. Here, he restricts himself to saying that the libertine's being-in-the-world is in itself intrinsically divided, with the moral law *qua* object remaining detached from the tormentor *qua* subject (651, 6). To the libertines, the law presents itself merely as an abstract 'point of emission', a disembodied voice, like a voice on the radio, which is heard but never seen, whereby they are simply committing themselves to executing what is being dictated.

Kant, however, continued to situate the object of the moral law outside the realm of sensory experience—a realm which Lacan, with reference to the *Critique of Pure Reason* (Kant, 1781/1998), calls the 'transcendental aesthetic' (651, 8)—and as not determined by it, even less so than the noumena of pure reason. Whereas the latter may still occasionally appear in the empirical world, the moral law is *imposed upon* the sensible world as a *super*sensible nature (Kant, 1788/1997: 38). Lacan argues that Kant may have also deemed it inconceivable for the moral law to impose itself upon the subject (a rational human being) as an object in its own right, because this type of object-law could have required the assumption of a God who is not just endowed with supreme intelligence (as the guarantee of its intelligibility), but also with less lofty features. After all, the moral law as a voice-object (and thus as something Other than the rational subject) could potentially detach itself from rationality, and become irrational, pathological, evil. As I explained above, the only object(ive) Kant was able to associate with the moral law is the highest good (the coincidence of virtue and happiness in the afterlife), whose intelligibility (because it is rational in its own right) only required the supposition of God as supreme intelligence. Like all good Christians, Kant did not wish to consider the possibility of God's enjoyment (*jouissance*, *Genuß*), in whose service a rational human being might be tempted to comply with the law, or whose paradisiacal sphere he may be looking forward to joining in the afterlife, provided he leads a virtuous earthly existence. And so he simply stated that a rational being who complies with the law will experience a certain "satisfaction with one's [own] existence", a kind of "contentment with oneself" (*Selbstzufriedenheit*), "in which one is conscious of needing nothing" (Kant, 1788/1997: 98–99). In this principle, Lacan (651, 9) recognizes an exaggeration of the Stoic *ataraxia* (ἀταραξία, lucid tranquility and detachment), which he designates as Kant's answer to a human being's earthly concern over the fact that God is but a faceless, supreme intelligence, who does not promise much enjoyment as a recompense for one's moral compliance, even in the afterlife (652, 1). And indeed, Kant was extremely skeptical of all religious beliefs in the possibility of a fusion with the divine nature, which he regarded as "monstrosities on reason according to the taste of each" and "enthusiastic *theosophical* dreams [*schwärmende* theosophische *Träume*]" (Kant, 1788/1997: 101–103). Without quoting this particular passage, Lacan speculates that, in this particular context, Kant was probably thinking of the mystic Jakob Boehme, his fellow countryman, who, in the best manicheistic tradition, had ascertained a duality in the divine nature between the first principle of 'God the Father' and the second principle of 'God the Son', whereby the first (which is also the generator of all subsequent things) was supposedly characterized by *Grimmigkeit* (bitterness, wrathfulness, harshness and contraction) (Boehme, 1618–1619/1909). For Kant, God was neither bitter nor joyous, neither wrathful nor happy, neither good nor bad, but simply intelligent perfection in his substance as the author of Nature.

Section 5

Embracing Kant's concept of *Schwärmerei*, Lacan now dispells these laconic reflections upon God's attributes, in order to concentrate on the typical being-in-the-world (*Dasein*) of the libertine tormentor or, as he calls it, "the function of presence in the Sadean fantasy" (652, 2).

At the end of *Philosophy in the Boudoir*, waiting for Madame de Mistival to regain consciousness, Dolmancé summed up what libertinage is all about: "If, as merely the blind instruments of its inspirations, nature ordered us to set the universe ablaze, the sole crime would be to resist! And all the scoundrels on earth are purely the agents of nature's caprices ..." (Sade, 1795/2006: 168). Echoing Dolmancé, Lacan avers that in the sadistic experience (*l'expérience sadique*), the presence of the executioner "is reduced to being no more than the instrument" of Nature's inspirations (652, 3). The sadistic fantasy of excess, which always comes at the expense of virtue, although it effectively requires virtue to be represented in the suffering target-subject (the one who has to bear the cross in the whole experience), is the libertines' response to what they believe Nature wants from them. In proceeding to realize this fantasy, they relinquish all common human feelings of sympathy, respect, compassion, shame, guilt and remorse—all those empirical objects and hypothetical imperatives that Kant would have designated as 'pathological'—in order to become both the reliable instruments of Nature's desire, and the invincible incarnations of supreme *jouissance*. Lacan writes that in the libertines' presence (in their being-in-the-world) *jouissance* becomes petrified (*s'y pétrifie*) and fixated (*s'y fige*), which makes them acquire the monstrous, threatening form of a 'black fetish' (*fétiche noir*) (652, 3)—a figuration similar to the power objects with which tribal people have traditionally worshipped and expressed their fear of the gods.

Yet although the libertines see themselves as gods, and relentlessly affirm their sovereignty and superiority in everything they do, they simultaneously have to admit that all the crimes they commit are but pale reflections of the ultimate criminal act they are so keen to perpetrate, and that the *jouissance* they experience is but a meager approximation of the eternal bliss they are looking for. Although the libertines' *jouissance* seems unrestricted, it is always to some extent insufficient and always somehow mediocre compared to the supreme state of limitless satisfaction they fantasize about. In Sade's libertine novels, hubris and despair are tightly woven together, and the more the libertines contemplate committing the most vicious crime, the more they are forced to accept their human limitations. The Sadean libertines can only conceive of the perfect crime and an unlimited *jouissance* in their fantasy, which they try to articulate in endless philosophical disquisitions. There are numerous examples in Sade's libertine novels of this relentless search for the 'crime of crimes', involving the largest number of victims being subjected to the widest range of criminal acts and suffering endlessly from the most extreme forms of pain. In the face of such high ambitions, and however divine they think they are, the libertines cannot but fail. As Lacan puts it: the libertine has to admit to "the humility of an act in which he cannot help but become a being of flesh and, to the very marrow, a slave to pleasure" (652, 5).

In this complex dynamic between the libertines' grand fantasy of eternal criminal bliss and their sorrowful earthly pleasures, Lacan detects an important reason as to why the 'sadistic experience' is never fully accomplished. Over and above the fundamental disparity between the enunciating subject (the tormentor) and the subject of the statement (the victim)—which Lacan calls "the subject's two alterities" here (652, 6)—in the formulation of the moral law, the sadist-executioners lose their grip on the whole situation every time their aspirational *jouissance* becomes reintegrated within the cycle of human sexual pleasure. If Nature's desire is to be situated in its cruel and brutal caprices, and the libertines hear the command to follow suit in Nature's voice, then their own interpretation of this command, which coincides with their 'will to *jouissance*' (*volonté de jouissance*) and their search for the ultimate crime, can never be fully realized, precisely because, when all is said and done, they are but imperfect human beings (652, 7).

Even when it is translated into a 'will to *jouissance*', libertine desire is governed by the law of pleasure, Lacan posits (652, 7), which implies that the expression of a 'will' is as close as the libertines will ever get to achieving their *jouissance*. The gradual increase in (sexual) tension and the promise of limitless bliss are being cut short by the occurrence of orgasm, which is but a moment of sexual pleasure and a return to a state of relative equilibrium or the "lowest threshold of tension" (652, 8). But this does not stop the libertines from pursuing their goal and seeking out new and better opportunities, whereby they even go so far as imagining the possibility of finding their supreme *jouissance* in the moment of their own death. As such, the most extreme reduction of tension is still being eroticized, death becoming intertwined with sex in the dramatic scene of the libertines' own execution as it appears in their fantasy. Lacan does not elaborate on this puzzling conjunction, but leaves it "to rest behind its Eleusinian veil", thus allowing the mystery to remain intact (652, 8).

In Kant's moral philosophy pleasure is but a human being's affective response to an empirical object, an arbitrary 'pathological' quality which can never constitute the basis upon which a formal moral law is issued, nor the incentive for, or the anticipated effect of, a rational being's compliance with this law. By contrast, for the Sadean libertines it is, as Lacan puts it, a "flagging accomplice" (652, 9), because it is simultaneously part and parcel of the *jouissance* they are seeking to attain, and a bleak shadow of the limitless satisfaction they have in mind. And in those moments when the libertines do attain some form of *jouissance*—when, for example, their carefully staged orgies allow them to reach one protracted orgasm after another—neither pleasure nor desire completely disappear, precisely because their fantasy of committing the supreme crime forces them to construct the experience as a mere (sexual) approximation of the ultimate criminal act.

In terms of the relationship between pleasure and pain, Lacan (653, 3) also points out that because the physiological cycle of pain is longer than that of pleasure, pain can be sustained for a more prolonged period of time, and thus in a sense constitutes a better approximation of *jouissance*. But even the cycle of pain reaches its 'natural end', either on account of the libertines transforming it back into pleasure, or on account of their target-subjects simply passing out. At the end of this section, Lacan stipulates that "in the sensory aspect of the Sadean experience" (653, 4), the libertines' fantasy will proceed from this possibility (of the victim passing out) in order to 'fixate' a desire—in Nature as well as in themselves, as the blind instruments of Nature's caprices—for an unassailable victim, someone who is the perfect incarnation of virtue, whose suffering can be infinitely extended, and who can be killed numerous times over. In the next section of the text, this will lead him to explore two paradoxical instances of libertinage in Sade's *Juliette*: Saint-Fond's incongruous belief in his victims' after-life, and the essential function of the so-called 'second death' in the system of Pope Pius VI (Sade, 1797/1968: 369–370, 771–772).

Section 6

To formalize the structure of the 'Sadean fantasy', which would be effectively restricted, here, to the 'sadistic' fantasy of Sade's libertines, Lacan proceeds from his own, 'most general' algebraic notation of the fantasy: $\$ \diamond a$ (653, 5). In representing the fundamental fantasy as $\$ \diamond a$, Lacan wants to problematize the relationship between subject and object, in a radical critique of the so-called 'object-relations'-movement in psychoanalysis, which continued to advocate the possibility of human beings establishing perfect, fully adequate relationships between themselves (as subjects) and others (as objects). For Lacan, the only way a divided subject can relate to an object (of desire) is via the fantasy, yet rather than instituting a harmonious relationship between subject and object, the fantasy re-confirms that there is no 'natural', pre-determined bond between subject and object, but only a fundamentally incongruous, disproportionate and deficient association between the two.

Applying this formula of the fundamental fantasy to the 'case' of Sade's libertines, Lacan (653, 10; Figure 6.1) proposes that the order of the two terms, $\$$ and a, should be inverted in accordance with two essential points he had made earlier, in Sections 5 and 3 of his paper. In Section 5, echoing

Dolmancé's explanation of the principles of libertinage, Lacan had suggested that, in their interpretation of Nature's capriciousness, which is acknowledged as the emblem of the desire they believe to detect in Nature's commanding voice, the libertine tormentors become the blind instruments, and thus the objects of Nature's "holy and immutable advice to enjoy" (Sade, 1795/2006: 65). Although they themselves cannot avoid being creatures of flesh and blood and, more importantly, divided subjects conditioned by the symbolic order of language, the libertines present themselves as objects in their own fantasy. As the chosen agents and executors of Nature's desire, which Lacan represents here with the letter *d* (653, 10), and which in a sense constitutes the true agency behind the entire construction, the libertines convey Nature's voice via their own, endlessly reiterated and rationally exposed 'will to *jouissance*', which Lacan in turn formalizes as *V* (654, 2). On the side of the libertine subject, the sequence can thus be summarized as: $d \rightarrow a \rightarrow V$ (see Figure 6.1).[4]

On the 'other side' of the libertines' fantasy, which Lacan also designates as "the side of the Other" (Lacan, S10, 1962–1963: 103), the target-subject *qua* victim always appears, or is forced to accept its status, as a divided subject, insofar as it is attacked and annihilated because of its strict compliance with a symbolic law of morality that promulgates dignity and respect, modesty and gratitude, pity and virtue. Whereas the libertine, as the "apparent agent" of the fantasy, "freezes with the rigidity of an object" (653, 7), the victim thus becomes the "$ of [Kant's] practical reason" (654, 2), a rational subject who remains strictly loyal to the dictates of its own moral law, despite the horrendous suffering that this moral obedience brings about. And so the conventional formula of the fundamental fantasy should be inverted: *a* ◇ $.

In the opening paragraph of Section 6, Lacan had already mentioned that the lozenge ◇ should be read as 'desire for', irrespective of the direction in which it is read, by which he had alerted his readership from the start that the formula's inversion, of *a* ◇ $, should not be taken to mean that in the libertines' fantasy the libertines now become the 'objects-being-desired', the target-victims occupying the position of 'desiring subjects'. The lozenge ◇, Lacan stipulates, is like the mathematical sign for identity =, to be read in the same way from right to left, with the proviso that the formula for the fantasy

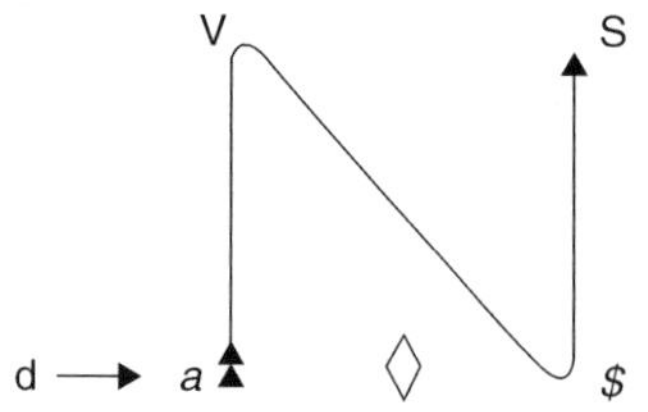

Figure 6.1 The Sadean fantasy

is based on "an absolute non-reciprocity" between the two terms of the equation (653, 5). However much the libertines' presumed right to *jouissance* may depend on the presence of suffering target-subjects, the latter do not constitute the ideal complement to the libertines' position as blind instruments of Nature's caprices. In the conventional fantasy, of $\$ \diamond a$, the object remains inadequate with respect to the subjective lack that has triggered the desire for it; in the libertines' inverted fantasy, of $a \diamond \$$, the divided subject on the side of the Other is equally by no means the perfect correlate of Nature's desire as expressed in the libertines' object-position or, for that matter, in their will to *jouissance*.

Lacan's argument is undoubtedly indebted, here, to Blanchot's work on Sade, although he himself never explicitly refers to it, at least not in '*Kant with Sade*'. In 'Sade's Reason', Blanchot had discerned an apparent contradiction in the libertine logic:

> When 'being the master of myself' means 'being the master of others', when my independence [as a libertine] does not come from my autonomy, but from the dependence of others on me, it is obvious that I forever remain connected to others and that I need them, even if only to obliterate them.
>
> (1949/2004: 23)

The fact that the libertines need their victims to assert their sovereignty is a problem, because it renders sovereignty impure, subservient, paradoxical. Yet Blanchot had also realized that in Sade's libertine universe the victims are but a means to an end. Although it may seem that the only thing the libertines want is to inflict as much suffering as possible on the greatest number of virtuous victims, this is not their final aim.

If it is not to capture, torment, mutilate and torture virtuous victims, what exactly is it, then, that the libertines want to achieve? According to Blanchot, it is a transcendental negation (Blanchot, 1949/2004: 26), a destructive act so grand that it swipes away all and everything: virtuous human beings, God and even Nature itself. According to Lacan, it is what he dubbed "the brute subject of pleasure" (*S sujet brut du plaisir*) which, following Kant, would of course be "the 'pathological' subject" par excellence (654, 2). How this undivided, raw, rough and uncut pleasure-subject should be interpreted is not at all clear from '*Kant with Sade*', yet this should not stop us from trying to understand what Lacan intends to convey. For one, it should be obvious by now that Sade's libertines have no intention whatsoever of generating pleasure in their victims, on the contrary. When Lacan refers to "the brute subject of pleasure", this should not be understood, therefore, as what the libertines hope to see taking shape, by way of transformative experience, in their victims. Second, "the brute subject of pleasure" should not be conflated with a subject (target-victim) that gives the libertines endless, unlimited pleasure, because this type of subject, assuming that it could be found and preserved—and, as I will demonstrate further on, the libertines are definitely doing whatever they can to maintain such a subject—would still be no more than a means to an end. What, in my opinion, Lacan is trying to capture with "the brute subject of pleasure" is what, in Freud's meta-psychological paper 'Instincts and their Vicissitudes' appeared under the name of a 'purified pleasure-ego' (*ein purifiziertes Lust-Ich*)—a pure, unblemished, undivided, complete subject of pleasure, which displays not a single flaw in its libidinal economy, because it has succeeded in expelling "whatever within itself becomes a cause of unpleasure" into the outside world, from which it has radically separated itself off (Freud, 1915/1957: 136). Needless to say, Freud was under no illusion that this type of *Lust-Ich* disappears with the advent of the reality-principle or, better still, that the possibility of the return to a state of purified pleasure once the ego has been re-transformed into a 'reality-ego' (*Real-Ich*), is but a neurotic illusion. When Lacan refers to "the brute subject of pleasure", without referring to Freud, he seems to have in mind, then, a primordial state of subjective being, of the kind that would have existed before the symbolic structure of language affected the human condition with its constraints and restrictions.

Like the image of the resplendent republic in the revolutionary pamphlet that Dolmancé is carrying with him when he arrives at Madame de Saint-Ange's boudoir, this libertine utopia is thus doomed to remain what it has always been: a fantasy. But this does not discourage the libertines from putting in 'some more effort' to make it happen. Sadly, their will to *jouissance*, if it does not prematurely run aground on their own experiences of pleasure, always has to pass through the divided subjectivity of their victims, which Lacan formalizes as: $V \rightarrow \$ \rightarrow S$ (see Figure 6.1).

Putting all of this together in a "quadripartite structure", Lacan thus produces a "didactic schema" (Figure 6.1) as a graphic modulation of the Sadean fantasy, which is to be interpreted, here, as the 'sadistic' fantasy of Sade's libertine heroes (653, 8). In a few extremely dense comments on this schema, Lacan defines the object *a* (the libertines' chosen position as the blind instruments of Nature's desire) as what operates in "the place of the cause" (654, 1), no doubt because, in a Kantian sense, it acts as the determining ground of the will to *jouissance*, which sets the whole fantasy in motion. The will to *jouissance* (*V*) itself he associates with the exclusive logical disjunction (in Latin, *vel*) of alienation, which he had discussed at length in his seminar on the four fundamental concepts of psychoanalysis (Lacan, S11, 1964: 203–215), and which "is supported only by the logical form of the union [in set theory]" (Lacan, *Position of the Unconscious*: 713, translation modified). It would take me too long, here, to explicate the intricacies of Lacan's exclusive logical disjunction of alienation.[5] Suffice it to say that, in '*Kant with Sade*', he intimates that the relationship between $\$$ and *S* should also be regarded as a forced choice between two options, whereby one option (*S*) is always by definition excluded, similar to the option of 'money' in the highwayman's prototypical question to his victim: "Your money or your life?" (Lacan, S11, 1964: 212). Although the libertines' will to *jouissance* aims to restore an original, pure experience of unblemished satisfaction (*S*)—a complete, sovereign being, in Blanchot's terminology—the only viable option is for them to please (and pleasure) themselves with a subject of non-*jouissance*, a moral subject in pain, a divided subject of practical reason (*$*) (654, 2). To the libertines' own chagrin, *S* is inconceivable without *$*, yet *$* is but a poor approximation of *S*, because it is *de facto* deprived of its own satisfaction, and ever so limited in the satisfaction that it can generate in the tormentors.

Lacan then posits that the curvy line (*la ligne sinueuse*) that runs from *V* to *S* via *$* "allows for a calculus (*un calcul*) of the subject" (654, 1). This may be interpreted in at least two different ways: whilst, on the one hand, the libertines devise, and literally calculate, extremely sophisticated torture arrangements for their victims, on the other hand they also compute, in the greatest detail, the size of genitals, the volume of sperm, the quantity of orgasms, the number of penetrations, and the amount of victims. Although commenting on Sade's own literary preoccupations rather than on the sexual practices of his libertine heroes, Francine du Plessix Gray hit the nail on the head when she wrote: "[T]his is a pornographer who often seems more interested in the sheer mathematics of sexuality … than in the carnal act itself" (du Plessix Gray, 2006: vii). As regards the victims, Blanchot highlighted how many of Sade's libertines greatly enjoy the thought, not to mention the act, of torturing a multitude of people or, failing that, of indefinitely prolonging their victims' pain. In '*Kant with Sade*', Lacan reiterates this observation when he writes that "there is a statics [a monotony] of the fantasy [in the libertines' philosophy of eroticized crime], whereby the point of *aphanisis* [of 'making disappear'] assumed to lie in *$*, must in one's imagination [i.e., in the libertines' vision of excess] be indefinitely pushed back" (654, 5). Despite the horrendous ordeals to which they are being subjected, many of the libertines' victims are indeed remarkably resilient and, as if transcending the very limits of their human existence, distinctively indestructible—the virtuous Justine being the prime example of someone who, time and again, manages to re-emerge more or less unscathed from the relentless onslaughts on her bodily and mental integrity, until she is finally killed by a flash of lightning (Sade, 1797/1968: 1190).

In many instances, the victims also inexplicably manage to preserve the exquisite delicacy of their physical features. Lacan is adamant that this incomparable and unassailable beauty has nothing to do with the libertines consistently selecting the most sexually attractive targets (654, 6), but rather with them erecting a last vestige against the satisfaction of their desire for absolute destruction, and thus against the unspeakable horror of seeing their criminal will come to full fruition. Beauty, as he had already put it in his seminar on the ethics of psychoanalysis (Lacan, S7, 1959–1960: 203, 216–217), is the second barrier (after 'goodness') against the object(ive) of *jouissance*, which would not only require the annihilation of humanity, God and Nature, but also of the libertines themselves. Rather than turning their victims into bleeding wrecks, the libertines thus prefer to see them being kept in a state of beautiful half-deadness or, as Lacan himself had called it, following his analysis of Sophocles' *Antigone*, in a zone "between two deaths" (Lacan, S7, 1959–1960: 270–287): dead to the world or dead in their inescapable fate as sacrificial objects of libertinage, but physically very much alive and well in the full radiance of their bodily splendour.[6] Fortunate as many victims may be when they are spared a terrible death as martyrs at the hands of their tormentors, their "hardly believable survival" (654, 5) evidently also plays into the libertines' fantasy, because the only thing they want is for their victims' suffering to be prolonged indefinitely.

Drawing on *Juliette* rather than *Philosophy in the Boudoir*, Lacan gives two other examples of the libertines' unquenchable thirst for infinite torments. The first, which had already been mentioned by both Blanchot (1949/2004: 23–24) and Klossowski (1967/1992: 75–77), concerns the minister Saint-Fond who, contrary to one of the cardinal principles of libertinage, reckons with the possibility that his victims, after they have been tortured to death, may still experience some form of bliss in a heavenly afterlife (655, 2). And so he is forced to confess to his friends—although not without shame and embarrassment, because he realizes all too well how much his belief contradicts the libertines' abhorrence of religion—how, in order to ensure that the victims' agonies will be everlasting in hell, he has come to adopt a rather idiosyncratic sexual practice:

> [I]n order to bar the victim from celestial joys, it is necessary to have him sign a pact, writ in his heart's blood, whereby he contracts his soul to the devil; next to insert this paper in his asshole and to tamp it home with one's prick; and while doing so to cause him to suffer the greatest pain in one's power to inflict.
>
> (Sade, 1797/1968: 369)

The second example, which Lacan may have borrowed also from Klossowski (1967/1992: 84–90), concerns the so-called 'system of Pope Pius VI', with whom Juliette has secured an audience (and a grandiose orgy) at the Vatican. Over a post-coital meal, the Pontiff, who also happens to be the most depraved libertine ever to occupy the Holy See, agrees to share his doctrine with his French companion. In essence, the Holy Father is convinced that in "all living beings the principle of life is no other than that of death: at the same time we receive the one we receive the other, we nourish both within us, side by side" (Sade, 1797/1968: 769). Yet he is also of the opinion that what is conventionally called 'death', that is, when a living being is no longer alive, this death is "only imaginary", because the now ostensibly inert matter that remains after the living being has 'died', constitutes in itself a new form of life, insofar as "it enriches the soil, fertilizes it, and serves in the regeneration of the other kingdoms as well as its own" (Sade, 1797/1968: 770). And so his Holiness concludes that whenever a human being is sacrificed on the altar of libertinage, this act only deprives the victim of his 'first life', and that to do justice to Nature's extreme cruelty, one would also need to be able to wrest away the 'second life', so that the decaying corpses are prevented from re-entering a new cycle of regeneration (Sade, 1797/1968: 771–772). Once again, Lacan notes the "incoherence in Sade's work" (655, 3), which is effectively twofold here: for one, libertines are not supposed to believe in a 'hereafter', even when they are the Pope—although one could probably argue that he believes in an 'after-death' rather than an 'after-life'—and second, it is difficult to see how a desire to kill life twice can be combined with a desire for suffering to be prolonged. From Pope Pius's doctrine, Lacan then distills the idea of the 'second death' (655, 3), which he had introduced previously in his seminar on the ethics of psychoanalysis, and which was designed to capture the "point at which the very cycles of the transformations of nature are annihilated" (Lacan, S7, 1959–1960: 248).

Section 7

Heeding Klossowski's reflections on the system of Pope Pius VI (Klossowski, 1967/1992: 89–90), Lacan (655, 4) compares the wish of the second death to Freud's controversial notion of the death drive (*Todestrieb*), which the founder of psychoanalysis had originally introduced in 'Beyond the Pleasure Principle', in an attempt to account for the manifestation of a 'compulsion to repeat' (*Wiederholungszwang*) in clinical cases of traumatic neurosis (Freud, 1920/1955). For Freud, the "dominating tendency of mental life, and perhaps of nervous life in general, is the effort to reduce, to keep constant or to remove internal tension due to stimuli" (Freud, 1920/1955: 55–56). Whereas he had initially associated this so-called 'constancy-' or 'Nirvana principle' with the pleasure principle, he subsequently argued that the latter is a modification of the former under the influence of the life-drive, so that the Nirvana principle (the mental tendency to reduce stimuli to nothing, or to keep levels of excitation as low as possible) should not be situated within the realm of the pleasure principle, but be conceived as operating exclusively in the service of the death drive (Freud, 1924/1961: 160).

At this point in his text, Lacan identifies Sade's, or rather Pope Pius' second death with Freud's death drive, yet without going so far as to rekindle the idea that Sade would be a precursor to Freud, and with the caveat that he exchanges Freud's biological foundation of the death drive (the natural cycle of all organic matter returning to an inorganic state) for a more abstract, symbolic setting. Indeed, from the mid 1950s, Lacan had designated the death drive as "the mask of the symbolic order", which "tends beyond the pleasure principle" and "beyond the limits of life" (Lacan, S2, 1954–1955: 326).

Apart from the Freudian death drive, the principle of the second death is, of course, also reminiscent of the Buddhist doctrine of Nirvana, as Lacan (655, 5) again repeats after Klossowski (1967/1992: 90). As an ostensibly nihilistic spiritual philosophy, Buddhism situates the supreme end of life and the height of perfection in a state of being that has transcended the cycles and constraints of individual existence as such. Ancient and widespread as these beliefs may be, Lacan indicates that it only takes some ignorant Western puppets (*fantoches*) to discard them as utter nonsense or, as had been the case with Freud's notion of the death drive, to radically dispute the ontological and clinical reality of the "pain of existence" (*douleur d'exister*) that lies behind a human being's wish to enter this state of absolute nothingness. Echoing Sartre (1943/1989), although without the humanist interpersonal touch, Lacan intimates that hell can be put back in its rightful place when it is confined to what human beings "traditionally inflict in this world" (656, 1). The thought, or the religious promise, of immortality is therefore far from appealing.

If the sociological, or the social psychological (interpersonal) perspective in psychoanalysis led to the dismissal of Freud's death drive, then it also contributed, Lacan continues, to a fundamental misunderstanding about the relationship between sadism and masochism, which shows that "the circles of those who have a surer experience of forms of sadism" (656, 4)—the social theorists who study interpersonal behaviour, rather than the clinicians, we need to assume—have not shed any light on the Sadean fantasy. Without specifying his sources, Lacan vehemently opposes a certain conceptualization of the "relation of reversion" between sadism and masochism, whereby the former would be the complement and mirror-image of the latter, and both would be working in tandem in a combined 'sado-masochistic' dynamic of domination and submission (656, 5). Instead of considering their social or clinical value, Lacan ridicules these views by referring to an old Polish joke: 'Under capitalism, man exploits man. Under communism, it's just the opposite' (656, 5). In the so-called sado-masochistic character, sadism and masochism are like capitalism and communism in the joke: they appear to be radically different, but underneath the surface they are exactly the same. Amusing as it may be, Lacan believes this outlook to be fundamentally flawed, although it was being disseminated in the psychoanalytic literature as if it were a serious and truthful explanation of the relation between sadism and masochism.

Putting these 'stupidities' aside, Lacan admits that "there are doctrinaires who strive for tidier appearances" (*une toilette plus soignée*), and go on to claim that the sadist "denies the Other's existence" (656, 7).[7] By way of antiphrasis, he 'concedes' that this is indeed what his own analysis of the Sadean fantasy might suggest, were it not for the fact that he had actually intended to show that sadism's Other (the target-victim), instead of being denied the right to exist, becomes the repository for the sadists' own pain of existence (656, 8). The sadists themselves seem keen to be transformed into Whiteheadian 'eternal objects'—immortal potentials and universals that exceed the boundaries of temporal existence (Whitehead, 1929/1978: 44). As I demonstrated above, the libertines evidently never completely succeed in evacuating their own pain of existence, insofar as their own ineluctable mediocrity vis-à-vis their grand project of radical destruction constantly imbues them with a new source of suffering.

Returning to Sade—the man and the author, rather than the work—Lacan proposes, then, that the creator of the most viciously brutal libertines was far from being duped by the sadistic fantasy he had impelled upon his heroes. Lacan insinuates, here, that Sade somehow knew very well that his libertines' desire for absolute destruction was *just* a fantasy, which allowed him not to be fooled or taken in by his own creative imagination. Although he equipped his libertine heroes with a sadistic fantasy, and may have fuelled his libertine novels with his own sexual fantasy, for Sade the Sadean fantasy remained essentially a literary, fictional universe, which did not take over his lived experience.

Section 8

Tacitly revisiting the long polemical tract Sade had inserted, more or less arbitrarily, under the title of '*Frenchmen, Some More Effort if You Wish to Become Republicans*' into the fifth dialogue of *Philosophy in the Boudoir*, and assuming that this "pamphlet within the pamplet" may indeed be more emblematic of Sade's own politics than any other part of the book, Lacan sets his readership an assignment. How does the fourfold structure of the Sadean fantasy, as graphically represented in section 6 of '*Kant with Sade*', and which is effectively an articulation of the 'sadistic' relationship between the libertines and their victims, relate to Sade's personal outlook on life? Using the logical sequence $a \rightarrow V \rightarrow \$ \rightarrow S$, is it possible to shed light on Sade's 'politics', his morals, his desire, his sexuality, and his social position, as the repeatedly incarcerated author of the most scabrous novels ever written?

The assignment set (656, 11), Lacan provides the reader with his own outline answer (656, 12). In sum, he proposes that the solution is to be found neither in a simple duplication of the first schema—Sade-the-man being a real-life replica of the 'sadistic' heroes that populate his libertine novels—nor in any kind of "symmetrical reversal along an axis or around some central point" (656–657)—Sade the wayward aristocrat and incorrigible fantasist only ever being made to suffer by the law enforcers and moral guardians of successive political regimes—but rather in a "90-degree rotation of the graph" (657, 1). This operation leaves the original sequence of the terms, $a \rightarrow V \rightarrow \$ \rightarrow S$, unchanged, but redistributes a and $\$$ to the 'side of the subject' and V and S to the 'side of the Other'. The new schema, which is designed to represent Sade's personal ideology, his morals and his life philosophy, in short his own 'practical reason' rather than that of his libertine protagonists, appears as follows (Figure 6.2):

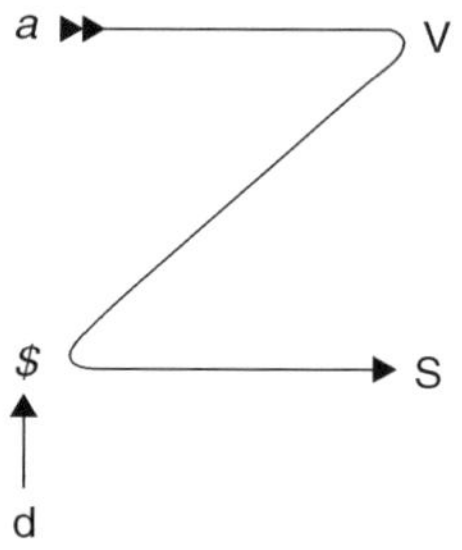

Figure 6.2 Sade's practical reason

By not merely reproducing the first schema when accounting for Sade's outlook on life, Lacan makes it clear that he does not think the mental economy of the man responsible for articulating the grand libertine fantasy of absolute destruction to be an identical blueprint of that of his characters. However, in not symmetrically reversing the first schema, Lacan also refuses to allocate Sade to the place of the passive victim, which would have involved his being deprived of any kind of sexual desire, or of his desire being systematically crushed under the barbaric *jouissance* of his own 'libertine' tormentors.

Lely's biography of Sade (Lely, 1952; 1957) would have taught Lacan that the Marquis was not exactly a paragon of virtue, and that long before he started devoting himself to writing he had already been imprisoned and sentenced to death for a series of sexual escapades. As a self-confessed libertine, Sade actively pursued all kinds of risky sexual adventures, involving beggars, prostitutes, chamber maids, cooks, valets and secretaries, not to mention his wife and sister-in-law, and there is no evidence that he enjoyed anything else but being the undisputed master of erotic ceremonies, even when he insisted on being whipped and sodomized. But Lacan would also have known that Sade was far from being a murderous sexual predator, and that he rarely went further than what would now be regarded as fairly elementary acts of bondage and domination, although within the legal context of eighteenth-century France these sexual activities would have been punishable as criminal acts, especially when they involved sodomy.

Does Lacan's '90-degree rotation' of his first schema imply, then, that we ought to approach Sade-the-man as a masochist? Lacan never goes so far as to categorize Sade as a masochist, and his reluctance to diagnose masochism in Sade is undoubtedly to his credit, because it stops the reader from seeing the complexity of Sade's *Weltanschauung* being reduced to a mere category of sexual psychopathology, which was moreover invented long after Sade's death, and with reference to another creative writer.

When glossing the newly distributed terms in the second schema, Lacan starts with *V* (657, 2), thus counter-intuitively avoiding the two obvious starting points, of $d \rightarrow \$$ and *a*. Much like in the first schema, *V* represents a will to *jouissance*, yet Lacan makes it immediately clear that this will is now stripped of its sexual overtones and enters the realm of absolute moral control, so that it conjures up Nietzsche's notorious 'will to power' (in French, '*volonté de puissance*'). Were the person who acts upon this will to experience any form of sexual satisfaction, it would be hidden behind an emotionless façade of sovereign authority. Reflecting upon Sade's 'politics', that is, his doctrine of the right to *jouissance* as the key to his utopian republic, Lacan recognizes this will to *jouissance* not in Sade himself, but rather in the figure of his stout-hearted mother-in-law, the unyielding *Présidente* de Montreuil, who saw it as her personal mission to ensure that the heinous husband of her eldest daughter would not escape his just punishment, and who even managed to obtain a series of so-called *lettres de cachet* from the French king, ordering for Sade's arrest and imprisonment—without trial, for an indefinite period of time, at the behest of the family, and by royal decree. Following his original sequence of terms, Lacan posits that the effect of Sade being on the receiving end of the Other's will to *jouissance* is tantamount to his subjective division, *\$*, which should be understood in this context as his physical disappearance from the scene of public life and from people's memories, and which would have been given the final stamp of approval when, during the early 1810s, the Emperor Napoleon Bonaparte (formerly known as the First Consul) personally signed two consecutive ministerial decrees to keep Sade locked up in the asylum of Charenton (Lely, 1957: 580; Lever, 1991/1993: 545–546; du Plessix Gray, 1999: 408; Schaeffer, 1999: 499–500) (657, 5).[8] But apart from Sade himself, the Other's will to *jouissance* also affected key figures in the Marquis' immediate environment, notably those who had decided to devote themselves unconditionally to his libertine cause, or who had continued to support him in his darkest hour (657, 4). Lacan singles out Sade's wife, his sister-in-law and his valet, and situates them in the place of *S*, firmly on the side of the Other, but fully sharing in his quandaries. Unlike the *S* in the schema of the Sadean fantasy, where it represents a pure experience of unblemished satisfaction, the *S* in the schema of Sade's practical reason is undoubtedly more fractured, but it still appears as a much more unchecked, and therefore blissful state of being than anything Sade himself would have lived through, if only because Sade's accomplices seem to have been more adept at escaping the wrath of Madame de Montreuil and her acolytes than the master they elected to serve. Lacan writes that those complicit with Sade's antics were "incarnating the heroism characteristic of the pathological" (657, 4), in the Kantian sense of their having been totally at the mercy of their passion. Of course, in the end they disappeared too—in provincial châteaux, consumed by illness, or swallowed up in the creases of history—but somehow they succeeded in getting away with the transgressions of libertinage relatively scot-free.

Without claiming that the Marquis had unconsciously orchestrated his own predicament, Lacan recognizes in Sade's division *cum* disappearance (*\$*) a corollary of his own desire as the author of *Justine*, *Juliette*, *Philosophy in* *the Boudoir*, and other libertine texts, hence the vector $d \rightarrow \$$ (657, 5). When *Justine* came off the press in 1791, the novel did not bear the name of its author; when *Philosophy in the Boudoir* was published four years later, the title page stated that it was a "posthumous work by the author of *Justine*", and when he released the ten volumes of *La Nouvelle Justine* and *Juliette*, Sade used the same subterfuge. Of course, the wish to remain anonymous could have stemmed from the simple aim to avert prosecution, but Sade was also in the habit of disowning his own works. Until his dying days, Sade vehemently denied that he was the author of the scandalous novels that had been attributed to him, and which had eventually been used as a pretext for punishing him 'administratively' and keeping him detained during the last thirteen years of his life (du Plessix Gray, 1999: 380–381). "[A]s a subject, it is through his disappearance that he makes his mark [*qu'il signe*]," Lacan (657, 5) writes, whereby he also alludes to the fact that no known portrait or likeness of Sade has survived, and that in the famous fifth clause of his last will and testament—drawn up at the asylum of Charenton in January 1806—he had insisted that "the traces of my grave may disappear from the face of the earth as I trust the memory of me shall fade out of the minds of all men" (Sade, 1806/1991: 157). Sade's ardent wish to be erased forever, to be killed off once more after his physical death, no doubt reminded Lacan of Pope Pius's fantasy of the second death, but he recalls instead how the chorus in *Oedipus at Colonus* had lamented the hero's tragic fate (657, 6): "Not to be born [*μὴ φυναι*] comes first by every reckoning; and once one has appeared, to go back to where one came from as soon as possible is the next best thing" (Sophocles, 1998: 547). Whereas for Oedipus, the chorus's invocation would allow him to ascend towards the gods, Sade's own invocation would eternalize his name in a different way, despite himself and against his own wishes, through the body of his works. And this is where Lacan locates the key to Sade's practical reason, and to the fantasy that presided over his life.

Indeed, what in Lacan's opinion occupies the place of the instrument, the black fetish and the object *a* in Sade's politics and morals is nothing more, nothing less than his writings (657, 6).[9] Although he would have been well aware of the fact that the *Présidente* de Montreuil's domineering will to *jouissance* had been unleashed by Sade's sexual mischief rather than his libertine novels, and that Sade's books had only landed him in jail some ten years after her assiduous persecution had come to an end, Lacan is adamant that the moral backlash had been sustained by the oeuvre (Sade as a text) rather than the man, whereby it had simultaneously elicited the most extreme of moral responses and secured his indestructibility and therefore his immortality. By way of illustration, he refers to an influential moralistic essay by the nineteenth-century critic Jules Janin, in which the author conceded (and deplored) that, whilst no one really dares to pronounce Sade's name, his libertine books are so ubiquitous—allegedly hidden, but ever so easy to find—that one may reasonably assume that most people have read them. Drawing on the transcript of the proceedings in the court case against Pauvert, Lacan further claims that whereas everyone (the judge, the solicitors and the witnesses; prosecutors as well as defendants) seems to agree that Sade's books are boring ["*Œuvre ennuyeuse*"], and that his literary style is weak, at the same time everyone also continues to be bothered and disturbed by it all (657, 7). In an attempt to account for this strange effect, he suggests that the Sadean fantasy, that is, the written discourse of Sade's libertine novels, confronts everyone with the issue of human desire, inasmuch as "it is asking you [the reader] … to square accounts with your desires" (658, 1).

One could no doubt detect in these words a faint echo of de Beauvoir's conclusion to 'Must We Burn Sade?', where she posited: "The supreme value of his [Sade's] testimony lies in its ability to disturb us. It forces us to re-examine thoroughly the basic problem which haunts our age in different forms: the true relation between man and man" (de Beauvoir, 1950–1951/1990: 64). However, Lacan's point is unquestionably more provocative, because it intimates that Sade compels us to re-examine a much more fundamental relationship than that between "man and man", namely the relationship we entertain with ourselves. Instead of interpreting the disturbing exhortation stemming from Sade's works as a demand for human beings to investigate the way they relate to each other, Lacan sees it as a demand for human beings to come to terms with themselves. In pursuing this point, Lacan enters into a tacit dialogue with Georges Bataille, who had defined human eroticism, and par excellence Sade's triumphant literary invocation of the violence of desire, as "the problematic part of ourselves" (Bataille, 1957/2001: 273). Indeed, Bataille's numerous influential texts on Sade, as well as his broader reflections on the intricate relationship between desire and the law, constitute the essential yet unacknowledged backdrop for Lacan's arguments in the following sections of '*Kant with Sade*', in which he embarks on a more general consideration of the status of human desire.

Section 9

At this point in his text, Lacan starts elaborating his own psychoanalytic theory of desire, pitting Sade against Kant, and arguing how neither the rationalist philosopher nor the libertine moralist had appreciated the strict inseparability of subjective desire and the moral law. Following in the intellectual footsteps of Bataille, yet without ever mentioning him by name, and extending a principle he had also ascertained in Freud, yet without referring to a specific text, Lacan argues that desire and the law are not antagonistic forces, but rather interdependent components of a single bipolar psychic system (658, 4). Reading Kant 'with Sade', he demonstrates how, despite Kant's great philosophical efforts, the emergence of a non-empirical formal law in a rational free will does not eradicate desire, but merely represses it, as a result of which it is simultaneously sustained and invigorated. Mutatis mutandis, reading Sade '*without* Kant', he shows how, despite Sade's grand libertine fantasy of an absolute, unrestrained liberation of 'natural' desire, there is no such thing as a raw, pure, 'natural' desire—even when it is being translated into an allegedly universal right to *jouissance*—but only ever a mediated desire, a desire that is dependent upon the symbolic Other of language and the law. The first part of this dual argument is developed in Sections 9 to 13 of '*Kant with Sade*', whereas the second part unfolds in Sections 14 and 15. For the first part, Lacan draws on a famous double apologue from the *Critique of Practical Reason*, whereas for the second part he probes deeper into the logic of *Philosophy in the Boudoir* and the constitution of the Sadean republic, as articulated in the book's "pamphlet within the pamphlet". The first stage of Kant's double apologue receives a critical airing in Sections 9 and 10, whilst the second stage is addressed in Section 11.

However, before properly exposing Kant to Sade, Lacan opens Section 9 with an arcane synthesis of the three key pillars upon which he had constructed his theory of desire during the 1950s and early 1960s, although not in chronological order of development, without listing them in a systematic fashion, and without making any concessions to those who had not participated in the process. They can be summarized as follows: 1. Insofar as desire is attached to an object, the latter continues to escape and therefore causes rather than satisfies desire; 2. Insofar as there is a subject of desire, the subject does not control, let alone possess his or her desire, but is rather subjected to and possessed by it, without knowing exactly where it is coming from and in which direction it is going; 3. Desire is not an autonomous force, but something conditioned by the Other's desire, although the latter remains equally opaque and can only be accessed via a fantasy, which therefore mediates between the subject of desire and the Other, as well as between the subject and the elusive object of desire.

Building upon the first pillar, Lacan suggests that the Sadean universe serves as a prime example of how the object of desire remains as "ungraspable as is the object of the Law according to Kant" (659, 2). As I explained earlier on, Kant formulated a moral law which operates without any reference to empirical objects, and whose sole object(ive) would be the realization of the highest good in the moment when complete virtuousness and complete happiness coincide. Because no rational being is intrinsically holy, this object is endlessly receding and can only maintain its function as a rational goal for moral action on the basis of the postulate of the immortality of the soul. Likewise, when the Sadean libertines conspire to realize their evil plan of transcendental destruction, they are constantly reminded of the restrictions imposed by their earthly existence. In order to realize their desire, they wish for nothing better than to relinquish the burden of their human bodies, but time and again they find themselves tragically constrained by the ineluctable limitations of life and the finite cycle of pleasure.

The Sadean libertines are a band of brothers and sisters who have chosen to obey a moral code that allows them to answer only to themselves, as instruments of Nature. If ethics, as Lacan claimed in *Seminar VII*, is about formulating a judgment on the nature of one's action (Lacan, S7, 1959–1960: 291), then the judgment made by the libertines, and the underlying question they repeatedly ask themselves, is not whether their action is of any consequence to anyone else, but whether it lives up to their ideal. Hence, whereas the repetitive alternation between philosophical disquisitions and sexual hubris in Sade's libertine novels may indeed elicit a sensation of boredom in the reader, the staccato rhythm of the narrative structure responds to the internal logic of desire, as something that is never fulfilled, that runs aground before it reaches its destination, that fundamentally fails to meet its object(ive) each and every time it ventures out on the pathway towards its realization. This is why Lacan situates the object of desire in the interstices, the pauses and the scansions of the Sadean fantasy, at those points when philosophy (theoretical exposition) turns into orgy (erotic performance), and when the orgiastic arrangements disband in order to give way again to philosophical reflections—at those points in *Philosophy in the Boudoir* when Sade included a stage direction such as "The arrangement breaks up".[10] As to the second pillar, Lacan echoes a fragment of the refrain of a 1943 poem entitled 'The Explanation of Metaphors' by Raymond Queneau: "But what's with all these metaphors ... and why?" (658, 7).[11] Queneau's poem presents human beings as creatures who are fundamentally lost, always in search of something to hold onto, but always failing to find their way, partly due to physical shortcomings but also on account of their disproportionate and contradictory efforts at finding a support that does not even exist. In Lacan's terminology, it is impossible for a subject to find his way in the desires that connect the molecules of life (658, 8). Like the farmer in Jean de la Fontaine's famed fable of 'The Peasant and the Snake', the subject will end up being betrayed every time he expresses his desire for kindness and charity towards an evil creature, who therefore does not deserve to be treated with dignity and respect, but at the same time it is by no means easy to distinguish the kind from the cruel.[12] In addition, as the ever-charming Monsieur Verdoux exemplified in Chaplin's eponymous 1947 film, one subject's love and devotion towards his disabled wife may very well coexist with the opposite desire to murder rich spinsters (658, 6). Alternatively, Monsieur Verdoux could have decided to sacrifice himself for the sake of his family, rather than killing wealthy women and stealing their money, whereby he would have emulated the Bodhisatta—the being destined to become the Buddha in his final life—who unselfishly ensured the survival of an emaciated tigress and her starving cub by offering himself up as a meal. Or Monsieur Verdoux could have applied the Kantian moral law before embarking on his criminal plan, which would have definitely forced him to abandon his strategy altogether. Regardless of the situation, Lacan argues, subjects' desires remain ambivalent and are largely based on what they believe the other desires—living comfortably, or food in order to survive—which also implies that they may be quite mistaken in thinking they know what the other wants (658, 9). In the end, the 'subject of desire' completely disappears as a command-and-control centre, insofar as it is reduced to the sound of a disembodied, signifying voice—Kant's 'voice of reason', or Dolmancé's 'voice of Nature'—which, according to Lacan, is "speaking nonsensically most of the time" ("*sans queue ni tête à ce qu'elle [la voix] dit le plus souvent*") (659, 3), and which reconfirms the subject in its status as a 'barred' function, $\$$.[13]

In addition, in Lacan's theory of desire, there is no such thing as a sovereign, autonomous, unmediated desire, and this is clearly borne out by Kant as well as by Sade. Repeating a formula he had invented during the early years of his teaching, and which was strongly indebted to Alexandre Kojève's reading of Hegel's *Phenomenology of Spirit*, Lacan emphasizes that the subject's "desire is the Other's desire" (658, 9), so that subjective desire can never be considered without pondering the impact of the Other, the symbolic structure of language and the law, or what, in Kant's book, is designated as the voice of Reason and in Sade's libertine ideology the voice of Nature. To complicate matters further, during the late 1950s Lacan had also come to the conclusion that the only way in which a subject can have access to the Other's desire is via a fantasy (658, 10), which is again perfectly illustrated in the Sadean universe, where the libertines' relentless speeches on the ruthless cruelty of Nature's desire—a discourse which functions, moreover, as the key impetus for their own desire and will to *jouissance*—is of course nothing more, nothing less than a precise articulation of the subjective side of their own 'sadistic' fantasies.

Armed with these principles, Lacan returns to the relationship between desire and the moral law, two seemingly opposing functions with the shared characteristic of being driven and maintained by an elusive object (659, 2). As we have seen, Kant detached the moral law and the fulfillment of duty from all empirical objects of desire, which he designated as pathological, and presented the human being as a conscious rational will who obeys an internal commandment for the pure sake of morality, regardless of subjective wishes and irrespective of the pain and unhappiness that this act of dutiful compliance might entail. Highlighting the ambiguity of the notion of 'freedom' (or liberty)—a notion which was as important for Sade as it was for Kant—Lacan (659, 5) sets out to unpack Kant's famous double apologue of the gallows, which had appeared in the *Critique of Practical Reason* just before the formulation of the categorical imperative. In Sections 9 and 10 of '*Kant with Sade*', he restricts himself to a critique of the first stage of the apologue, which Kant presented as follows:

> Suppose someone asserts [*vorgibt*] of his lustful inclination that, when the desired object and the opportunity are present, it is quite irresistible to him; ask him whether, if a gallows were erected in

> front of the house where he finds this opportunity and he would be hanged on it immediately after gratifying his lust, he would not then control his inclination. One need not conjecture very long what he would reply.
>
> (1788/1997: 27)

The point of Kant's example is clear: whatever someone may claim, 'lustful inclinations' are not irresistible at all, because a rational human being will immediately renounce his sexual desire and the promise of gratification if he knows that his life is at stake. Faced with the choice between sex and certain death, or life without sex, a rational human being will not hesitate to opt for the latter. Hence, the death penalty functions as an effective deterrent, strong as someone's inclinations may be. In '*Kant with Sade*', Lacan surmises that for Kant's example to work in his favour, it is necessary to assume that the human being in question is an "ideal bourgeois" (660, 1), someone who would not dare to stoop so low as to become the victim of his own passions, someone whose passions are not as irresistible as he claims, someone whose uprightness of character allegedly commands unconditional respect. But it is entirely possible, Lacan argues, that a different kind of person, and not necessarily a 'hoodlum' ("*le mauvais garçon*") (660, 2), would be more truthful than this ideal bourgeois about the irresistibility of his inclinations, so much so that he would be prepared to testify about his lust under oath, and would as a "partisan of passion" (660, 2) react to his impending execution with utter contempt, or with an even stronger desire to follow his propensities.

Of course, punishment is not synonymous with the symbolic Law, but even when the Law is present in full force—as Lacan recognizes in Sophocles' *Antigone*, notably when Creon decrees that political traitors such as Polynices should not be granted a proper burial—it still does not prevail over desire, but only reveals itself as sustaining desire and as being fundamentally supported by it (660, 3). Without referring to a specific text, but undoubtedly recalling a line of argument by Freud in *Totem and Taboo* (Freud, 1913/1955: 30–31), Lacan states that "Law and repressed desire are one and the same thing" (660, 6), and so he can boast that merely by virtue of Professor Freud, he is already "ahead at half-time" (660, 6), that is, halfway through his discussion of Kant's double apologue.

Section 10

At this point, Lacan feels that he is definitely one up against Kant, and without having required the support of Sade, nor the doctrine of human rights and its underpinning principles of freedom of thought and self-governance ("*ton corps est à toi*"), nor the "daring deeds" of courtly love (660, 7). Drawing on a chessboard metaphor, he attributes his intellectual victory purely to the pawns (the infantry), as epitomized by the Freudian offensive in the previous

Section, but still proceeds to demonstrate how the first part of Kant's double apologue can be dismantled in other ways too.

Putting Sade in the place of Kant's 'ideal bourgeois', Lacan contends that the threat of death may not *de facto* compel a person to renounce his desire. In the case of Sade, it would be too simple to claim that he could not have foreseen the disastrous consequences of his actions when, on Easter Sunday 1768, he decided to amuse himself with Rose Keller, or when, in June 1772, he proceeded to stage an orgy with his valet and four local girls, or when, throughout the 1790s, he carried on writing inordinately obscene novels of massive proportions. Did he feel invulnerable, invincible, above the law? Or was he quite simply naïve? Whatever his motives, Lacan intimates that Sade's compulsion to write, much like his 'lustful inclination', was definitely not alleviated by the menace of his incarceration or execution, and may even have been exacerbated by them.

Of course, in saying and doing so, Sade was considered a criminal, and by four successive political regimes no less, yet Lacan does not think that the Marquis' principles and inclinations warranted this label, nor does he accept that Sade suffered from what early nineteenth-century alienists, in the wake of Philippe Pinel's 'visionary' observations on the nature and treatment of mental illness, had come to be designated as 'moral insanity'—a type of madness that only perturbs a person's affective faculties, leaving reason, judgment and intelligence intact (661, 1). Taking his lead from Foucault's recently published *Folie et déraison* (Foucault, 1961), Lacan is distinctly sceptical of Pinel's new clinical doctrine on mental illness. For although it may have freed the mentally ill from their chains and from the solitary confinement of their dungeons, it also introduced a much more insidious and potentially much more exploitative power structure, insofar as it established a new, absolute form of authority—incarnated by the alienists and the hospital administration—which reduced the patient to a silent object of medical investigation and social exclusion. "Willy-nilly", Lacan claims, "he [Pinel] supported the destruction [*l'abattement*], on the right and the left, by thought of the freedoms that the Revolution had just promulgated in the very name of thought" (661, 1).

As to the issue of human rights, Lacan (661, 2) suggests that Kant's 'ideal bourgeois' would not be infringing upon the personal rights of his beloved when acting upon his lustful inclination, but merely take advantage of the situation to indulge in an act of consensual sex, and could therefore feel justified in pursuing his desire by relying on article 4 of the very first *Declaration of the Rights of Man and of the Citizen*, upon which the anonymous author of the revolutionary pamphlet in *Philosophy in the Boudoir* had also drawn. Although this declaration was not signed until one year *after* the publication of the *Critique of Practical Reason*, and only in France, Kant's thought-experiment could thus be interpreted as violating an essential human right, much like Sade's 'administrative' punishment for being the author of *Justine* and *Juliette* effectively contradicted article 11 of the same Declaration. Of course, Lacan is very much aware of the fact that a declaration of human rights, including the 'universal' one that was passed in 1948, does not always translate into concrete, emancipatory actions, much less into substantially improved living conditions for all human beings, even in those countries that pledge their allegiance to its principles. Insofar as they constitute a Law, the truth of human rights, Lacan posits, is that they generally "boil down to the freedom to desire in vain" (661, 2), because they generally increase hopes and aspirations rather than fulfilling them. As a type of Law, a declaration of human rights articulates the fundamental human needs that have to be respected and satisfied, yet in doing so it contributes, more than anything else, to the creation and preservation of desire (661, 4). Adding a more controversial note to the discussion, Lacan points out that, were Kant's 'ideal bourgeois' *not* to renounce on his desire, but to remain truthful to his allegedly irresistible, transgressive inclination, and thus offer himself up for subsequent execution, this in itself could be understood as an illegal or reprehensible act of self-governance. For in doing so, the 'ideal bourgeois' could be seen as re-claiming his right to consciously, voluntarily give up his life, that is, to autonomously assert his individual right to die, which is not inscribed in any declaration of human rights, no doubt because it is not seen as partaking of human needs. Nonetheless, Lacan implicitly advocates, here, the legal recognition of suicide as the ultimate personal freedom.

Finally, Lacan (661, 5) disputes the validity of the first half of Kant's double apologue with reference to a more lighthearted concept, that of the medieval ethic of courtly love. Without giving the reader any details as to how this critique should be understood, he indicates that it requires not only erudition but also a "sense of comedy" (661, 6), something on which neither Kant nor Sade are known to have placed much value. To follow what Lacan had in mind, here, one needs to divert one's attention to *Seminar VII*. As part of a lengthier analysis of Kantian ethics, he had argued there that the overvaluation of the inaccessible Lady in the practice of courtly love could very well have prompted a lover to prefer a night of passion over his own life, now that his exalted 'feminine object' was finally available. "All of which leads to the conclusion", Lacan asserts, "that it is not impossible for a man to sleep with a woman knowing full well that he is to be bumped off [*zigouillé*] on his way out, by the gallows or anything else" (Lacan, S7, 1959–1960: 109).

Section 11

And so Lacan (661, 8) moves to the second part of Kant's double apologue, in order to demonstrate that here too the philosopher had been too rash in predicting the outcome of his thought-experiment. Kant wanted the first part of the apologue to prove how a rational human being would gladly renounce his lustful inclination, irresistible as it may be, because of his love of life. For the second part, he intended to show how this very love of life may itself be renounced in favour of the preservation of the categorical imperative, so that the latter appears as ruling both over transitory empirical pleasures and over the most fundamental empirical quality of a rational being's earthly existence—the conscious experience of life itself. Here is what Kant wrote:

> But ask him [the same rational being who featured in the first part of the apologue] whether, if his prince demanded, on pain of the same immediate execution [*unter Androhung derselben unverzögerten Todesstrafe*], that he give false testimony against an honorable man whom the prince would like to destroy under a plausible pretext, he would consider it possible to overcome his love of life, however great it may be. He would perhaps not venture to assert whether he would do it or not, but he must admit without hesitation that it would be possible for him. He judges, therefore, that he can do something because he is aware that he ought to do it and cognizes freedom within him, which, without the moral law, would have remained unknown to him.
>
> (1788/1997: 27–28)

Kant suggested that bearing false witness can never constitute a universally applicable rule of conduct, which implies that the rational human being is left with no other option than to forfeit his own life. In this case, the weight of the moral law frees the rational subject of his love of life, and allows him to accept his own death for the sake of the categorical imperative.

Lacan agrees with Kant that bearing false witness could never qualify as a universally applicable practical law, but at the same time he identifies a confounding factor: the act of bearing false witness is instructed by an unscrupulous ruler and results in an innocent person losing his life. What if the person against whom one is asked to testify were to be put at risk of losing his life because of a truthful testimony, the truth about this person being exactly what the ruler would be looking for in order to condemn him to death? Bearing true witness would definitely be admissible as a universally applicable practical law, but what if it is done to incriminate one's fellow man in the service of a repressive authoritarian agency? If telling the truth is a fine Kantian maxim, what if it is merely an act of self-preservation, or an act of cowardly compliance with authority, leading to someone else's human rights being violated? Were Kant's example to be changed into a command that the individual bear true witness in order to give the ruler a reason for executing his adversary, would the philosopher still argue that the categorical imperative must prevail? In '*Kant with Sade*', Lacan intimates that in his fervent ambition to articulate a purely formal law, which is devoid of all content, matter and empirical references, Kant had been too quick in discarding certain options as determining grounds for the will, and had failed to appreciate the fact that acting upon one's desire, when freed from any 'pathological' considerations such as pride, contentment or self-interest, can *also* be constructed as doing one's duty in accordance with the moral law (662, 3). If someone really does have irresistible inclinations and decides to act upon them, in spite of the awkward circumstances and the lethal consequences, then this is a good Kantian ethical act. If someone decides to counter a tyrant's demands, irrespective of the type of testimony that is being called for, because he believes that no one has the right to usurp legitimate sovereignty for the sake of absolute power or, as Lacan put it, "to enslave the Other's desire" (662, 3), and despite the risks associated with this opposition, then this is surely a good Kantian ethical act too.

Sections 12–13

Mainly drawing on Freud and Sade, Lacan concludes that the Kantian law of practical reason is not nearly as pure as the philosopher had wished it to be. Although Kant had been at great pains to articulate a purely formal categorical imperative, devoid of any reference to empirical objects, stripped of all subjective experiences of pleasure, and liberated from the 'pathological' faculty of desire, the moral law surreptitiously sustains desire, and therefore runs aground on an idealization, which is also why Kant needed to introduce the postulate of the immortality of the soul. Only in the afterlife will it be possible for a rational human being to become holy, to enter a state of perfect compliance with the moral law, to achieve the highest good—as the only true object(ive) of the law—and to experience the convergence of virtue and happiness.

Emphasizing his point, Lacan now reminds his readership of Kant's definition of happiness in 'Theorem II' of the first chapter of the *Critique of Practical Reason*: happiness is "a rational being's consciousness of the agreeableness [*Annehmlichkeit*] of life uninterruptedly accompanying his whole existence" (Kant, 1788/1997: 20). If this is indeed what happiness consists of, then it can only be conceived in terms of a complete renunciation of the "pathway of desire" (663, 5), because desire is strictly incompatible with the conscious experience of uninterrupted agreeableness. Drawing once more on Freud and Sade, Lacan argues that in advocating a complete renunciation of desire—and thereby of pleasure, as the satisfaction of desire—the Epicureans, the Stoics and Kant had not only failed to acknowledge "the subject's truth" (663, 5), but also misjudged the effect of this renunciation on the rational being's state of mind. In an effort to question psychoanalytically the viability of a dispassionate, virtuous existence or, in the case of Kant, the consistency of a purely formal categorical imperative, Lacan summarizes Freud's views on desire, pleasure and repression. Mapping his own concepts onto Freud's work, he states that psychoanalytic experience had discovered how an unconscious desire is generally repressed because its realization is likely to elicit a sensation of unpleasure at the level of the reigning set of conscious representations in the ego (663, 3). In wanting to preserve its integrity against the emergence of an incompatible desire, the ego enforces its law and represses the desire, as a result of which the desire becomes unconscious, and the ego maintains a certain degree of pleasure. Yet rather than sinking into a sphere of inactivity, the unconscious desire returns with a vengeance, thus creating pleasure in terms of the mechanisms presiding over the unconscious, but also a new experience of unpleasure as far as the ego is concerned. When this intra-psychic dynamic is applied to the Epicurean and Stoic conceptions of happiness—as the inner state of tranquility stemming from the renunciation of the passions—it becomes immediately clear that happiness is but a philosophical illusion, because the superior pleasure associated with the renunciation of the inferior desires will be diminished by the constant return of the repressed desires striving for satisfaction. Lacan writes that the notion of *ataraxia* had "deposed their [the Stoics'] wisdom" (663, 5). And implicitly referring to the fact that the Stoics regarded a human being's full compliance with the cardinal virtues as indicative of someone's voluntary acceptance of the laws of Nature, he adds that in this respect the Stoics did not deserve praise for degrading desire either, because in doing so they had not so much elevated the (symbolic) Law (of Nature), but rather cast it aside, given that Nature's Law—as Sade's libertines tend to repeat *ad nauseam*—is also, and perhaps primarily, characterized by the very capriciousness of desire, especially in its most brutal manifestations of absolute cruelty. As to Kant, because his categorical imperative is also based upon a renunciation of the 'pathological', its formal impact will be equally contaminated by the material objects of the faculty of desire.

In his libertine novels, Sade had advanced a radically different ideology of desire and happiness. Much like the Stoics, Sade's libertines campaign for the recognition of Nature as the supreme sovereign authority. Yet unlike their Greek and Roman counterparts, they do not believe that Nature is driven by virtue, neither in the form of justice, courage, wisdom or temperance, nor in the shape of any other mechanism that might contribute to progress and development. As we saw earlier, for Sade's libertines, the ultimate goal in life is the realization of a state of absolute destruction, which goes so far as to include self-immolation and the annihilation of Nature itself, and for which—in accordance with the spirit of libertinage—they deem the liberation of desire to be an essential precondition (663, 6). In their libertine philosophy, Sade's heroes want to set a rational being's desire free from the burden of religion, morality, and all social institutions that are aimed at curtailing its ferocious potential. By implication, they therefore also require their republic to be based on a limited framework of policies, rules and regulations, and a minimal set of laws. Although his ethical system was very much the opposite of Kant's, Sade shared Kant's belief in the insuperable antagonism between desire and the law. In order to set desire free, in order to ensure that desire instills freedom in the citizens of the republic, the law itself needs to be set free, that is, it needs to be unpacked, unleashed and allowed to disappear to the point where but the smallest remnant of its regulatory power remains intact.

Lacan writes that at exactly the right point ("*là où il faut*") Sade had taken up Saint-Just (663, 6), one of the main political leaders during the French Revolution, and one of the chief architects of the so-called Reign of Terror, when thousands of purportedly anti-revolutionary elements lost their head under the guillotine. And indeed, although Sade never referred to Saint-Just in any of his libertine novels nor, for that matter, in the political pamphlet that was inserted in *Philosophy in the Boudoir*, the latter's legendary opposition to extensive, detailed laws chimes with Sade's anti-legalistic political philosophy. "We require few laws. Where there are many, the people are slaves," Saint-Just noted in his own doctrine for a revolutionary republic (Saint-Just, 1794/2004: 1136). Both for Saint-Just and for Sade's libertines, reinforcing this principle came at the cost of mass murder, but it was squarely implemented in the service of freedom, equality and fraternity.

Returning to what he had written at the very beginning of '*Kant with Sade*', Lacan asserts that Sade had fractured "the ancient axis of ethics" (663), because insofar as happiness remains an ethical goal and the highest good in Sade's system, it is no longer regarded as of communal benefit, but as intrinsically selfish—pervaded by self-interest rather than an altruistic concern over the equal well-being of all citizens. Sade professes another kind of happiness, which Lacan had described in the opening page of his text as "happiness in evil" ("*bonheur dans le mal*") (645, 3), and which not only imposes a reconsideration of the precise status of desire, but also a re-examination of the right to *jouissance* that is allegedly derived from this desire (663, 8).[14] This is the task to which Lacan will devote himself in the next section of '*Kant with Sade*'.

Section 14

In essence, Lacan contends that despite his grand literary fantasy of ruthless libertines 'setting the universe ablaze' on the basis of a self-proclaimed right to *jouissance*, Sade had failed to liberate desire from the constraining, regulatory force of the law. As he had already suggested in Sections 5 and 6 of his text, this structural failure first of all expresses itself in the discourse of the libertines themselves, who time and again admit to the mediocrity and inadequacy of their exploits. Adding to this, Lacan avers in Section 14 that Sade's failure to fully execute the principle of the right to *jouissance* can also be identified at the level of his own writing. "I have conceived everything conceivable in that [libertine] genre," Sade disclosed to his wife as early as 1781 (Sade, 1997: 229), but this admission did not stop him from carrying on inventing and describing more radical, more sinful and more ferocious criminal acts, in an endless spiral of widening and deepening literary excess, which suggests that something resisted the full realization of his devious plan.

Lacan opens Section 14 with a question: "How far does Sade lead us in the experience of this *jouissance*, or simply of its truth?" (664, 3). If he does not give the solution straight away, or even contemplates giving any kind of straightforward, unequivocal response, his remarks all converge upon a simple answer: not very far, not far enough, not as far as Sade would have wanted it to be led, only as far as it showed itself to be ineluctably constrained by the cycles of pleasure, desire and the law. In deciding to commit the most detailed descriptions of the most ghastly atrocities to paper, Sade had somehow managed to cross the limits of his own fantasy—the one ruling over his desire in real life—but Lacan does not believe that this new fictional space of the 'Sadean fantasy' was therefore a fully accomplished, limitless arena of *jouissance*. In two highly lyrical paragraphs, Lacan compares Sade's exceedingly complex sexual installations—as depicted in the numerous illustrations accompanying his libertine novels—to the baroque fountains at the famous *Villa d'Este* in Tivoli, near Rome, but whereas the latter derive part of their splendor from the spectacular flow of water, Lacan wonders what exactly was flowing in Sade's "human pyramids" (664, 4). In these depictions, which have not been reproduced in any of the English editions of Sade's libertine novels, Lacan recognizes "unpredictable quanta by which the love-hate atom glistens in the vicinity of the Thing from which man emerges through a cry" (664, 5), that is, a force-field whose elements of combined love and hate may have their energy increased or decreased in ways that cannot be foreseen, which makes them approximate the fundamentally unknowable Kantian thing-in-itself, or even the fundamental strangeness of the Freudian and Heideggerian 'Thing' (*das Ding*) in its appearance as both materiality and void, and from which the participants re-emerge either with the scream of voluptuous orgasm or the cry of deadly expiration. Whatever it is, Lacan claims, it is not supposed to have anything to do with desire and the fantasmatic structure sustaining it. Insofar as Sade's work may indeed be considered an outline, a sketch or a blueprint ("*épure*") (664, 7) of his actual, real-life fantasy, he would have had to transcend the latter's boundaries in order to conceive *everything* in the libertine genre. Yet at the same time, this literary Sadean fantasy would have remained attached to Sade's real-life fantasy and therefore subjected to the latter's limitations, following the interlocking dynamic of desire and the law.

All in all, Lacan identifies four instances of Sade not having succeeded in lifting the experience of *jouissance* above the realm of desire and the law at the level of his own writing. Starting with *Philosophy in the Boudoir*, he claims that for all the transcendental wickedness Sade had attributed to the Supreme Being in Saint-Fond's libertine theology (Sade, 1797/1968: 399), one is left wondering about Eugénie's "modulations of the heart" (664, 9). If wickedness reigns supreme, why does Eugénie admit, in an echo of her two main instructors: "I'm crazy about my father, but I feel that I hate my mother" (Sade, 1795/2006: 21). Second, and without going so far as to suggest that *Philosophy in the Boudoir* should be dismissed as a bad piece of writing, Lacan feels that the work suffered from excessive preachiness (664, 11), combined with "dreary" historical information, and anatomo-physiological descriptions of the human body and its sexual functions that would not be misplaced in a mediocre medical textbook. Third, Lacan points out that for all Sade's attempts at celebrating the prosperities of vice, there is not a single example to be found in all his libertine novels of virtue being truly corrupted. One year before she is invited to Madame de Saint-Ange's boudoir, the delightful young Eugénie made the Madame's acquaintance at a convent, and although Saint-Ange tells her libertine friends that nothing happened back then, they are also assured of the fact that Eugénie has a certain "natural aptitude" (Sade, 1795/2006: 8). In Sade's works, virtue is never transformed into vice, which is what prompts Lacan to write that, when all is said and done, it is not just the misfortunes but also the "triumph of virtue" (665, 5) that is paradoxically being confirmed there. Finally, Lacan (665, 6) recognizes another instance of Sade's failure to liberate desire from the constraints of the law in his scanty use of witticism—a stylistic technique which would have allowed him to criticize more effectively not only the doctrinal principles against which his libertines were rallying, but also the laws of the genre and, most importantly, the syntactic and semantic laws of language as such. As we saw from our discussion of Section 3 of '*Kant with Sade*', Lacan did acknowledge the black humour and the satirical elements in Sade's works. Here, too, he points towards the occasional funny twist, such as the one occurring at the very end of Sade's posthumously published 'Dialogue between a Priest and a Dying Man', where the priest, instead of converting the libertine dying man to good Christian values, is said to have become "a man corrupted by Nature—and all because he had been unable to explain what he meant by Corrupted Nature" (Sade, 1782/2008: 160). Alluding to Alexander Pope's influential 'An Essay on Criticism' (Pope, 1709/2008), in which the great British poet had suggested that wit constitutes one of the three essential qualities of good criticism, Lacan wishes Sade had spiced up his writings with some of the piquancy of Ernest Renan's classic and hugely controversial *Life of Jesus* (665, 8). In this study, the French orientalist and philosopher, to whom Lacan had already referred in Section 7 of '*Kant with Sade*', had portrayed Jesus as a master-provocateur, who goes about launching round after round of scathing invectives against the Pharisees, and who regularly draws on mockery and irony to drive his critique home (Renan 1863/1991: 169–173) (665, 9). Endorsing Renan's outlook, Lacan remarks that the effect of Jesus' wit on Pharisaism could not have been better: before long an Apostle (the Apostle Paul) emerged from their ranks, and in the end proper Pharisee values such as righteousness and humility prevailed (666, 2).

In sum, Sade had not succeeded in overcoming the massive challenges associated with the ambition of conceiving and saying everything, partly because he remained subjected to the symbolic law of language, partly because the symbolic language of the law, and its corollaries of crime and punishment, may very well have elicited and sustained his ambition in the first place. Persistent as he may have been, he had not managed to move outside the sphere of desire and the law, into an unblemished experience of *jouissance*. According to Lacan, this is what gave Sade's work its "somber beauty" (666, 3), and what opened up its tragic dimension, both in terms of the cathartic effects resulting from its radical crossing of fear and pity, and in terms of a certain conjunction of "bewilderment and shadows" (666, 4), which he opposed to the "bewilderment and illumination" Freud had considered to be characteristic of the joke.[15] However, qualifying his own point, Lacan also designates Sade's works as "feeble tragedy" (*tragique gâteux*), which was allegedly only a stone's throw away from "noble tragedy" (666, 5). In doing so, he alludes to the lengthy literary analysis of Paul Claudel's Coûfontaine-trilogy—*L'otage* (1911), *Le pain dur* (1918) and *Le père humilié* (1920)—which he had conducted in May 1961, as part of *Seminar VIII* (Claudel, 1911–1920/1945; Lacan, S8, 1960–1961: 263–325). Intermittently referring to Sade, Lacan had argued there that, in portraying a woman who feels forced to 'voluntarily' engage in the 'law of marriage' for the mere sake of rescuing the Pope and who ends up sacrificing herself for the greater good of humankind, Claudel's distinctly Christian take on tragic drama had taken classical tragedy—as represented, for instance, in the stories of Oedipus and Antigone—beyond the conventional imposition of a legal or divine order, and thus beyond its historical constraints (Lacan, S8, 1960–1961: 276).

Section 15

After he himself had acknowledged the tragic aspects of Sade's project, connecting them to the Christian thematic of Claudel's trilogy, Lacan feels encouraged to delve deeper into Klossowski's arguments, especially those pertaining to the status of the neighbour.[16] He agrees with Klossowski that the Sadean fantasy "is better situated among the stays [*les portants*] of Christian ethics", and posits that this is what his own "structural reference points" had confirmed (666, 8). How these reference points should be understood, here, is not entirely clear. Lacan may have been involuntarily reminded of the pervasive dimension of redemption and sacrifice in Sade's libertine novels. Sade's libertine heroes are forced to sacrifice virtuous boys and girls, in order to position themselves as instruments of Nature, yet in the end they often proceed to sacrificing themselves, or dream of being sacrificed for the pure purpose of bringing their vision of absolute destruction to fruition. In all probability, however, he is thinking of how Sade's libertines explicitly position themselves vis-à-vis the Law, and more specifically with respect to the commandment "Thou shalt love thy neighbour as thyself", which is considered to be one of the central tenets of Christian doctrine. With Klossowski, Lacan highlights the importance of Sade's vehement protest against the Christian ethic, but he disagrees over the precise meaning of the opposition. Whereas for Klossowski, it paradoxically signalled Sade's implicit love of God, for Lacan it is indicative of his retreat from the sphere of *jouissance*, and of his ongoing attachment to the dialectic between desire and the Law (667, 3).

To understand Lacan's point, one needs to consult his remarks in *Seminar VII* on Freud's own critique of the Biblical commandment, in the fifth chapter of *Civilization and its Discontents* (Freud, 1930/1964: 109–112). Questioning the rationale, the meaning and the feasibility of the injunction, Freud formulated a whole string of arguments against it, the strongest one referring to the fact that the neighbour is not particularly deserving of my love if it turns out that he is not at all like me, that he does not present me with an ideal image of myself, or that he does not show any kind of love and consideration for me. "If the commandment had run 'Love thy neighbour as thy neighbour loves thee'", Freud conceded, "I should not take exception to it" (Freud, 1930/1964: 110), but since in most cases the neighbour is a complete stranger, and one who is not particularly well disposed towards me, but rather appears as my enemy, it is absurd to expect of me that I give him my unconditional love. Whereas one cannot fully comply with the commandment, Freud nonetheless understood its source and origin:

> The element of truth behind all this ... is that men are not gentle creatures who want to be loved ...; they are, on the contrary, creatures among whose instinctual endowments [*Triebbegäbungen*] is to be reckoned a powerful share of aggressiveness.
>
> (1930/1964: 111)

And in what sounded almost like an uncanny echo of Sade's pamphleteer, Freud concluded that the commandment "is really justified by the fact that nothing else runs so strongly counter to the original nature of man" (Freud, 1930/1964: 112). Of course, this is only an echo of Sade inasmuch as Freud too believed that the 'original nature of man' or the 'laws of nature' were intrinsically violent, brutal and cruel. Whereas for Freud, man's natural aggressiveness justified the commandment—much like the law of the incest-prohibition is justified *because of* the 'natural' desire to commit incest—for Sade the 'cruel nature of man' made the commandment unjustifiable. Apart from this, Sade and Freud would no doubt also have agreed that the commandment remains absurd, and needs to be exposed in all its fallacious assumptions.

When commenting on these passages in *Seminar VII*, Lacan made three important observations. First, he pointed out that the commandment not only governs the relationship between 'man' and 'fellow man' (the '*Nebenmensch*', who is not identical to me, but someone who is in the position of a stranger), but also the relationship of 'man' to himself. Second, he argued that Freud's scepticism about the neighbour's good intentions should also be applied to the subject who stands before this neighbour. If evil is found to dwell in my neighbour's heart, then there is no reason to think that it would not also dwell in mine (Lacan, S7, 1959–1960: 186). Third, following Freud's argument about the interdependence of the Biblical commandment and the 'natural' cruelty of man, Lacan articulated a new, paradoxical interpretation of why human beings (Sade, Freud and no doubt quite a few others) back away from it: "The resistance to the commandment 'Thou shalt love thy neighbour as thyself' and the resistance that is exercised to prevent his [the human being's] access to *jouissance* are one and the same thing" (Lacan, S7, 1959–1960: 194). This is a paradoxical interpretation, because one may reasonably expect someone to oppose the commandment in order to reclaim the right to cruelty. In this vein, Sade's pamphleteer would reject it, because he wants to reinstate the right to *jouissance*. Lacan's reading is counter-intuitive, here, because it proposes that in rejecting the one (the commandment), one also rejects the other (what the commandment is designed to regulate and deplete, the 'natural cruelty', which Lacan conceptualized as *jouissance*). Whereas the opposition to the commandment may be perceived as stemming from a human being's desire to see the 'law of nature' being recognized, Lacan thus inverted the dynamic.

In '*Kant with Sade*', Lacan conveys these ideas in two highly condensed paragraphs. He first of all states that Sade "refuses to be my neighbour" (666, 9)—as exemplified in the pamphleteer's rejection of the commandment—and then indicates that this refusal, which Sade shared with Freud, originates in the fact that he "does not have neighbourly enough relations with his own malice [*méchanceté*] to encounter his neighbour in it" (666, 10). In light of Lacan's observations in *Seminar VII*, the latter point can be re-phrased as Sade being unable to accept the command because he could not face the naked reality of his own cruelty. And this also explains why the pamphleteer was adamant "to wipe out forever the atrocity of capital punishment" (Sade, 1795/2006: 119)—not so much, as he himself put it, because it is unjust with reference to the reigning law of Nature, and ineffective with regard to the prevention of crime, but because the death penalty is an essential correlate of the Christian doctrine of Charity (the love of one's neighbour). Hence, rather than being truthful to his proposed liberation of desire, in the uncompromising expression of a ruthless will to *jouissance*, Sade had once again failed to achieve his goal, remaining stuck "at the point where desire and the law become bound up with each other" (667, 3).

Bringing his paper to a close, Lacan contends that the law from which Sade wanted to liberate desire, and which he found himself perpetually reconfirming, is not just an external legal principle, but also, and primarily, an internal law, which operates as the necessary precondition for the emergence of desire, and allows the prohibited object (the inaccessible Thing) to become invested with the fantasy of limitless *jouissance*. Alluding to Saint Paul's epistle to the Romans, he endorses the thesis that the presence of the law makes sin "inordinately sinful" (667, 4); it is only by virtue of the law that sin acquires "an excessive, hyperbolic character" (Lacan, S7, 1959–1960: 84). Whether through his endlessly repeated paeans to crime, or in his carefully choreographed sexual installations, which are ideally designed to integrate as many sacrilegious acts as possible, Sade is time and again compelled to accept the Law or to reinstate a figuration of the Supreme Being. It is not that his flesh is weak, Lacan comments (667, 5), but that his spirit is too willing "not to be deluded" by the idea that the abolition of the law would truly liberate desire. If Sade, through the mouth of his libertine heroes, professes a radical belief in the inexhaustible force of 'mother Nature', then this is no more than a "typical dream of potency" (667, 7), in which we would be foolish to place our faith. And this is what Lacan also recognizes in the final scene of *Philosophy in the Boudoir*, at the point where Eugénie takes a "huge needle and a thick, red, waxen thread" (Sade, 1795/2006: 171) and starts sewing up her mother's vagina, after the latter has been dutifully infected with syphilis by Dolmancé's servant Lapierre. Without shunning away from a certain degree of psychoanalytic reductionism, Lacan (667, 9) interprets the scene as Eugénie resolving her penis envy—more specifically, the hatred towards her mother instilled by the fact that she blames her for not having a penis—by sending her mother off on the path of a painful yet certain death, and as proof of the fact that, when all is said and done, "the mother remains prohibited" ("*Noli tangere matrem*"), raped and sewn shut" (667, 10).[17] Lacan writes that Sade's decision to replace Diotima—the Maninean priestess who initiated Socrates into the mysteries of love, according to Plato's *Symposium* (Plato, 2004: 41–56)—with Dolmancé as the main instructor evidently did not help when it came to 'closing the affair', not in the least because Dolmancé is known to have the strongest repulsion for "the usual orifice" (the vagina) (667, 10). Yet as to Eugénie's penis envy, he seems to ignore the fact that before sewing up her mother's vagina, and Dolmancé subsequently doing the same to her anus, Eugénie penetrates her mother with a massive dildo, which would effectively contradict the idea that the mother remains off limits. Indeed, apart from the fact that at the end of '*Kant with Sade*', Lacan engages in a fairly crude type of psychoanalytic reductionism, it is not quite true that in the final scene of *Philosophy in the Boudoir* the maternal body appears as fundamentally prohibited, because Madame de Mistival is only sewn shut *after* she has been penetrated and infected. It would be more accurate to say that the closure of her orifices serves the purpose of ensuring that she really does meet her end, in a 'sadistic' reversal of the healing function of the suture. In addition, as to the entire scene being submitted to the law, Lacan could have tried to substantiate his argument by referring to the fact that the libertines feel all the more permitted and encouraged to immolate Madame de Mistival, because they have actually received a letter of approval from Eugénie's father. Yet in this respect, the paternal law does not really 'close the affair', but opens it up to libertine intervention—rather than prohibiting access to the maternal body, the paternal law enables and facilitates the process (Sade, 1795/2006: 158–159, 172).

Nonetheless, Lacan states that Sade's works contain little or nothing by way of a treatise on desire in its pure form (667, 11), that is, in its naked detachment from the law. At the most, they include some rational declarations on the status of desire, and some reasons for the inseparability of desire and the Law, as it manifests itself in the eroto-philosophical encounters between a loose band of ferocious libertines and a largely interchangeable succession of virtuous victims (667, 12).

Conclusion

On 29 October 1974, Lacan was in Rome for a conference of his *École freudienne de Paris*. Questioned by an Italian journalist about his purportedly Kantian concept of the real, he responded: "I have written only one thing about Kant, which is my short paper entitled '*Kant with Sade*'. To be quite frank, I make Kant into a flower of sadism [*fleur sadique*]. No one paid the slightest attention to that article. Some second-rate fellow commented on it somewhere, and I don't even know if his commentary was ever published. But no one has ever sent me any remarks on that article. It is true that I am incomprehensible" (Lacan, 1975/2013: 83). I am not quite sure who Lacan had in mind, here, when he referred to the 'second-rate fellow'. Maybe he was thinking of the anonymous author of the *Paraphrase de "Kant avec Sade"*, which had indeed been published in 1970, notably in Lacan's own journal *Scilicet* (NN, 1970). If so, the designation 'second-rate' was definitely justified, partly because the text was effectively no more than a loose paraphrase, written in so convoluted a style that Lacan's own essay reverts back into 'light reading', partly because it only re-stated a very small portion of Lacan's original essay.

The only essay that was published during Lacan's lifetime in which the author explicitly engaged with '*Kant with Sade*' is by Sollers (1977), yet his remarks only cover the last three sections of the text and do not address Lacan's reading of Kant nor, for that matter, the two schemas, the complex dynamic between desire and the Law, and the problematic relationship between Sade (the man, the author) and his 'Sadean fantasy'. As such, it is fair to say that throughout Lacan's lifetime '*Kant with Sade*' was completely ignored by Sade-scholars, philosophers and psychoanalysts alike. Maybe the Sade-scholars believed that Lacan was too much of a psychoanalyst and not enough of a literary critic to be taken seriously. Maybe the philosophers thought that Lacan was too much of a Sade-scholar and insufficiently versed in the Kantian tradition to be given credit for his work. Maybe the psychoanalysts felt that Lacan's paper was too literary–philosophical, and lacking in concrete clinical applications to be given serious consideration. Maybe all of them agreed that '*Kant with Sade*' was simply unreadable, either because this is what they had heard, or because this is what they had discovered through personal experience. And after all, Lacan himself had admitted that the text was incomprehensible ....

Ignored and neglected by one and all, '*Kant with Sade*' nonetheless received a great deal of attention by Lacan himself, more in fact than most of his other essays in *Écrits*. Lacan returned to '*Kant with Sade*' on a regular basis in his seminars, not only in the context of his yearlong seminar on *The Logic of the Fantasy* (Lacan, S14, 1966–1967), but equally in further elaborations of his theory of desire, and in advanced conceptual developments of the interrelations between *jouissance*, desire and truth. "As to '*Kant with Sade*', I've written things that are actually pretty good," he admitted to his audience in March 1974, "things no one evidently understands …" (Lacan, S21, 1973–1974: session of 19 March 1974). Of the thirty-four essays that were included in *Écrits*, '*Kant with Sade*' comes third in Lacan's tally of references to his own work, after the seminal '*Rome Discourse*' (Lacan, *The Function and Field*) and the 1955 paper on '*The Freudian Thing*' (Lacan, *The Freudian Thing*), although the latter paper received only one more mention than '*Kant with Sade*' (Le Gaufey et al., 1998: 66). If '*Kant with Sade*' had been published ten years earlier, or some time during the 1950s—but it would undoubtedly have been a very different text—Lacan would have had more time to re-engage with his essay, and it may very well have come out top of the list. Unlike his contemporaries, including those philosophers and psychoanalysts attending his seminar, Lacan thought extremely highly of '*Kant with Sade*' and did not let an opportunity go by to remind his audience of what he had accomplished in it—incomprehensible as it may have been.

Since Lacan's death in 1981, '*Kant with Sade*' has received more extensive critical attention, both in France and in other parts of the world, yet compared to some of Lacan's other adventures in the world of literature, such as the essay on E. A. Poe's 'Purloined Letter' (Lacan, *The Purloined Letter*), the seminar sessions on Antigone (Lacan, S7, 1959–1960: 241–287), and the yearlong seminar on Joyce (Lacan, S23), '*Kant with Sade*' is by no means a household reference in contemporary explorations of the so-called 'literary Lacan'. This is all the more remarkable since one of Lacan's main arguments in '*Kant with Sade*', which set him apart from mainstream psychoanalytic interpretations of literary texts, is that there is no strict correspondence between authors and their work, between the author's subjective fantasy and the literary fantasy that appears in the space of creative imagination. Indeed, over and above Lacan's claim that Sade had revealed Kant's truth—insofar as he had demonstrated how a purely formal law, which excludes all considerations for empirical objects and dispels pleasure and emotion as mere pathological motives for dutiful compliance, does not by definition facilitate the advent of the highest good, but may easily descend into the sphere of radical evil—'*Kant with Sade*' offers a truly innovative perspective on the status and function of creative writing, which does away with conventional psychoanalytic reductionism.

Finally, whereas with few exceptions Lacan's text continues to be ignored by Kant- and Sade-scholars alike, since Lacan's death psychoanalysts and psychoanalytically inclined philosophers and cultural critics have been more responsive to its message. Unfortunately, this has not always implied that the subtleties and intricacies of Lacan's arguments have been properly appreciated, nor that the text has been given the close reading that it most definitely requires and deserves. To add insult to injury, psychoanalytic commentators have often injected concepts and ideas into Lacan's paper that seem most alien to it. The most striking example concerns the notions of perversion and sadism. The former only appears once in Lacan's entire text, in the very first paragraph, and in a fairly trivial context. If the latter appears more frequently, Lacan always seems to qualify its meaning, never goes so far as to advance a psychoanalytic theory of sadism, does not conflate the 'Sadean fantasy' with the clinical category of sadism, and radically avoids mapping the 'Sadean fantasy' onto Sade's subjectivity. Purely relying on Lacan's text, it is impossible to say that it deals with perversion, sadism or sado-masochism, much less with Sade's sadism. Remarkably, this has not stopped even the most astute commentators from claiming that '*Kant with Sade*' is an essay on perversion, on the perverse fantasy, or on fantasy in perversion (Miller, 1998: 74). Were Lacan to have wanted to conceive his essay as a psychoanalytic contribution to the study of perversion, then there is no doubt in my mind that he would have said so, or that he would have used the requisite terminology. And the same may be said for other notions that are undoubtedly related to the scope of Lacan's text, but that do not appear within its texture, not even implicitly: the Real, the Symbolic and the Imaginary, anxiety, the phallus, the Oedipus complex, the Name-of-the-Father, identification. In many ways, '*Kant with Sade*' still remains to be discovered and properly evaluated in its implications for the status of Kantian moral philosophy, the style and scope of Sade's libertine novels, the psychoanalytic conceptions of desire, *jouissance*, fantasy and the Law, and the power of creative writing as literary fantasy.

Notes

1 I should also inform the reader that my critical analysis, here, has been distilled from a much more detailed and comprehensive commentary, which also elucidates all of Lacan's allusions in the essay, and which has been published previously as a scholarly monograph (Nobus, 2017).

2 Lacan writes 'delight in evil' ("*bonheur dans le mal*") in quotation marks yet, as will become clear from my discussion of Section 3 of Lacan's text, not everything placed in quotation marks in 'Kant with Sade' is *de facto* a quote. The literary work which most closely echoes Lacan's 'delight in evil' (*bonheur dans le mal*), is Barbey d'Aurevilly's short story '*Le bonheur dans le crime*' (Barbey d'Aurevilly, 1874/1985), but the expression *bonheur du Mal* had also already been used by Blanchot in '*La raison de Sade*' (Blanchot 1949/1986: 28; 1949/2004: 18), where it has been translated as 'the pleasures of Evil'. In the last paragraph of Section 13 of 'Kant with Sade', Lacan refers to "another happiness … whose name I first uttered" (664), by which he presumably alludes to the 'delight in evil' from the opening section of his text. Taking Lacan at his word, here, this would suggest that Lacan himself coined the phrase in question. Also, when Lacan writes at the end of the previous

paragraph (645) that one should add "another sixty years before one could say why [Freud's path had become passable]", this is most likely an allusion to his own work. Indeed, Lacan's seminar on the ethics of psychoanalysis, on which 'Kant with Sade' is based, took place in 1959–1960, almost exactly 160 years after Sade released the last of his scandalous novels—the monumental *La nouvelle Justine ou les Malheurs de la vertu, suivie de L'histoire de Juliette, sa sœur*, which appeared in no less than ten volumes.

3 The difference between the 'enunciating subject' and the 'subject of the statement' is even clearer in the English translation, because Fink has placed additional quotation marks both at the end of the first clause, and at the beginning of the second clause of the law of *jouissance*, thus making it unambiguous that there is another sentence of direct speech within the spoken statement.

4 The letter V is evidently taken from the French '*volonté de jouissance*', a notion also invoking '*volonté de puissance*', which is the French translation of Nietzsche's concept of '*Wille zur Macht*' (will to power). Given that the English translation of this notion is 'will to *jouissance*', one could argue that, here and elsewhere in the English version of 'Kant with Sade', the V should be changed into a W. However, as I shall explain later, Lacan also interprets the V as the first letter of the Latin word *vel* (which means 'or'), representing the lower half of the ◇, which he then regards as a certain type of logical disjunction, for which the conventional notation in propositional logic is v. As such, there are good reasons for maintaining the letter V in English.

5 Because Lacan will draw again on the logical disjunction (*vel*, V) of alienation, in section 8 of 'Kant with Sade', as an operation that is based on the principle of the union (*réunion*) in set theory, I should nonetheless explain that Lacan's point has to do with the fact that the truth table of the inclusive disjunction in a propositional calculus follows the definition of the union in set theory: the union of two sets is made up of those elements that belong to one *or* the other set, *and* those elements that belong to both, whereas the inclusive disjunction is valid when one *or* the other of two propositions is true, *and* when both are true.

6 In this context, Lacan also refers to *Antigone* in 'Kant with Sade' (654, 6), whereby he quotes (although with a misspelling that has been reproduced in the English version) the famous first line (781) of the Chorus' response to Creon's decree that the eponymous heroine be buried alive: Ἔρως ἀνίκατε μάχαν (Love invincible in battle) (Sophocles, 1998: 77). What he has in mind, though, is not so much this particular line, but three subsequent lines (795–797), in which the Chorus sings ἐναργὴς βλεφάρων ἵμερος εὐλέκτρου νύμφας, which can be translated as "the visible desire that comes from the eyes of the beautiful bride" (Sophocles, 1998: 79). Lacan thus intends to remind his readership of how Sophocles, prior to Antigone reappearing on the scene to hear her sentence and being taken away to her cavern, had also highlighted both her beauty and the radiant splendour of her desire.

7 At this point in his text, Lacan employs a number of sartorial metaphors, which have unfortunately disappeared in Fink's translation. Lacan states that amongst those who strive for "tidier appearances" (*une toilette plus soignée*), and argue that the sadist "denies the Other's existence", some may draw on the "*bon faiseur existentialiste*" and others on the "ready-made *personnaliste*". The expression '*bon faiseur*' does not refer to a 'do-gooder', as Fink has rendered it, but to a 'good tailor', as opposed to the mass-market, factory-produced clothing of the *ready-made*.

In addition, '*existentialiste*' and '*personnaliste*' are the adjectives rather than the nouns, so that the expressions should be rendered as "existentialist custom tailoring" and "personalist ready-made".

8 The footnote in which Lacan expresses this point has been misplaced in Fink's translation, thus giving the reader the impression that Lacan was somehow referring to Sade's manservant.

9 Bizarrely, this crucial link between Sade's works and the object *a* in the second schema has completely disappeared from Fink's translation. In the original, Lacan wrote: "*sa malédiction moins sainte que celle d'Œdipe, ne le porte pas chez les Dieux, mais s'éternise:* a) *dans l'œuvre*", whereby "a) *dans l'œuvre*" is the start of a new paragraph. In Fink's translation, we read in one and the same paragraph: "Sade's curse is less holy than Oedipus', and does not carry him toward the Gods, but is immortalized in his work" (657, 6). As such, the algebraic notation *a*) is no longer there, and the only reason I can think of to explain this omission is that '*a*)' was interpreted not as indicative of the object *a*, but as the beginning of a list of things—a), b), c), etc.—and was eventually dropped, because b) did not follow and so *a*) was seen as a confusing and superfluous marker.

10 In French, the stage directions read "*La posture se défait*" and "*La posture se rompt*" (Sade, 1795/1998: 96 & 108), whereby '*posture*' refers to the sexual combinatory the characters have been 'performing'. In his text, Lacan quotes the latter sentence, which Wainhouse and Seaver have translated as "They dissolve their position" (Sade, 1795/1965: 293), and Neugroschel has rendered as "The arrangement breaks up" (Sade, 1795/2006: 101). In his translation of Lacan's text, Fink has opted for "Change of positions" (658, 2)—despite referring the reader to Wainhouse and Seaver's version of *Philosophy in the Boudoir*—which wrongly suggests that the characters are about to change their sexual positions, and which fails to capture the crucial meaning of things breaking up, coming apart, becoming undone.

11 Like his earlier 'quote' from Jarry's *Ubu Rex*, Lacan's line is a free adaptation of the original, which reads (in translation): "—Unreal in fact. So, one will likely ask, / What is the meaning of this metaphor: / 'Thin as a hair, wide as the light of dawn'/ And why these less than three-dimensional hands?" (Queneau, 1943/2008: 131). However, as was the case with the quote from *Antigone* in Section 6 of his text (654, 6), this particular line from Queneau's poem is actually not directly relevant to Lacan's argument, and is merely intended as the placeholder for the general spirit of the poem. In other words, as with the quote from Antigone, the significance of Lacan's reference to Queneau needs to be sought outside the quoted line.

12 Again, Lacan abbreviates and adapts the final lines of La Fontaine's fable, which in full read as follows: "Charity is a virtue, but toward whom? / Best choose the ones you show it to! / As for ungrateful cads, none are there who, / sooner or later fail to meet their doom." See La Fontaine (1668/2007: 142–143).

13 Lacan writes that in the symbol of the 'bar' (/), "the signifier *\$* bastardizes him [the subject]" (659, 3), by which he alludes to the fact that in heraldry a diagonal band running from the viewer's upper right (dexter) to the lower left (sinister) of a shield, and which is called 'bend sinister' in English, is believed to be associated with bastardy. In French blazon, this type of band is also known as '*barre*'—the same word Lacan utilizes to designate the divided subject.

14 Because Fink has translated Lacan's "*bonheur dans le mal*" as "delight in evil" at the beginning of 'Kant with Sade' (645, 3), the connection between "another

happiness" ("*un autre bonheur*") at the end of Section 13 and the programmatic "happiness in evil" from the beginning of the paper is no longer evident from the English translation of Lacan's text.

15 In *Seminar VII*, Lacan had reminded his audience of a line (1449b, 26–27) from Aristotle's *Poetics*, in which the philosopher had referred to catharsis as what is accomplished δι' ἐλέου καὶ φόβου (literally, "through pity and fear") (Aristotle, 1995: 46). In Lacan's interpretation, it was

> in connection with this power of attraction that we should look for the true sense, the true mystery, the true significance of tragedy—in connection with the excitement involved, in connection with the emotions and, in particular, with the singular emotions that are fear and pity, since it is through their intervention, δι' ἐλέου καὶ φόβου, through the intervention of pity and fear, that we are purged, purified of everything of that order [of desire].
>
> (S7, 1959–1960: 247–248)

As to "bewilderment and illumination" (*Verblüffung und Erleuchtung*), this is the sequence of reactions singled out by the Dutch psychologist Gerardus Heymans in a 1896 paper, as typical for the effect of a joke, and which Freud adopted in his 1905 study *Jokes and their Relation to the Unconscious*. See Heymans (1896: 36) and Freud (1905/1960: 12–13).

16 Although this is the first time Lacan explicitly refers to Klossowski's work in 'Kant with Sade', it is definitely not the first time he draws inspiration (and examples) from it. As I pointed out earlier in my exposition of Sections 6 and 7 of 'Kant with Sade', Lacan no doubt borrowed the examples of Saint-Fond's paradoxical belief in the afterlife, Pope Pius VI's vision of a 'second death', and the latter's relationship with Buddhism, from Klossowski's texts.

17 The sentence "Raped and sewn shut" translates Lacan's "*V … ée et cousue*" and thus closes the ellipsis by interpreting V … ée as *Violée* (raped). However, at least two other interpretations are possible, and Lacan clearly wants the reader to consider all of these: *Vérolée* (infected with syphilis) and *Voilée* (veiled).

References

Adorno, T. W. and Horkheimer, M. (1944/1997) *Dialectic of Enlightenment*, trans. J. Cumming, London/New York: Verso.

Arendt, H. (1963/2006) *Eichmann in Jerusalem: A Report on the Banality of Evil*, London: Penguin Books.

Aristotle (1995) *Poetics*, trans. S. Halliwell, Cambridge, MA/London: Harvard University Press.

Barbey d'Aurevilly, J. (1874/1985) 'Le bonheur dans le crime', in *Les Diaboliques*, Paris: Librairie générale française, pp. 113–176.

Bataille, G. (1957a) *La littérature et le mal*, Paris: Gallimard.

Bataille, G. (1957b) *L'érotisme*, Paris: Minuit.

Bataille, G. (1957/2001) *Eroticism*, trans. M. Dalwood, London: Penguin.

Blanchot, M. (1949/1986) 'La raison de Sade', in *Sade et Restif de la Bretonne*, Paris: Complexe, pp. 7–66.

Blanchot, M. (1949/2004) 'Sade's Reason', in *Lautréamont and Sade*, trans. S. Kendall and M. Kendall, Stanford, CA: Stanford University Press, pp. 7–41.

Boehme, J. (1618–1619/1909) *The Three Principles of the Divine Essence*, trans. J. Sparrow, London: L. N. Fowler & Co.

Breton, A. (1939/2009) *Anthology of Black Humour*, trans. M. Polizzotti, London/San Francisco, CA: Telegram Books.

Claudel, P. (1911–1920/1945) *Three Plays (The Hostage/Crusts/The Humiliation of the Father)*, trans. J. Heard, New York: Howard Fertig.

de Beauvoir, S. (1950–1951/1990) 'Must We Burn Sade?', trans. A. Michelson, in Marquis de Sade, *The 120 Days of Sodom and Other Writings*, trans. A. Wainhouse and R. Seaver, London: Arrow Books, pp. 3–64.

du Plessix Gray, F. (1999) *At Home with the Marquis de Sade*, London: Chatto & Windus.

du Plessix Gray, F. (2006) 'Introduction', in Marquis de Sade, *Philosophy in the Boudoir*, trans. J. Neugroschel, London: Penguin, pp. vii–xvi.

Foucault, M. (1961) *Folie et déraison. Histoire de la folie à l'âge classique*, Paris: Plon.

Freud, S. (1905/1960) 'Jokes and their Relation to the Unconscious', in J. Strachey (Ed.), *The Standard Edition of the Complete Psychological Works of Sigmund Freud*, Vol. 8, London: The Hogarth Press and the Institute of Psycho-Analysis.

Freud, S. (1911/1958) 'Formulations on the Two Principles of Mental Functioning', in J. Strachey (Ed.), *The Standard Edition of the Complete Psychological Works of Sigmund Freud*, Vol. 12, London: The Hogarth Press and the Institute of Psycho-Analysis, pp. 213–226.

Freud, S. (1913/1955) 'Totem and Taboo', in J. Strachey (Ed.), *The Standard Edition of the Complete Psychological Works of Sigmund Freud*, Vol. 13, London: The Hogarth Press and the Institute of Psycho-Analysis, pp. 1–162.

Freud, S. (1915/1957) 'Instincts and their Vicissitudes', (1915), in J. Strachey (Ed.), *The Standard Edition of the Complete Psychological Works of Sigmund Freud*, Vol. 14, London: The Hogarth Press and the Institute of Psycho-Analysis, pp. 109–140.

Freud, S. (1920/1955) 'Beyond the Pleasure Principle', in J. Strachey (Ed.), *The Standard Edition of the Complete Psychological Works of Sigmund Freud*, Vol. 18, London: The Hogarth Press and the Institute of Psycho-Analysis, pp. 1–64.

Freud, S. (1924/1961) 'The Economic Problem of Masochism', in J. Strachey (Ed.), *The Standard Edition of the Complete Psychological Works of Sigmund Freud*, Vol. 19, London: The Hogarth Press and the Institute of Psycho-Analysis, pp. 155–170.

Freud, S. (1927/1964) 'Humour', in J. Strachey (Ed.), *The Standard Edition of the Complete Psychological Works of Sigmund Freud*, Vol. 21, London: The Hogarth Press and the Institute of Psycho-Analysis, pp. 159–166.

Freud, S. (1930/1964) 'Civilization and Its Discontents', in J. Strachey (Ed.), *The Standard Edition of the Complete Psychological Works of Sigmund Freud*, Vol. 21, London: The Hogarth Press and the Institute of Psycho-Analysis, pp. 57–145.

Garçon, M. (1963) *L'affaire Sade. Édition complète avec l'arrêt de la Cour d'appel*, Paris: Jean-Jacques Pauvert.

Heine, M. (1932/1950) 'Une thèse de doctorat sur le marquis de Sade', in *Le Marquis de Sade*, texte établi et préfacé par Gilbert Lely, Paris: Gallimard, pp. 105–110.

Heine, M. (1950) *Le Marquis de Sade*, texte établi et préfacé par Gilbert Lely, Paris: Gallimard.

Heymans, G. (1896) 'Ästhetische Untersuchungen in Anschluß an die Lipps'sche Theorie des Komischen', *Zeitschrift für Psychologie und Physiologie der Sinnesorgane*, 11, pp. 31–43, 333–352.

Jarry, A. (1896/1968) 'Ubu Rex', in *The Ubu Plays*, trans. C. Connolly and S. Watson Taylor, London: Methuen & Co., pp. 17–73.

Kant, I. (1781/1998) *Critique of Pure Reason*, trans. and ed. P. Guyer and A. W. Wood, Cambridge: Cambridge University Press.

Kant, I. (1785/2012) *Groundwork of the Metaphysics of Morals*, trans. M. Gregor and J. Timmermann, Cambridge: Cambridge University Press.

Kant, I. (1788/1997) *Critique of Practical Reason*, trans. M. Gregor, Cambridge: Cambridge University Press.

Klossowski, P. (1947) *Sade mon prochain*, Paris: Éditions du Seuil.

Klossowski, P. (1967/1992) *Sade my Neighbour*, trans. A. Lingis, London: Quartet Books.

Krafft-Ebing, R. von (1901) *Psychopathia Sexualis. Mit besonderer Berücksichtigung der conträren Sexualempfindung. Eine medicinisch-gerichtliche Studie*, 11th edition, Stuttgart: Ferdinand Enke.

Lacan, J. (1966–1967) *Le Séminaire XIV, La logique du fantasme*, unpublished.

Lacan, J. (1973/1994) *The Seminar. Book XI: The Four Fundamental Concepts of Psycho-Analysis* (1964), trans. A. Sheridan, ed. J.-A. Miller, Harmondsworth: Penguin.

Lacan, J. (1973–1974) *Le Séminaire XXI, Les non-dupes errent*, unpublished.

Lacan, J. (1975/2013) 'The Triumph of Religion', in *The Triumph of Religion, preceded by Discourse to Catholics*, trans. B. Fink, Cambridge: Polity, pp. 53–85.

Lacan, J. (1978/1988) *The Seminar. Book II: The Ego in Freud's Theory and in the Technique of Psychoanalysis* (1954–1955), trans. S. Tomaselli, Cambridge: Cambridge University Press.

Lacan, J. (1986/1992) *The Seminar. Book VII: The Ethics of Psychoanalysis* (1959–1960), trans. D. Porter, ed. J.-A. Miller, New York/London: W. W. Norton & Company.

Lacan, J. (2001/2015) *The Seminar. Book VIII: Transference* (1960–1961), trans. B. Fink, ed. J.-A. Miller, Cambridge: Polity.

Lacan, J. (2004/2014) *The Seminar. Book X: Anxiety* (1962–1963), trans. A. R. Price, ed. J.-A. Miller, Cambridge: Polity.

Lacan, J. (2005/2016) *The Seminar. Book XXIII: The Sinthome*, trans. A. R. Price, ed. J.-A. Miller, Cambridge: Polity.

La Fontaine, J. de (1668/2007) *The Complete Fables of Jean de la Fontaine*, Champaign, IL: The University of Illinois Press.

Le Gaufey, G. et al. (1998) *Index des noms propres et titres d'ouvrages dans l'ensemble des séminaires de Jacques Lacan*, Paris: E.P.E.L.

Lely, G. (1952) *Vie du Marquis de Sade. Tome 1: De la naissance à l'évasion de Miolans (1740–1773)*, Paris: Gallimard.

Lely, G. (1957) *Vie du Marquis de Sade, avec un examen de ses ouvrages. Tome 2: Des années libertines de La Coste au dernier hiver du captif (1773–1814)*, Paris: Gallimard.

Lever, M. (1991/1993) *Sade: A Biography*, trans. A. Goldhammer, New York: Farrar, Straus and Giroux.

Marty, É. (2011) *Pourquoi le XXe siècle a-t-il pris Sade au sérieux?* Paris: Éditions du Seuil.

Miller, J.-A. (1998) 'Sobre "Kant con Sade"', in *Elucidación de Lacan: Charlas brasileñas*, Buenos Aires: Paidós, pp. 201–280.
Miller, J.-A. (2003) 'Une incroyable exaltation', in J.-A. Miller (Ed.), *Lakant*, Paris: Navarin-Seuil, pp. 27–41.
NN (1970) 'Paraphrase de "Kant avec Sade"', *Scilicet*, 2/3, pp. 283–324.
Nobus, D. (2017) *The Law of Desire: On Lacan's 'Kant with Sade'*, Basingstoke: Palgrave Macmillan.
Origen of Alexandria (2013) *Against Celsus* (248), trans. F. Crombie, Grand Rapids, MI: Ex Fontibus Co.
Paulhan, J. (1945) 'Le marquis de Sade et sa complice ou les revanches de la pudeur', *La table ronde*, 3, pp. 95–136.
Paulhan, J. (1945/1990) 'The Marquis de Sade and his Accomplice', in Marquis de Sade, *Justine, Philosophy in the Bedroom, and Other Writings*, trans. R. Seaver, New York: Grove Weidenfeld, pp. 3–36.
Pauvert, J.-J. and Beuchot, P. (Eds.) (1999) *Sade en procès*. Paris: Mille et une nuits.
Plato (2004) *Symposium*, trans. R. Waterfield, Oxford: Oxford University Press.
Pope, A. (1709/2008) 'An Essay on Criticism', in *The Major Works*, Oxford: Oxford University Press, pp. 17–39.
Queneau, R. (1943/2008) *Eyeseas (Les Ziaux)*, trans. D. Hurezanu and S. Kessler, Boston, MA: Black Widow Press.
Renan, E. (1863/1991) *The Life of Jesus*, Buffalo, NY: Prometheus Books.
Roudinesco, É. (1993/1997) *Jacques Lacan*, trans. B. Bray, New York/London: Columbia University Press.
Sade, Marquis de (1782/2008) 'Dialogue between a Priest and a Dying Man', in *The Misfortunes of Virtue and Other Early Tales*, trans. D. Coward, Oxford: Oxford University Press, pp. 149–160.
Sade, Marquis de (1795/1965) *The Complete Justine, Philosophy in the Bedroom, and Other Writings*, trans. A. Wainhouse and R. Seaver, New York: Grove Press.
Sade, Marquis de (1795/1998) La Philosophie dans le boudoir, in *Œuvres*, vol. 3, Paris: Gallimard Pléiade, pp. 1–178.
Sade, Marquis de (1795/2006) *Philosophy in the Boudoir*, trans. J. Neugroschel, London: Penguin.
Sade, Marquis de (1797/1968) *Juliette*, trans. A. Wainhouse, New York: Grove Press.
Sade, Marquis de (1806/1991) 'Last Will and Testament of Donatien-Alphonse-François Sade, Man of Letters', in *Justine, Philosophy in the Bedroom, Eugénie de Franval, and Other Writings*, trans. A. Wainhouse and R. Seaver, London: Arrow Books, pp. 155–157.
Sade, Marquis de (1904) *Les 120 journées de Sodome, ou l'École du libertinage*, publié pour la première fois d'après le manuscrit original, avec des annotations scientifiques par le Dr Eugène Dühren, Paris: Club des bibliophiles.
Sade, Marquis de (1997) *Lettres à sa femme*, Arles: Actes Sud.
Saint-Just, A.-L. de (1794/2004) 'Institutions républicaines', in A. Kupiec and M. Abensour (Eds.), *Œuvres complètes*, Paris: Gallimard, pp. 1085–1147.
Sarfati, S. (1930) *Essai médico-psychologique sur le Marquis de Sade*, Lyon: Bosc Frères et Riou.
Sartre, J.-P. (1943/1989) 'No Exit' ('*Huis clos*'), in *No Exit and Three Other Plays*, trans. S. Gilbert, New York/London: Vintage, pp. 1–46.

Schaeffer, N. (1999) *The Marquis de Sade: A Life*, Cambridge, MA: Harvard University Press.
Sollers, Ph. (1977) 'Lettre de Sade', *Obliques*, 12/13, pp. 213–217.
Sophocles (1998) *Antigone, Women of Trachis, Philoctetes, Oedipus at Colonus*, ed. and trans. H. Lloyd-Jones, Cambridge, MA: Harvard University Press.
Whitehead, A. N. (1929/1978) *Process and Reality: An Essay in Cosmology*, corrected edition, ed. D. R. Griffin and D. W. Sherburne, New York: The Free Press.

7

THE SUBVERSION OF THE SUBJECT AND THE DIALECTIC OF DESIRE IN THE FREUDIAN UNCONSCIOUS

Fabio Vighi

Context

Jacques Lacan's famous text '*The Subversion of the Subject and the Dialectic of Desire in the Freudian Unconscious*' (henceforth *Subversion*), usually regarded among the most impenetrable of all his *Écrits*, was presented at the conference '*La Dialectique*' ['*The Dialectic*'], organized by Jean Wahl and held at Royaumont, France, on September 19–23, 1960. It can be argued that this complex text is organized around three overarching themes which Lacan presents and elaborates in different directions. First, Lacan claims that his psychoanalytic method should be granted scientific status as it is rooted in praxis. Second, he argues that the analytic field allows for a thorough critique of the limitations of modern science and philosophy by expanding on the Freudian discoveries in relation to knowledge, subjectivity and desire. Finally, he contends that the subject of psychoanalysis is divided by the intervention of the signifier (language), which brings about desire while reconfiguring the function of the drives. In conjunction with this last contention, *Subversion* marks a major shift in Lacan's thought by reframing the function of desire as presented in *Seminar VII* (*The Ethics of Psychoanalysis*, 1959–1960).[1] Especially in the second part of the text, the dialectic of desire is connoted as a protective mechanism which allows the subject of the unconscious to confront and partly neutralize the threat represented by the inconsistent / lacking status of the Other (the symbolic order of signification). By contrast, the Freudian drives are re-elaborated by Lacan against the background of symbolic castration and are thereby accorded a new role in relation to the non-existence of Other itself.

The title of the conference offers Lacan the opportunity to establish from the outset the central theme of the essay, namely the subversion of the subject as related to the psychoanalytic dialectic of desire. It soon becomes apparent that Lacan intends to set up his understanding of the dialectic against two dominant epistemological fields of his day, namely Hegelian philosophy and the scientific discourse. Throughout his intervention Lacan uses considerable irony to debunk the pretenses of epistemological self-assurance driving those discourses on subjectivity that he sees as opposed to the psychoanalytic praxis. As is well known, Lacan's reading of Hegel's dialectic was heavily influenced by Alexander Kojève (see Roudinesco 1993/1997: 88–106). This influence undoubtedly transpires through *Subversion*, where Lacan seems to target polemically the widely shared reading of dialectical progress in Hegel understood as leading to a synthetic and panlogicist apprehension of the coincidence of knowledge and truth. Similarly, he is eager to debunk the Cartesian foundations of scientific empiricism. To put it bluntly, the subject of science only *thinks* he knows what he is doing, ignoring the centrality of that 'point of ignorance' (*Subversion* 672, 2) on which Lacan's entire edifice, as we shall see, is based. In order to counter Hegelianism and scientific discourse, Lacan from the outset of *Subversion* introduces the insubordinate dimension of the subject of the unconscious in its relation to knowledge. The irony, in this respect, is unmistakable. What it targets is the paradox of 'knowing without knowing' that, according to Lacan, qualifies both the Hegelian and the scientific accounts of the subject.[2] Hegel, particularly, is a recurrent reference in the opening pages of *Subversion*. In Lacan's eyes, despite the centrality of negation in his dialectic, Hegel is ultimately the philosopher of metaphysical closure, the thinker whose system of tireless *Aufhebung* (sublation) relies on the fact that "the subject knows what he wants" (679, 9).[3] In truth, from the outset Lacan specifies that his reference to Hegel is "entirely didactic" and serves the purpose of showing "where things stand regarding the question of the subject such as psychoanalysis properly subverts it" (672, 4). In this essay I will not attempt to explore or challenge Lacan's reception of Hegelian dialectics, as this task would take me beyond the remit of my commentary. I will limit myself to note that, while Lacan here marks his departure from Hegel, at the same time he uses the structural composition of Hegel's dialectic as a springboard to both develop his own dialectic of desire and find a way of engaging with an audience that, as he puts it in the opening paragraph – and not without a touch of sarcasm – "is supposed to be philosophically sophisticated" (671, 1).

Commentary on the text

Analytical praxis

Lacan's introduction of the subversion of the subject is supported, initially, by repeated references to the practical justification of psychoanalysis, which are meant to distance his analytical method from philosophical thought as such, as well as from scientific empiricism. Indeed, Lacan has often referred to his own work as being, in essence, anti-philosophical, if only because driven by the reference to a recalcitrant dimension of the human psyche that resists theoretical capture. Lacan introduces this point with a reference to the centrality of structure ("A structure is constitutive of the praxis known as psychoanalysis", 671, 1) followed by the claim that the subject is conveniently situated on the basis of its relationship to knowledge. In this respect, the specific aim of *Subversion* is to outline the ambiguity upon which the rapport between subject and knowledge is established in psychoanalysis.

As anticipated, the ironic reference to science (671, 6–7 and 672, 1–2) allows Lacan to reassert the primacy of psychoanalytic praxis. First, he claims that what qualifies him to follow the psychoanalytic path is "my experience of this praxis. What made me decide to do so [...] is a failure of theory coupled with abuses in its transmission, which, while presenting no dangers for praxis itself, result, in both cases, in a total absence of scientific status" (672, 5). While claiming that contemporary theory lacks scientific status, Lacan also conveniently appeases his audience of philosophers with the following remark: "Nevertheless, I shall take advantage of your kindness in assuming we agree that a science cannot be conditioned upon empiricism" (672, 8). Here we arrive, indirectly at least, at a definition of a 'psychoanalytic science' which is sustained by analytic experience but refuses blind empiricism. If anything, this is one way of defining the ambiguity of the relationship between subject and knowledge as understood by Lacan, while also introducing the central theme of the essay, namely the *subversion* of the subject. The empirical method of modern science is also the object of Lacan's scorn in his subsequent references to psychology, which he claims he challenges

> precisely because, as I will show, the function of the subject, as inaugurated by Freudian experience, disqualifies from the outset what, going by the name 'psychology', merely perpetuates an academic framework, no matter how one dresses up its premises.
>
> (672, 9–10)

Later he will confirm this view by referring to "the Philistines of general psychology" (695, 4).

Lacan's position is thus clear from the start. It is both assertive and polemical, in as much as it challenges "the unity of the subject" (673, 1) as a presupposition of both philosophical enquiry and psychology. In Philippe Van Haute's words:

> According to Lacan, academic psychology can provide no solace here; for it assumes the unity of the subject whose various properties and functions it studies, without pausing even for a moment to consider the scientific validity of this assumption. The emphasis on the unity of an essentially "knowing" subject goes together with the idea that the psyche has to be understood as a functional double (*doublure*) of the organism. The psyche must assist the organism in

> its attempt to adapt itself to reality. Just like psychoanalytic orthodoxy, academic psychology believes that psychic life must be understood primarily and fundamentally as "adaptation", or in terms of an "adaptive" problematic.
>
> (2001: xxviii–xxix)

The criticism Lacan levels against the academia can legitimately be regarded as an anticipation of the University discourse, which he introduced in the late 1960s. In a similar vein, Lacan decries the attention given by "a whole body of traditional thought" (673, 2) to empirically verifiable states of consciousness supposed to represent the limitless or the ineffable which, he adds with proud conviction, find no room in 'Freudian practice' (673, 4). He refers specifically to "the states of enthusiasm described by Plato", namely states of inspired consciousness that find expression in acts of ecstasy and rapture; "the degrees of samadhi in Buddhism", where consciousness becomes completely absorbed in the object of meditation; and "the experience (*Erlebnis*) one has under the influence of hallucinogens" (673, 2), where the use of the German word *Erlebnis* (translatable roughly as 'immediate lived experience') is intended as a reference to phenomenology. What is hereby confirmed is the seemingly "heretical" status of Lacan's method of enquiry, at once rooted in analytic praxis and yet eschewing empiricism. The reason for this is immediately and, dare I say, intuitively obvious: the praxis of which Lacan speaks in his "return to Freud" concerns unconscious formations rather than self-evident facts, sensory experience or the above-mentioned hypnoid states of mind (673, 4–7 and 674, 1). And the unconscious, as Lacan here confirms, "speaks", that is, it is made of language:

> I have some difficulty in getting across – in a circle infatuated with the most incredible illogicality – what it means to interrogate the unconscious as I do, that is, to the point at which it gives a reply that is not some sort of ravishment or takedown, but is rather a 'saying why'.
>
> (673, 8)

In the unconscious, Lacan adds, one can detect 'a sort of logic' in the form, for example, of "an interrogative voice or even the development of an argument" (673, 9).

Freud's Copernican turn

After his polemically charged introduction, Lacan turns to Freud's so-called Copernican turn, that is to say, the discovery of the unconscious as the central agency of subjectivity (674, 2). However, he immediately warns against any facile appropriation of such metaphor: the very positing of a gravitational centre, whether earth or sun (whether consciousness or the unconscious), is at risk of generating "a lure": "by exalting the center, heliocentrism is no less of a lure than seeing the earth as the center", while "the existence of the ecliptic probably provided a more stimulating model of our relations with truth" (674, 4). At the core of Lacan's argument lies the notion of *disavowal*, which should be considered the very staple of his dialectic of desire. He makes the meaning of disavowal clear with a mention to Darwin: it is not because men have been told that they originate from monkeys that they stop believing that they are "the best among the creatures, for it is precisely of this that he [Darwin] convinces them" (674, 5). In other words, it is precisely because we know that we are not by natural right at the centre of the universe (as we originate from monkeys) that we are easily lured into believing that we are superior creatures, for instance by way of cultural acquisition. Here Lacan is claiming that the relativization of truth through scientific knowledge paradoxically ends up strengthening the *effect* of truth, since the latter has a chance, as it were, to operate stealthily – or, to use the obvious term, unconsciously. This is what Lacan refers to as "the doctrine of double truth", where knowledge shatters old religious beliefs while at the same time providing a new "regime of truth" (674, 8). Along these lines, we could argue that it is not because we know that our adaptation to the socio-symbolic order never fully succeeds that we stop acting as if we were perfectly adapted.

Without Lacan stating it explicitly, the above point can also be deployed in relation to what is commonly referred to as 'ideology critique'. To put it in a nutshell: beliefs have a chance to operate more effectively when one is convinced that there is nothing worth believing in – when all the evidence that would justify belief is rationally dismantled.[4] It is in this sense that the discovery of the subject of the unconscious – a subject guided by a logic that remains radically disavowed – acquires political weight. Starting from *Subversion*, and especially throughout the 1960s, Lacan becomes increasingly aware that the psychoanalytic discourse offers a uniquely powerful arsenal of critical tools to confront what he regards as the central lure of modernity. His argument can be summarized as follows: despite the impact of the discourse of scientific objectivity, with its demolition of the ancient metaphysical truths and concurrent attempted abolition of the subject, 'things' (the insertion and manipulation of the subject within the socio-symbolic network) keep functioning efficiently *through belief*. The paradox that psychoanalysis has a chance to express is that without explicit ideological parameters ideology thrives all the better. Put differently, psychoanalysis testifies to the presence of "a new seism" (675, 2) occurring at the border between knowledge and truth – a seism that science cannot register. Here Lacan dedicates a long paragraph to Hegel's dialectic, criticizing it as a system of thought where "what is disturbing about truth is constantly reabsorbed" (675, 3). In Lacan's view, the dialectic is defined by its thrust toward an absolute knowledge where the symbolic (i.e. knowledge) connects with "a real from which nothing more can be expected", giving shape to "a subject finalized in his self-identity" (675, 3).

Psychoanalysis, however, as well as "the history of science itself", presents a different picture, one where "the thesis / antithesis / synthesis dialectic" is constantly proved implausible (675, 4).

Far from establishing a perfect and seamless conjuncture of knowledge and truth, then, psychoanalysis draws attention to "a number of creaks", reminding us that "it is elsewhere that the moment of truth must sound for this field of knowledge as for others" (675, 5). This psychoanalytic truth is thus akin to a return of the repression of truth in Hegel's "absolute subject" and in science's "abolished subject" (676, 2). In the Freudian field, Lacan continues, what emerges is "the skewed relation that separates the subject from sex" (676, 3), in other words the predominance of the subject of the unconscious as opposed to the predominance of the subject of consciousness characterizing psychology as well as phenomenology. By the same token, the unconscious cannot be defined via the negation of consciousness (676, 4), but is instead a "chain of signifiers that repeats and insists somewhere [...] interfering in the cuts offered it by actual discourse and the cogitation it informs" (676, 5). At this stage in his teaching, Lacan is keen to insist on the linguistic composition of the unconscious ("the crucial term is the signifier", 676, 6), going some distance in his attempt to link Freud's 'Copernican turn' with a structuralist agenda that he believes Freud anticipated (given the centrality in Freud of linguistic tropes such as metaphor and metonymy) but could not fully embrace owing to the self-evident historical gap with modern linguistics.[5] But aside of this question, the central theme for Lacan here is that of the signifier and its relevance for the subject of the unconscious. Crucially for him the signifier does not reflect a pre-existent reality, but it creates meanings out of its combinations with other signifiers. Signifiers are independent from the reality they structure.[6]

Now, for Freud the unconscious is not made of language because it exists independently of reality. This is what Lacan also states by claiming the opposite to what Freud claims, that is, that the unconscious is constituted by a chain of signifiers (677, 1–2). In both Lacan and Freud, then, the unconscious does not have to do with (historical) reality. The difference between the two is that Freud conceives of language as inextricably linked to the reality it refers to, whereas for Lacan language (the signifier) is in its deepest connotation remains autonomous from reality, it intersects and signifies. It is Lacan's view that language at its most elementary is unconscious, and as such independent of the historical context while representing the very deadlock of history itself. Because the Lacanian unconscious is made of language, it obeys the linguistic patterns of metaphor and metonymy rather than condensation and displacement as Freud had thought (677, 1–2).

The split subject of the unconscious

After this clarification, Lacan is ready to ask the question that no doubt is central to his intervention: "Once the structure of language is recognized in the unconscious, what sort of subject can we conceive of for it?" (677, 2). He claims that if the 'I' qua grammatical subject of the statement (or of the enunciated) represents the speaking subject, at the same time it "does not signify him" (677, 3–4). In other words, the 'I' is what linguists know as a shifter, a signifier whose role is to 'anchor' or 'root' the sentence by attributing a subject to it (677, 3). In itself, however – that is to say, irrespective of the enunciated content – it does not signify anything, let alone a speaking subject. To the question 'Who is speaking?', then, we can only answer: a divided subject (the unconscious subject of the enunciation as opposed to the subject of the enunciated); a subject who undergoes a fading, and who therefore leads us to a frontier, or a cut, where something is elided, decreeing the fundamental opacity concerning what the signifier 'I' actually stands for. To demonstrate how the subject of the enunciation can make its appearance in the statement in different ways than as the shifter 'I', Lacan uses here the example of the expletive *ne* in French, a signifier considered superfluous by grammarians, but whose elision would reduce the emphasis of the enunciation that carries its message. By eliminating the expletive *ne* from a polemical sentence (exemplified by Lacan's own polemical attack against grammarians), the same sentence would turn into an impersonal assertion deprived of its crucial caustic or mocking edge (677, 4).

In an explicit reference to Freud, Lacan reminds us of how slips of the tongue, jokes and so on provide clear evidence for the 'insistence' of this divided subject, to the extent that, as he puts it in another polemical innuendo, this time to Heidegger's philosophy, "we are astonished the hunt for Dasein hasn't made any more of it" (678, 1). Lacan clarifies how the unconscious subject of the enunciation emerges unexpectedly in the cut of discourse, as "a bar between the signifier and the signified" (678, 2). Only via this cut, Lacan specifies, are we able to locate the subject:

> The cut made by the signifying chain is the only cut that verifies the structure of the subject as a discontinuity in the real. If linguistics enables us to see the signifier as the determinant of the signified, analysis reveals the truth of this relationship by making holes in meaning the determinants of its discourse.
>
> (678, 3)

More succinctly put: the psychoanalytic discourse endorses modern linguistics' affirmation of the priority of the signifier over the signified, but only insofar as such priority reveals the truthfulness of the failed connection between the two terms. And the subject stands precisely for such short-circuiting of signifier and signified.

Insofar as we are talking about the subject of the unconscious, or of the enunciation, the subjective agency in question is never in complete control of the statement. Quite on the contrary, the subject is spoken by its statement, in the precise sense that the subject materializes the cuts (contradictions, failures, gaps, etc.) produced by the statement itself. This is what causes the fading of the 'I' in the grip of "an ever purer signifier" (678, 1) – a signifier that reveals its autonomy from the signifed. In *My Teaching* (Lacan, 2005/2008: 36), Lacan states that the subject of the enunciation is "the subject not insofar as it produces discourse but insofar as it is produced [*fait*], cornered even [*fait comme un rat*], by discourse". This inversion of the rapport between subject and enunciation is of extraordinary importance if we are to grasp Lacan's discourse theory. The central issue at stake can be summarized as follows: it is not that the subject constructs a discourse which is by definition ambiguous in relation to its truth-value – from Lacan's angle, this is the misplaced starting point of any traditional epistemology. Rather, Lacan asserts that any discourse by definition comes from 'out there' (from the Other), being structured around an ontological cut whose name is 'subject'. This means that we are by definition alienated in the Other: there is always something intrinsically fake in our discourse, since it is always-already operative outside ourselves, and it reproduces itself through our being radically split.

While our identity is moulded by the Other, then, the subject as such, the subject of the unconscious, makes its appearance in those gaps, inconsistencies and contradictions (cuts) produced by discourse (language) as it informs subjectivity. For this precise reason the cut of which Lacan speaks intersects both objectivity and subjectivity. For Lacan, Freud's famous motto *Wo Es war, soll Ich werden* owes its significance to this subject of the unconscious causing the fading of the 'I'. In Lacan's interpretation, which updates his previous ones by centering on language, the *Ich* ('I') as signifier has a chance to "come into being by disappearing from the statement" (678, 6). It is worth noting that Lacan refers to Freud's motto as a "pre-Socratic gnome" (678, 4), in other words a maxim or aphorism that he associates with the wisdom of the pre-Socratic tradition, where being and thinking were considered reciprocal and inseparable.[7]

How else can we grasp this paradoxical disappearing of the 'I' from and through the statement? Lacan offers a suggestive definition when he says that it happens "through an enunciation that makes a human being tremble due to the vacillation that comes back to him from his own statement" (679, 2).[8] This means, in essence, that the truth of any message is the fading of the 'I', its disappearance in/from the statement, for the simple reason that the 'I' as signifier is always-already dead – like the 'dead father' from the famous dream related by Freud that Lacan here refers to –[9] but sustains itself precisely on its ignorance concerning his non-existence. The 'I' "comes on the scene as a subject who is conjugated with the double aporia of a veritable subsistence that is abolished by his knowledge, and by a discourse in which it is death that sustains existence" (679, 5). Here is the double (dialectical) aporia of which Lacan speaks: on the one hand, there is the psychoanalytic knowledge about the 'I''s radical inconsistency (the cut embodied by the subject of the unconscious) which deprives the 'I' of its "veritable subsistence"; on the other hand, there is a discourse, in which the function of desire is nestled, that sustains the 'I' by preventing it from encountering its psychoanalytic truth, namely the fact that it is always-already dead.

It is important to grasp this central Lacanian topos of the mortifying intervention of language, whose dialectical function is to bring life (sense, communication, intersubjectivity, desire, etc.) *through death*, that is, by enforcing the mortification of being via the statement. What is dialectical is precisely this overlap of existence-through-desire and death: we become 'desiring subjects' by dying to our being. The desire that sustains us is correlative to a deadly cut – the cut of the signifier. Here the novelty of *Subversion* comes to full fruition: far from leading us straight to the subject of the unconscious – the pure and tragic desiring subject of which Lacan speaks in *Seminar VII* apropos Antigone – desire is connoted as a mortifying and alienating agency, always-already characterized by the deadly spell it carries and with which it envelops the subject, determining the content of its subjectivity. Lacan identifies in this understanding of desire the key difference between Freud and Hegel: "in Hegel's work it is desire (*Begierde*) that is given responsibility for the minimal link the subject must retain to Antiquity's knowledge [*connaissance*] if truth is to be immanent in the realization of knowledge" (679, 9). In Freud's work, on the other hand, such desire to know is always the Other's desire (679, 11), that is to say it is bound up with the alienating logic through which subjectivity emerges. The elementary paradox at stake here is the formation of subjectivity (self-consciousness) through what Bruce Fink (2004: 108) calls "a constitutional inscience": the horizon of knowledge emerges for us as the other side of our constitutive lack of knowledge; knowledge as episteme is the effect of our ignorance about the ontological inconsistency of our being. This means that our desire is first and foremost the cipher of our alienation, the mark of our being dead while believing we are alive, which in turn sustains our self-consciousness. Put differently, it is the alienating acquisition of desire that gives us subjective life, while preventing us from realizing that we are always-already dead, mortified by the signifier.

Drive and revolution

At this point (679, 13), Lacan hastens to bring in the death drive as that crucial psychic component of human subjectivity which, as it were, allows us to get in touch with our own 'being dead', that is, with "the margin beyond life that language assures the human being of due to the fact that he speaks" (680, 1). Lacan is very precise here: it is language that makes us aware of a "margin beyond life"; only language leads us to the death drive. It is therefore "in the metaphor of the return to the inanimate" (680, 1) that we encounter the truly revolutionary dimension of Freud's thought, namely his discovery of the centrality of the death drive (*Todestrieb*) as that which lies beyond the pleasure principle, which is why "to evade the death instinct in his [Freud's] doctrine is not to know his doctrine at all" (679, 13). The Freudian drive, Lacan avers, brings into contention a *savoir* that cannot be articulated as *connaissance* (680, 3). Lacan conveys the significance of *savoir* by evoking the figure of the messenger-slave from ancient Greek who "carries under his hair the codicil that condemns him to death" – of which he "knows neither the meaning nor the text, nor in what language [*langue*] it is written, nor even that it was tattooed on his shaven scalp while he was sleeping" (680, 3). Slavery, like death, is a central metaphor in Lacan, insofar as it is linked to the intervention of the signifier, thereby implying that each one of us is enslaved to a *savoir* – the unconscious chain of signifiers – which 'condemns us to death', in the exact sense that it splits us, triggering the emergence of the subject of the enunciated. As Lacan underscores in another famous text, *The Function and Field of Speech and Language in Psychoanalysis*, "we analysts deal with slaves who think they are masters" – who (slavishly) believe in their ego-centric mastery (242). Lacan's point is that there is no escaping our condition of slavery, which is inaugurated by the arrival of the signifier and the logic of desire it installs.

It is at this level that we should detect the novelty of Freud's Copernican revolution, which, as Lacan warns, should not be seen in mere correspondence to heliocentrism: the subject proper is the unwanted, accidental *effect* of the intervention of language (discourse) on the speaking being, in as much as this effect also belongs, originally, as a discursive cut, in the Other (bearing witness to the fact that 'there is no other of the Other'). Revolution, in the specific meaning of 'celestial revolution' (i.e., as for planets, bodies returning to the point of departure by completing the rotation on their axis), is a word Lacan uses twice in this essay, in connection with Freud's discovery of the breach between truth and knowledge, as opposed to (what he believes to be) Hegel's closure of this breach. He clearly assigns fundamental significance to this understanding of revolution, as it will become evident at later stages in his teaching, and perhaps nowhere more significantly than in *Seminar XVII*.[10] Revolution effectively implies for Lacan locating and identifying with the point of incongruence between conscious knowledge and unconscious truth. This incongruence is "the mobility out of which revolutions arise" (679, 10). And it is highly significant that Lacan links this understanding of revolution to what Freud had designated by death drive. So what does the death drive designate in Lacan? Simply put, that conscious signification is sustained by the holing of meaning it causes, the margin or surplus of sense (corresponding to "the inanimate") that, at one and the same time, it attempts to repress in order to function. It is the existence of this hole that the death drive makes manifest, and ultimately embodies. More precisely, this hole is "the margin where this being places in signifying position, not only those parts of his body that lend themselves to this because they are exchangeable, but the body itself" (680, 1). The death drive becomes activated as the unconscious libido that emerges in the signifying chain, materializing the cut or impossibility that signals the presence of the subject. It is for this reason that Lacan refers polemically to the supposed relationship between psychoanalysis and physiology (680, 4–6). Since its inception, he claims, psychoanalysis has contributed nothing to physiology, for the psychoanalytic concern with the real of the body and its "imaginary mental schema" (680, 6) cannot be integrated within a doctrine whose interest lies in the developmental constitution of the body. In such doctrine, the developmental stages "function first and foremost like elements of a heraldry, a heraldry of the body. This is confirmed by the use that is made of them in reading children's drawings" (680, 3). Lacan's polemical target here would seem to be object-relation theory, where the developmental (psychogenetic) perspective is confirmed by the observation that the subject's relation to the partial objects is progressively assimilated within the relation with the body as a whole – hence the reference to children's drawings, which would confirm such theory.

The first graph of desire

Yet, in order to grasp the full significance of the drive, Lacan needs first to introduce desire in its relation to the subject of the signifier. Again, the aim is to reject the accusation that his psychoanalytic theory has been "lured by a purely dialectical exhaustion of being" (681, 2), since he clearly endorses "desire's irreducibility to demand", which is "the very mainspring of what also prevents it from being reduced to need" (681, 3). In fact, it is the awareness of desire's intrinsic aporia – its being articulated but also its not being fully articulable – that, as we shall see, will lead Lacan to validate what we could call an ethics of the drive. Desire, in other words, is from this point on conceived as intimately connected to the drive. It is at this stage that Lacan introduces his topology (Figure 7.1).

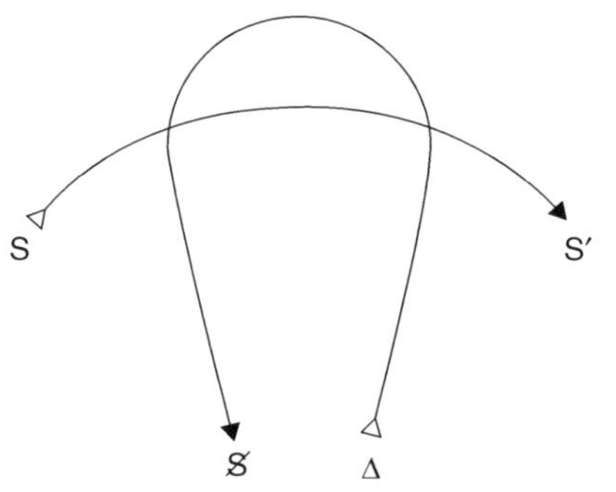

Figure 7.1 Lacan's Graph 1

The first formulation of his graph of desire (its "elementary cell"; 681, 5) "will serve here to show where desire is situated in relation to a subject defined on the basis of his articulation by the signifier" (681, 4). Such formulation, which Lacan had already built up in two seminars of the late 1950s (*Seminar V* and *Seminar VI*), and which he will continue to develop in the late 1960s (*Seminar XVI*), is fairly straightforward. It consists, simply put, of the intervention of language upon the indeterminate, pre-linguistic flux of life in which the subject is immersed. We thus have the signifying chain, represented by the vector S→S' (left to right), and the "fish-hook" or "horse-shoe" vector of subjectivation Δ→*\$* (right to left). The key point to underline when looking at the elementary cell of the graph is that the body on its own does not produce any meanings whatsoever; in order to do so, it has to be intercepted by a signifying chain – by language and the symbolization it carries. Furthermore, this sense-creating intervention is ultimately enabled by the signifier qua *point de capiton*,[11] that is, the loop caused by the signifier that halts the otherwise infinite sliding of the signifying chain (681, 5). The living trajectory of the being of needs (Δ), who merely seeks satisfaction, is intercepted by language, and it is through this linguistic/cultural capture that biological needs will be transformed into desires. Thus, the subject of desire, insofar as it is the subject of the signifier, is irreducibly split, 'out of joint', never transparent or coincidental with itself (*\$*).

Evidence of the alienating grafting of language on the body is the fact that linguistic signification works retroactively through the *point de capiton* (682, 1). To give an example of this retroactive function, Lacan mentions the signification obtained by a sentence through its last term (682, 2): it is only thanks to the choice of a term that puts an end to a given sentence that the latter can, retroactively, secure a meaning. While the definition of the diachronic (retroactive, or "negatively oriented" 682, 1) working of language is relatively unproblematic, synchronically things are more complicated (682, 3). To understand what allows the signifying chain to begin and sustain its course, we must return to the initial operation by which the signifier is raised to its proper function.

Lacan uses as an example the way in which the child deals with a signifier by disconnecting it from its symbolic attributions, an operation which makes room for "the sophistics of signification" (682, 3) precisely by bringing the signifier to its 'zero level', its original emptiness. What is at work here is not metonymy, which functions diachronically, but metaphor:

> It is metaphor insofar as the first attribution is constituted in it – the attribution that promulgates 'the dog goes meow, the cat goes woof-woof,' by which, in one fell swoop, the child, by disconnecting the thing from its cry, raises the sign to the function of the signifier and reality to the sophistics of signification, and in his contempt for

> verisimilitude, makes necessary the verification of multiple objectifications of the same thing.
>
> (682, 3)

Here the meaning of metaphor in Lacan's synchronic conception of the signifier comes to full fruition. Initially, and fundamentally, metaphor means nothing but the power to disconnect from its apparently self-evident attributions in order to bring to the surface the emptiness of the signifier, its *purely literal function*: originally, the signifier means nothing but itself, the materiality of its own 'letter'. And metaphor at its purest, as evidenced by the child's disconnecting skills, makes manifest the absolute self-referentiality of the signifier. Thus the child effectively 'begins from the beginning', from the zero level of signification, returning the signifier to its constitutive meaninglessness. As Van Haute (2001: 65–66) puts it, underscoring the founding role of metaphorization in the subjective construction of reality:

> A child who says that a dog meows and a cat barks disconnects the sound that imitates the cry (onomatopoeia) from the object (dog, cat), and in this way it breaks through the univocal relation between the sound and the object to make the sound into a signifier. [...] from now on the child can freely signify reality without taking account of what reality announces at first sight or 'naturally' [...]. This break is therefore equiprimordial with the process of metaphorization. For in the metaphor, new meanings forever arise from the mere substitution of one signifier by another, independent of any founding reference to a reality that might motivate this substitution.

A signifying chain, Lacan tells us, cannot sustain itself without this hidden presupposition. That is to say, the constitutive emptiness of the signifier is the synchronous condition of possibility of the diachronous character of signification; such emptiness cannot be eliminated, since it secretly 'props up' any signification. The elementary function of the signifier is that of *representing the space of representation itself*: it opens up such space with its empty presence. This is what Freud intended to signal with the expression *Vorstellungrepräsentanz*, translated as "ideational representative" in the Standard Edition of his work. It is in this hidden or disavowed function that Lacan situates the subject proper. As such, the subject does not represent (the supposition of) knowledge – which we find in the Other qua "rubbish dump of the representatives representing the supposition of knowledge" (S9, 1961–1962, session 15 November 1961) – but rather it represents *representativeness itself*, embodying the very condition of possibility of symbolic representation.

By now it should be clear that Lacan departs from Ferdinand de Saussure's conceptualization of the sign by detaching the signifier from the signified, and giving priority to the former. Crucially, it is at the level of the signifier that he locates the subject. However, which signifier? As it will be further clarified in the first Seminars of the 1960s, the signifier in question is the unary trait, which owing to its structural necessity precedes the formation of the subject. See, for example, the following statement from *Seminar X*:

> There is no conceivable appearance of a subject as such than starting with the first introduction of a signifier and of the simplest signifier [...] the unary trait. The unary trait is before the subject. In the beginning was the word means in the beginning there was the unary trait.
> (Lacan, S10, 1962–1963: 21)

So here Lacan affirms, *in nuce*, the fundamental necessity, yet also ambiguity, of the unary trait, which later he will define as master signifier: it creates meaning by halting the signifying chain, but at the same time it is the radically empty and meaningless (*insignifiante*) signifier which secures the identification of the subject of the unconscious (683, 1). A successor of Freud's ego-ideal, the unary trait is for Lacan strictly necessary for the emergence of the subject of the unconscious. In this respect, the Other as "treasure trove of signifiers" (682, 5) is the locus where signifiers can be found and collected according to a simple logic of opposition, since no signifying chain is therein initially constituted.

Lacan (682, 5) emphasizes the dissymmetry between A (the Other) and *s*(A) (the signification emerging through the Other via the *point de capiton*, the mechanism whereby meaning is created out of infinite signifying possibilities or differentiations). These are the two points where the subjective vector intersects the signifying chain in the first graph. It is in the trajectory covering these two points that the subject effectively "submits to the signifier" (682, 8), though this submission never completely works out. First, the subject encounters A as the "treasure trove of signifiers": language in its disconnected, uncoordinated status, the locus where signifiers exist outside signification and yet, by simply being there, function as a break with the real (think, again, of the child's utterly baffling first encounter within language). It is only through this self-distancing of the Real, effected through the encounter with signifiers, that the possibility of/from signification, and truth, begin to materialize. Then, we have the second encounter with the signifying vector in the form of what, as Lacan states, is not a locus (a place), but "a moment (a scansion, rather than a duration)" – in other words it embodies a different temporality (682, 6). This second encounter, which retains a retroactive value inasmuch as it casts meaning upon the first intersection with the signifying chain, corresponds to the precarious temporal point at which language begins to make sense; as such, it corresponds to "the punctuation, in which signification ends as a finished product" (682, 5).

The subject's submission to the signifier, then, is completed when the subject encounters the signifier qua *point de capiton*, whose strength lies, paradoxically, in both *embodying* and *negating* the fundamental meaninglessness of the signifier itself as initially encountered in the first stage of the trajectory of subjectivation. What we should note here is Lacan's conviction that meaning arises not from the connection between language and reality, but, strictly speaking, between language and itself – that is, from the very articulation of the signifiers, which as such is not predicated upon the direct signification of external reality. The basic ambiguity of this operation can be described as follows: on the one hand, the existence of the subject depends on the encounter with the signifiers; on the other, such encounter will never return a fully consistent subjectivity, since the subject will never fully coincide with the Other. Ultimately, the movement between A and *s*(A) cannot be completed owing to its being profoundly tautological, that is, founded on nothing other than itself (it has only itself as guarantee of its production of sense). And the subject inhabits the very inconsistency that underlies the process of subjectivation.

Circular retroactivity

Lacan at this stage adds a significant twist to his argument by claiming that the movement between the two points of interception is not only retroactive, but circular, for meaning is formed "in the circuit that goes from *s*(A) to A and back from A to *s*(A)" (682, 8). The emphasis on retroactivity is clearly aimed at stressing the profoundly illusory character of signification, which relies on the ruse whereby language erases the traces of its own ontological inconsistency, that is to say it closes the gap initially opened by the signifier itself when attempting to inscribe a break in the meaningless continuity of the real. However, while the movement from *s*(A) to A captures the birth of signification through the 'necessary imposture' of the concealment of lack, the second movement, from A to *s*(A), is equivalent to a sort of 'sealing' of such signification, insofar as with that movement the subject erases the traces of retroactivity and identifies with the (falsely) linear, chronological formation of meaning.

It is interesting, in the context of Lacan's aforementioned critique of Hegelian dialectics, to observe how this circular movement effectively consists of a sort of 'double illusion', which corresponds to Hegel's notion of 'negation of negation'[12] the third moment in the dialectic. While the second intersection – *s*(A) – is equivalent to a first negation of the status of the signifier ('the signifier is/was not meaningless'), it is only with the attempt at squaring the circle that we get the 'negation of negation', which truly bolsters signification while creating an unconscious 'surplus of sense'. For this second negation does not merely assert that the signifier *was not meaningless*, but, rather, *it negates the very possibility of meaninglessness* by constructing the illusion that the signifier was always-already inserted in a consistent signifying chain. The second negation, that is, the movement 'back forward' from A to *s*(A), is thus the truly generative moment, for it allows the subject to gain a distance from the traces of meaninglessness that still haunted the first negation (inasmuch as meaninglessness was still a predicate, albeit in a negative modality). However – and this is the key Hegelian issue at stake – the whole point of Lacan's insistence on the double movement constitutive of signification is that it produces, ultimately, the opposite of what it seeks to produce: the very deadlock of signification; in other words, it creates the inconsistency that affects language, thus thwarting any communication, and ending up splitting the subject (since $ is the end result of the double intersection of subject and language).

To recapitulate: the subject first encounters language in its uncoordinated meaninglessness (A), and yet to be in a position to perceive such meaninglessness as antagonism or deadlock it has to assume the burden of signification, which is what takes place with the intervention of the *point de capiton* and consequent determination of *s*(A). Only at this stage does negativity truly surface (as with Hegel's 'negation of negation'): the attempt at squaring the circle by 'sublating' a given predicate (the meaninglessness of the signifier) opens up the abyssal inconsistency that the predicate alone could not represent.

In Lacan, then, the fundamental ambiguity concerning the rapport between 'subject' and 'signification through the Other' is of the dialectical kind: on the one hand, to form an identity the subject must submit to language; on the other hand:

> [t]his squaring of the circle is nevertheless impossible, but solely because the subject constitutes himself only by subtracting himself from it and by decompleting it essentially, such that he must, at one and the same time, count himself here and function only as a lack here.
>
> (683, 3)

What Lacan alludes to here is the paradox of 'including oneself out', which captures perfectly the dialectic at work in the formation of subjectivity. The subject of the unconscious, in other words, is the very lack or gap within signification that must be excluded (or rather, included out) if signification is to emerge. The question of the simultaneity of the signifier qua lack and the endless shifting of signification is therefore confirmed here as central to Lacan's theory of the subject. Put differently, the 'passage through the Other', with its potentially endless shifting significations, is the necessary move that enables us not only to begin to form our subjectivity, but also to apprehend such subjectivity as deeply antagonized by the subject at its heart, which incarnates the impossibility to 'square the circle'. This means that the structural consistency obtained at the subjective level via the detour through the Other is predicated upon the ultimate meaninglessness of the signifier. Although what we get back from the immersion in the battery of signifiers is the precious gift of signification, the key point underscored by Lacan is that such gift is strictly co-terminus with the signifier as the foundational lack of signification, which materializes in the unconscious – thus confirming that the subject is at once included in and subtracted from the signifying chain itself.

To feign feigning

In this way Lacan effectively does away with any psychological notion of depth, since he tells us that the formation of our subjectivity, inclusive of its unconscious underside, takes place through a process of radical externalization, or self-ejection. It is from the Other that we acquire those significations that determine us insofar as they are, as it were, suspended upon the signifier, whose meaninglessness is constitutive of the process of signification while also making such process deeply inconsistent and destined to fail. The importance of the Other cannot be underestimated and is repeatedly highlighted by Lacan (683, 4–5), particularly when he claims that it plays the role of "Truth's witness" (683, 6). Why? Because what makes the Other the ultimate guarantor of signification is that *it redoubles the deception of language*, working as the fictional (mythical) framework where all available signifiers are supposed to be found. As such, the very fact that we speak is turned into the ultimate truthful horizon of the human condition.[13]

Here, again, it is impossible not to notice the radical ambiguity of Lacan's contention. While the Other is the lure that secures meaning, by the same token (that is, precisely because it is a lure) it also captures the intrinsic instability of language. This ambiguity is inscribed in famous Lacanian propositions such as 'there is no meta-language' or 'there is no Other of the Other.' While asserting that there is no alterity sustaining our linguistic (fictional) essence effectively establishes such essence as necessary, at the same time it makes it deeply inconsistent: it makes truth and inconsistency coincide. In other words, language is truthful in its radical inability to secure meanings. Yet another way of reading Lacan's formulation regarding the Other is by saying that it frames us by framing the language that frames us; what is at stake in the functioning of the Other is therefore a double frame which turns the very act of framing enforced by language into self-framing. While alienating us, language is always-already self-alienated, immersed in its own intrinsic and therefore unsurpassable otherness. The Other works as a sort of detached background (akin to the eye of a witness) to the deceptiveness of language, without which the "the deceptiveness of Speech would be indistinguishable from the feint" (683, 6). This means that if language promotes and sustains the formation of subjectivity through alienation, at the same time there is no alternative to such alienation, inasmuch as language is rooted in the form of its otherness alone, the unwritten symbolic presupposition (witness) of language's efficacy. Lacan's point is that reality for us emerges as a result of an illusion (language qua fiction) sustained only by its own fictional horizon. The feint, for humans, is always redoubled in the feigning of the feint, which is what makes the Symbolic the true horizon of our lives.[14]

In brief, the Other's function is, as Lacan puts it, to "feign feigning" (683, 6)[15] – every deception at the level of the statement is a pretense of deception, since the signifier by definition lies at the level of the statement (or enunciated) but tells the truth insofar as this lie is always-already part of the symbolic lure designated by the Other. It is exactly through its role as that which redoubles deception into a pretense of deception that the Other functions as the locus of truth, for if there was only the first (linguistic) deception, then the truth would be elsewhere. This is why, as Lacan states, the signifier "requires another locus – the locus of the Other, the Other as witness, the witness who is Other than any of the partners – for the Speech borne by the signifier to be able to lie, that is, to posit itself as Truth" (684, 1). Again, it is only as a fiction inserted in a fictional structure that language accomplishes its task – in order to work, it has to rely on this Other qua fictional repository of all signifiers: "Truth draws its guarantee from somewhere other than the Reality it concerns: it draws it from Speech. Just as it is from Speech that Truth receives the mark that instates it in a fictional structure" (684, 2).

The second graph of desire

At this point, Lacan proceeds to introduce the second stage of the graph of desire (Figure 7.2), where the fish-hook vector of subjectivity, which indicated the passage from the subject of needs to the barred subject (Δ→$), is replaced by a vector (also negatively oriented) that signals the move from the barred subject to the ego-ideal as the first substantial identification of the subject ($→I(A)). As ego-ideal, the matheme I(A) stands at the point of symbolic identification outside myself, where I see myself from another's point of view.[16] Lacan specifies that what is described in this second graph "is a

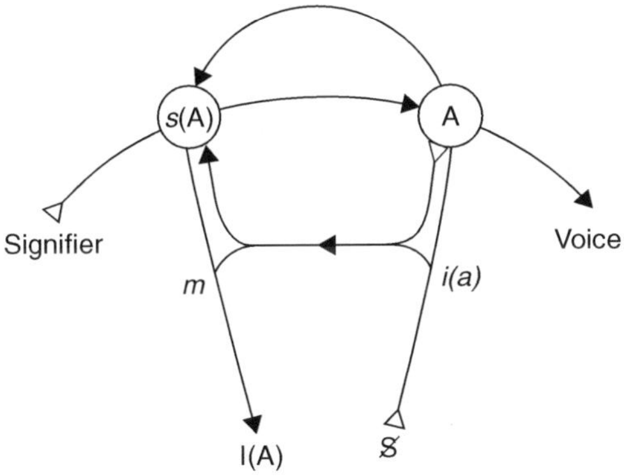

Figure 7.2 Lacan's Graph 2

retroactive effect by which the subject, at each stage, becomes what he was (to be) [*était*] before that, and 'he will have been' is only announced in the future perfect tense" (684, 6). We are dealing with symbolic identification, which the subject catches a glimpse of by looking back upon itself after arriving at *\$* as described in the first graph.

The main novelty of the second graph, therefore, is the outlining of the imaginary capture, which supplements the founding role of language in the formation of subjectivity. It is important to note how, by 1960, the imaginary dimension, which had been Lacan's central category in the 1930s and 1940s, comes in after the elementary symbolic capture (first graph), the latter having concerned Lacan throughout the 1950s. This means that by the time of *Subversion* Lacan views the role of the Imaginary as secondary with respect to that of the Symbolic. The Imaginary is recast as a determination of the Symbolic; it plays its role in the formation of the ego only as a consequence of the initial, founding intervention of language qua untranscendable symbolic horizon. This is why apropos his second graph Lacan claims: "Here arises the ambiguity of a misrecognizing that is essential to knowing myself [*un méconnaître essentiel au me connaître*]" (684, 7). Effectively, the graph tells us that the split subject (*\$*) looks back and all he can be sure of "is the anticipated image – which he had caught of himself in his mirror – coming to meet him" (684, 7).

Without rehearsing his theory of the mirror stage, which occupies the lower part of the second graph, Lacan reminds his audience that, insofar as it established the imaginary dimension of the initial formation of the ego, that theory was meant to debunk the psychoanalytic belief in the autonomy of the ego that was prevalent at the time in American ego-psychology.[17] For our purpose we shall recall that Lacan's mirror theory is built on an inerasable ambiguity: while the mirror provides for the child an image of the precarious unity of its biological body – *i(a)*, that is to say the ideal ego as imaginary projection of the ego, which brings comfort by anticipating a sense of selfness, at the same time this unity is perceived as detached, external to the child's body and its actual sensations. Apropos this reassuring yet failed or illusory identification between the body and its image, Lacan in his famous 1949 paper on the mirror stage had spoken of a "primordial Discord" (78) affecting the human being's relation to itself as well as to nature. Hence the fundamental Lacanian assertion that any self-knowledge is accompanied, or is equivalent to, a misrecognition. Despite promoting identification, the ideal ego is the bearer of an essential misrecognition which will never be eliminated.

Lacan is particularly unequivocal about the (inevitable) narcissistic consequences of accepting the ideal ego as the first image of one's consistent self:

> what the subject finds in this altered image of his body is the paradigm of all the forms of resemblance that will cast a shade of hostility onto the world of objects, by projecting onto them the avatar of his narcissistic image, which, from the jubilation derived from encountering it

> in the mirror, becomes – in confronting his semblables – the outlet for his most intimate aggressiveness.
>
> (685, 2)

In short, Lacan confirms Freud's theory of aggressiveness as deriving from narcissistic (primary) identification – whether the aggression is directed against others or is turned against the ego itself. Because any relation to others is predicated upon imaginary identification, the subject is by definition at odds with these others, prone to aggressive behavior; by the same token, the externalization of such aggressiveness provides evidence of the "primordial Discord" pertaining to the subject's relation with his/her own reflected image. A whole range of affects, from jealousy to love, hatred, fear, pity and so on are thus strictly related to imaginary misrecognition.

All this leads Lacan to assert that the ego is "a function of mastery, a game of bearing, and constituted rivalry" (685, 3). It is, in other words, a battlefield where the signifying material garnered from the Other attempts to mask its own duplicity, which is none other than the duplicity of the signifier inasmuch as it does not correspond seamlessly to the signified. It is a mistake, according to Lacan, to assume that consciousness is "immanent in the ego", for instead it functions transcendentally via the ego-ideal – I(A) – qua unary trait (684, 3–4). The imaginary contribution to the process of ego formation, then, consists of the mirror stage as indicated by the vector linking *i(a)* and *m* (for the French *moi*, the ego). It is important to underline that, at this stage in his teaching and in the development of the graph, Lacan claims that this imaginary vector is doubly inscribed in the dialectics of ego formation. First, it subsists as a "short circuit" of the wider vector of identification that goes from $\$$ to I(A); second, and most importantly, it functions as a "return route" of the upper vector from A to *s*(A), thus crucially attempting to secure meaning for the subject *after* the subject's first encounter with language: "This shows that the ego is only completed by being articulated not as the *I* of discourse, but as a metonymy of its signification" (685, 4).

As a short circuit which bypasses the encounter with the Other, in other words, the vector of mirror-like imaginary identification by definition fails. Instead, imaginary identification takes its cue from the "treasure trove of signifiers". As exemplified correctly by Van Haute (2001: 92), one should think of an infant carried in front of a mirror by a parent who accompanies the infant's imaginary identification with sentences such as "Isn't John lovely?", "What a big boy you are!" Here we witness a clear conflation of symbolic and imaginary identificatory processes, which captures nicely the functioning of the imaginary in Lacan's second graph. The other, in this case a parent, is not merely a mirror-like image of the child; rather, the parent qua Other possesses the ability to satisfy the child's needs and therefore retains a symbolic authority that is key to the achievement of the ego-ideal. It is indeed difficult to overestimate the importance of language even in primary identification: it is thanks to those uttered significations – whether real or imagined – that the infant is able to secure for him/herself a place in the symbolic order. For this reason, the verbal tense that defines the subject is, as Lacan emphasizes, the future perfect. Each one of us effectively 'will have been', in the sense that *we become what we were for others*; the formation of the traits of our subjectivity is strictly correlated with what we heard from others about us before we gained any sense of who we are.

What we should reiterate here is the centrality of I(A) qua unary trait as the signifier in the Other that secures the acquisition of meaning in the subject:

> Take just one signifier as an insignia of this omnipotence, that is, of this wholly potential power, of this birth of possibility, and you have the unary trait which – filling in the invisible mark the subject receives from the signifier – alienates the subject in the first identification that forms the ego-ideal.
>
> (684, 4)

The crucial signifier is, as we have seen, often insignificant, and yet it marks that part of the other (e.g. the parent) without which the other would not have any real influence on the subject. The child, for instance, tends to insist on a detail that allows him/her to identify with the other, and recognize the other as an authoritative source of signification. A child might want – or even insist on wearing – shoes that are "just like mummy's" (or indeed mummy's own shoes); another might start imitating a small, almost imperceptible gesture habitually made by the father. In short, subjectivation through the Other is necessarily tied to a process of *metonymical identification* which functions as a sort of anchoring point for the formation of subjectivity and the formulation of the subject's desires. To put it in a somewhat oversimplified way, it is not enough to say that we are the products of our socio-historical circumstances. What we need to add is that, insofar as we are the flawed outcome of our encounter or intersection with the Other (A in graph 2), we anchor our being in some metonymical element (I(A) in graph 2) which opens up for us the possibility of signification.

Imaginary identification could be said to work as an attempt to compensate for the lack brought about by the subject's encounter with language. Since the body is never 'fully covered' by language, the imaginary register intervenes to attempt to provide an answer (the image of its own unity) to the discord experienced in language. As Van Haute (2001: 98) notes, the imaginary vector runs counter to the symbolic one above it:

> For in the imaginary register, the subject structurally *fails to recognize* the transcendence of its origin; it fails to recognize that it borrows its identity from the Other. It believes, rather, that it is master of itself, and it is blind to its alienation in the symbolic.

What ensues is the conflict between ego-ideal (the *trait unaire* as "symbolic introjection"; Evans, 1997: 52) and the ideal ego (the totalizing outcome of imaginary identification). While, logically, alienation through the ego-ideal in the Other comes first, such symbolic process, at this stage, runs up against what it itself engenders, namely the potential for countless imaginary (immanent) identifications which risk overwhelming the alienating (transcendental) character of symbolization. This explains why, at the end of this process, we arrive at what Lacan indicates as I(A), namely identification through the ego-ideal in the Other. So when Lacan states that "the ego is only completed by being articulated not as the *I* of discourse, but as a metonymy of its signification" (685, 4), he refers to that metonymical identification with the ego-ideal which "provides a vantage point or a fixed point (even a *point de capiton*) outside the ego that gives the ego its unity" (Fink 2004: 118), and is therefore the decisive aspect of subjectivation.[18]

We should not overlook how, at this stage, the process of subjectivation is only completed through imaginary identification. This is what Won Choi (2012) remarks in his critique of Žižek's reading of the graph in question:

> Although, or precisely because, the symbolic law arrives in advance and thus is experienced by the subject prematurely, it is not experienced in a symbolic way, but merely in an imaginary way. The genuine symbolic identification, which is exactly what is meant by the 'secondary (Oedipal) identification,' only comes after the child experiences the 'castration complex,' as Lacan later shows in his essay. The primary identification that precedes such a secondary Oedipal identification is, of course, the imaginary identification whose effect is twofold: the formation of the i(a) and that of the I(A). Both formations are the two results of the same process of the identification which is imaginary.

Although I(A) stands for symbolic identification, that is, identification through language qua Other, at this stage it is still very much dependent on imaginary capture, namely i(a). The above-mentioned example used by Van Haute (the child in front of the mirror with parents talking about him/her) perfectly conveys this early dependence of the symbolic on imaginary identification: language qua I(A) works precisely because of the imaginary dimension that sustains it.

Master and slave

Before proceeding any further, let us see how Lacan tackles the Hegelian narrative of the struggle between Master and Slave, since this is no doubt one of the most significant objections Lacan makes to Hegel. As reiterated throughout the essay, Lacan understands Hegel's 'cunning of reason' as the way in which self-consciousness manages to establish "its impersonal reign" (686, 1). It is the rigour of Hegel's rationality that Lacan finds at fault – a rigour now attributed to the understanding that slavery is supposed to inaugurate, in Hegel, "the road to freedom" (686, 2). This, for Lacan, provides evidence that Hegel's notion of self-consciousness as presented in the *Phenomenology of Spirit* is deeply misleading. More precisely, what emerges in that concept is something "blatantly symptomatic", that is, "indicative of repression" (686, 6), which Lacan relates by way of analogy to the aggressiveness that typifies imaginary capture (686, 3). This allows us to infer that Lacan's Hegelian reference addresses the central shortcoming of imaginary identification. What Hegel omits when telling the story of the struggle between Master and Slave against the background of death – a struggle which inaugurates the dialectic of self-consciousness – is that death itself is always-already symbolized. Hegel's point is that the Master prevails due to his readiness to embrace the risk of death. However, Lacan adds, death is not supposed to take place, as that would bring the dialectic to a halt. As he states,

> a pact always precedes violence before perpetuating it, and what I call the symbolic dominates the imaginary, allowing us to wonder whether or not murder really is the absolute Master. For it is not enough to decide the question on the basis of its effects: Death. We need to know which death, the one that life brings or the one that brings life.
>
> (686, 4–5)

The death involved in the Hegelian struggle between Master and Slave is clearly, according to Lacan, an imaginary one, and therefore it will not lead to the liberation or emancipation of the slave through the assumption of work (686, 7) – as much of the Marxist readings of the dialectic have tended to argue. In fact, "[t]here can be no more obvious lure than this, politically or psychologically. Jouissance comes easily to the slave, and it leaves work in serfdom" (686, 6) – that is to say: the more the slave works, the more he enjoys, and the more he remains a slave. As Mladen Dolar (2006: 132) has put it:

> it is the slave's enjoyment that comes surprisingly easily, and which presents an obstacle to the slave's liberation. [...] Indeed, enjoyment appears as the one thing that one can never be rid of. It is recalcitrant to negation, and its negation produces a surplus.

Lacan's point, then, is that the struggle between Master and Slave takes place against the disavowed background of a symbolic pact that has always-already been stipulated between the two actors. This is one way of claiming that, within Hegel's dialectical logic of self-consciousness, the Symbolic precedes the Imaginary and yet it is not recognized. In this respect, the slave, Lacan argues, situates himself on the side of the Other, simply waiting for something to happen, "thus eliminating all risk to himself – especially the risk of a joust – in a 'self-consciousness' for which death is but a joke" (687, 1).

Lacan adds further criticism by observing how the use of the cunning of reason is typical of the obsessive's forma mentis, which is particularly ripe among the intelligentsia (686, 7). In this respect, both philosophy and psychology, for Lacan, continue to neglect "the enigmatic traumas" of the Freudian discovery, having instead opted to embrace "a practice which has degenerated into an educative banality that is no longer even redeemed by its laziness" (687, 3). What we have here is another foretaste of that critical assessment of the University discourse that Lacan will unleash a few years later. The obsessive banality of modern education, which has eliminated the last vestiges of potential self-sabotaging – which Lacan here identifies in "laziness" (687, 3) and "humor" (687, 5) – already marks the advent of a new form of mastery based on the hyper-valorization of life itself, inclusive of its "cultural / educational" side, which Lacan refers to as "the contraband flag of 'culturalism'" (688, 4). The "Freudian discovery" (687, 4), on the other hand, allows him to place significant emphasis on a recalcitrant surplus of sense that by definition rejects being turned into a value – that is to say, it resists what Lacan takes to be the Hegelian 'cunning of reason'.

The defiles of the signifier

Once again, however, we need to stress how it is in its linguistic composition that the unconscious defies valorization, thus rejecting the principle of equivalence. As it emerges at different points in *Subversion*, Lacan firmly opposes a transcendentalization of the unconscious, its being imagined, seductively, romantically even, as the abyssal and ineffable 'stuff' of some mysterious sensory experience. Instead, he detects in Freud clear indications of the fact that the unconscious belongs to an immanent plane, while preserving there its radical alienness. It is for this reason that Lacan is constantly at pains to reassert the centrality of linguistic structures in establishing the division of the subject, for instance by claiming, against psychology, that need (*besoin*), demand (*demande*) and desire (*désir*) all pass through "the defiles of the signifier" (687, 7): it is by submitting to the signifier that they come to represent the irredeemable contradiction embodied by the unconscious (687, 6).

Needs, Lacan states, pass over into the diversified register of desire, a process that takes place not only through the contingency of traumas, but most importantly thanks to the intervention of linguistic structures (687, 8–9). Lacan mentions "the somatic ananke of man's inability to move" to stress that if the fate (ananke) of the human being at birth is its inability to move independently, this does not allow anyone to ignore that "this dependence is maintained by a universe of language" (687, 8). By encountering language, needs are transubstantiated, inasmuch as they are filtered through networks of cultural references which uproot, multiply, diversify and most crucially elevate them beyond matters of biological functionality (687, 9). And as soon as the signifier allows desire to emerge, thus forcing the subject out of its primitive biologism, frustration also sets in, for language institutes a margin beyond the biological body that by definition alienates the subject, precluding forever the possibility of complete satisfaction through biological gratification alone. In Fink's words (2004: 118–19):

> A young bear is given honey to eat by its mother, gorges itself, and lies down for a nap, sated. We receive the blanket we demand from our mother and then dream about cars and dolls and world domination. For us there is always something more to be desired.

Although the first two graphs of desire do not deal directly with desire as such, this is because Lacan wants first to clarify the extent to which the subject is dependent on the signifier, and then how desire itself is borne out of this dependence. Desire is therefore not merely submitted to, and dependent upon, the ebb and flow of historical contingency, the supposedly natural development of humanity. Its force, as well as its actual definition, derives rather from its being necessarily subjected to jarring symbolic structures. Lacan includes "moralists", "theologians" and, more recently, "Sartre – desire, a useless passion" (687, 8), in a long list of thinkers who have dealt with the paradoxical and precarious status of desire in its dependence on language. When he mentions Sartre, he paraphrases a well-known phrase from *Being and Nothingness*, first published in 1943: "Man, a useless passion" (Sartre, 1943/1992: 784). Lacan insists that there is no such thing as a natural or spontaneous desire, since all desires acquire their status via the signifier – something which Freud understood when he admitted that "sexuality had to bear the mark of some hardly natural flaw" (688, 1).

Need, demand, desire

Even the Oedipus myth for Lacan signifies nothing but the centrality of language in matters of sexual conflict. For if the father in this myth is in fact "the dead father" (688, 3), as Freud had attempted to demonstrate, Lacan emphasizes how this status should be seen in symbolic terms. He emphasizes this by introducing the term "Name-of-the-father" (688, 3), which is meant to draw attention to the symbolic metaphor established by the theme of the dead father. Otherness itself is nothing but the place of the signifier: "Let us begin with the conception of the Other as the locus of the signifier. No authoritative statement has any other guarantee here than its very enunciation, since it would be pointless for the statement to seek it in another signifier, which could in no way appear outside that locus" (688, 7). This preludes to and clarifies Lacan's well-known motto according to which "there is no metalanguage that can be spoken, or, more aphoristically, [...] there is no Other of the Other" (688, 7). Ultimately, the law itself owes its authority to its enunciation alone – there is no moral or theological grounding principle that the law might successfully appeal to; yet "the Law itself is not an impostor, nor is he who authorizes his actions on its basis" (688, 8).

At this stage in the discussion, Lacan introduces the figure of the Mother as "the subject who is led to really occupy the place of the Other" (688, 9), despite the Father's attempt at installing the authority of the law. This in turn allows Lacan to develop his central definition of desire as the desire of the Other (689, 3), which, since the Other is a conflicted battleground, takes on multiple meanings. Lacan introduces his definition of desire as what

> begins to take shape in the margin in which demand rips away from need, this margin being the one that demand – whose appeal can be unconditioned only with respect to the Other – opens up in the guise of the possible gap need may give rise to here, because it has no universal satisfaction (this is called 'anxiety').
>
> (689, 5)

Let us try to unpack this complex statement. First, we must say that, unlike what happens with animals, human needs for Lacan can only be met or answered by another human being, or group of them. Second, demands arise when the infant realizes that beyond the satisfaction of bodily needs, he/she requires also the other's love or affection. It is when the child realizes that demands have no universal satisfaction – that is, when demand emerges out of need as something different from it, in that it can never be fully satisfied – that desire makes its appearance. Let us say that a child needs food qua biological function, and is appeased when the other provides it; then, the child begins to demand love (a different kind of food) from this other, but realizes that such demand is problematic since it never achieves full satisfaction; it is at this stage that desire develops out of demand's difference from need.

The mother's breast, for instance, provides satisfaction of the child's need (when he/she is hungry), but it is also an object through which the child measures the (m)other's readiness to respond to his/her demand for affection: in this sense, the breast becomes an object that signifies the child's demand for the (m)other's unconditional love, that is to say for recognition. It is at this stage that symbolic structures start playing a part in the child's development, in that they radically alter the significance of the object (the breast) whose initial function was 'merely' that of satisfying a physiological need. For as soon as the breast becomes the catalyst of the subject's demand for love, it begins to be uprooted from its functional role in order to be inscribed into a symbolic structure where its meaning is decided metonymically, that is, by the shifting of the signifier that represents it. This means that suddenly the breast is inserted in a signifying chain – in the flow of language – whose chief feature, however, is that it lacks the signifier that would square the circle and guarantee the full satisfaction of the demand for love. This is precisely when desire emerges out of the jarring of need and demand. By ripping away from need via the alienating encounter with the signifier, demand opens up the abyssal dimension of lack, which desire strives (in vain) to fill through the endless shifting and diversification of the object itself.

From anxiety to desire

Things here become more interesting, but also considerably more complicated. The unconditional nature of the demand that develops out of need's encounter with symbolic structures, Lacan says, also brings in anxiety, which, in terms of the child's awareness, implies being exposed to the enigmatic desire of the first other, who is therefore perceived as omnipotent. Since in the eyes of the child the (m)other is the bearer of a thoroughly enigmatic and capricious will, the child's automatic reply to this enigma ('what does she want, *especially* from me?') is to imagine that he/she is the missing object of the (m)other's desire. The risk involved in this identification is particularly high, namely that of reducing the child to being a mere object whose function is to satisfy the mother's desire.

This 'becoming the object of the other's desire' is precisely what qualifies Lacan's understanding of anxiety as that which arises out of demand's splitting off from need. And desire is what, normally, is produced by this deadlock, namely the attempt to gentrify or diffuse the situation whereby I posit myself as the object that fills in the lack in the other. Let us take the following example: a child who insistently demands sweets is not simply trying to satisfy a need; more than that, he/she articulates a somewhat absolute demand that, as such, exposes the child to the threat of anxiety. Why? Because what resonates in that unwavering request is the unconditional form of demand, which, by presupposing the omnipotence of an other who is supposed to satisfy the demand, objectifies the child in relation to that other. Thus, by asking insistently for the same object, the child effectively gives him/herself up to the other. As such, this persistence speaks for the child's failure to articulate the logic of desire, which is built on the fantasy of an autonomous subjective position vis-à-vis the proliferation of different objects.

The child, then, places plenty of expectation on the other, including what Lacan calls its "phantom of Omnipotence" (689, 5). This point is worth pondering: the fantasy of omnipotence is not on the side of the uncoordinated child, as Freud had surmised, but on the side of the other as seen with the eyes of the child. It is precisely from this fantasy that arises "the necessity that the Other be bridled by the Law" (689, 5). The obvious case in point here are Freud's two fathers as described in *Totem and Taboo*: the *Urvater*, who enjoys fantasmatic status as the omnipotent one, and the father as representative of the law, who intervenes to 'bridle' his own excess. Desire, Lacan tells us, "reverses the unconditional nature of the demand for love, in which the subject remains in subjection to the Other, and raises it to the power of absolute condition (in which 'absolute' also implies 'detachment')" (689, 6). Given the Latin root of 'absolute' (*absolvere*, i.e. 'to free'), Lacan suggests that the acquisition of desire as the untranscendable condition of being human is predicated upon the detachment from the unconditional, anxiety-laden dimension of demand (689, 7). Put differently, by articulating desires the child is able to find a way out of that 'desperate' demand for the (m)other's love which, inevitably, kept him/her at the mercy of the mother's enigmatic and unfathomable whim. And the law that brings in desire is language itself, the signifier. More precisely, the signifier introduces that lack (the rift that disarticulates the unconditionality of demand) which, in turn, gives the subject a chance to develop a desiring relationship vis-à-vis the other. Thus, the order of the law coincides with the order of language, in as much as language symbolizes the lack already experienced at the level of the Imaginary (demand), thereby gentrifying it, turning it into something that can potentially be filled by metonymically different objects.

Lacan notes, in passing, that one of the first manifestations of the object of desire is what has been identified by British psychoanalyst Donald Winnicot as the "transitional object" (for instance, "the shred of blanket or beloved shard the child's lips or hands never stop touching", 689, 7), whose role is to mediate between a subject still in the thrall of the (m)other and the outer world of objects. The transitional object, in other words, provides some much-needed respite from the threat of anxiety, inasmuch as it embodies an otherness that is not the (m)other qua terminus of an unconditional demand for love. Insofar as it emerges through a process of metaphorization (i.e. of signification), the transitional object for Lacan is emblematic of the child's encounter with the symbolic order, which on the one hand opens up the possibility of freeing oneself from the clutches of demand, but on the other delivers the subject to the infinite sliding of the signifier – and therefore to the frustration that typifies desire. The outcome of this process of detachment from the mother as first "representative of representation" (Freud's *Vorstellungrepräsentanz*), that is, the one who provides the very framework for the possibility of representation (meaning), is the dialectic of desire, whose roots are off-limits as they belong in the unconscious (689, 8).

Emancipation from demand, then, is achieved through desire, whose cause remains radically excluded from the subject's knowledge. While the object of desire can be isolated and, strictly speaking, known, the cause of such desire remains foreclosed.[19] In other words, while the object of one's desire can be a positive and identifiable object, the cause of that desire is the very 'thing' the object masks, namely the lack embodied by the unconscious in its radical alterity. In this sense, Winnicot's transitional object and Lacan's *object a* can be seen to fulfill the same function, that of delivering the subject from the unconditionality of demand. At this point, having asserted how desire characterizes itself by its attachment to an object-cause that remains unconscious, Lacan proceeds to explain, in line with the driving emphasis of his intervention, that such unconscious roots of desire do not actually dwell within us, but concern the Other – the Other in its utterly enigmatic status.

Desire is the other's desire

Lacan's famous maxim about desire is as follows: "le désir de l'homme est le désir de l'Autre", "man's desire is the desire of the Other" (690, 2). The ambiguity of this definition rests with the interpretation of the French preposition *de* (of) in *de l'Autre*. As an "objective determination" (690, 1) such preposition indicates that desire has to do with the otherness, that is to say the enigma, in/of the Other. This is the most intuitive and to an extent commonplace understanding of desire as something which is triggered by what the subject finds elusive and therefore fascinating in the Other. However, this also amounts to a superficial reading which needs to be taken into a different direction if we are to grasp the actual reflexivity of desire, the fact that it does not point to something innate but rather acquired. Lacan quickly adds that the preposition *de* should also be understood as a "subjective determination" (690, 2) meaning 'possessed by the Other', which implies that desire takes on a reflexive significance charged with ambiguity. This means that far from being natural, our desires are alien to us, inasmuch as they are borne out of our necessary encounter with the symbolic order that splits us by creating a lack embodied by the unconscious. Our desires, then, are testament to the mark that the Other leaves on us in the form of a division into conscious and unconscious knowledge. And it is precisely the invasion of the 'alien' signifiers forming the unconscious which, ultimately, determines our desires and therefore shapes our existence, unbeknownst to us. The desires rooted in the signifying chain of the unconscious follow a path that, by definition, has no pre-established object, in the sense that the ever-shifting objects of desire are so many (infinite) answers to the unbridgeable rift inscribed in subjectivity by the signifier.

First, then, *le désir de l'homme est le désir de l'Autre* means that our desire is a desire for the recognition of the Other. As we have seen, the terminus I(A) in the second graph stands for our identification with the gaze of an other, the ego-ideal, from which we see and recognize ourselves. This means that we desire to be acknowledged by a signifier outside ourselves; we desire to be desired. At this level, desire is the first embodiment of the rift inscribed in demand and, to an extent, it overlaps with the latter; desire emerges from the deadlock of the demand for unconditional love. Second – and it is here that we can gauge the originality of Lacan's position – desire as the other's desire also signifies a 'second-hand' desire, a 'desired desire': ours is always-already the desire that belongs to/in the Other. Put simply, we desire what (we suppose) the Other desires, that is, we learn to desire through the Other. This reading adds a new layer of complexity to the initial interpretation of *de* as an "objective determination": when we desire the other in its fascinating elusiveness, we are in fact asking questions about what the Other desires. As Lacan (1967/2008: 38) will put it later on in a lecture: "Desire full stop is the desire of the Other. Which basically means that we are always asking the Other what he desires." It can therefore be seen how Lacan strips the concept of desire of its supposed authenticity, laying bare the fact that what we believe to be the most intimate and genuine locus of our subjectivity is in fact borrowed from the Other, something that was already out there even before we came into the world. Also intended as a question ('What does the Other want (from me)?'), the subject's desire is violently deprived of its supposed autonomy and authenticity.

Chè vuoi?

For this reason Lacan claims that "the Other's question [...] which takes some such form as 'Chè vuoi?,' 'What do you want?,' is the question that best leads the subject to the path of his own desire" (690, 3). Lacan takes the phrase from the eighteenth-century novel *Le diable amoureux* (The Devil in Love, 1772), by Jacques Cazotte, and uses it for the first time in *Seminar IV*, where it is meant exactly as in Cazotte's novel, namely as a question that the Other (the Devil) asks the subject. In *Seminar VI*, however, Lacan turns around the direction of the question, which now, as in *Subversion*, is posed to the Other (see also Pluth, 2007: 69–72). Lacan's point is that the child who is asked what he/she wants, unconsciously tends to answer such a question by questioning the asker, that is, by attempting to answer the following question: 'what does this person who is interrogating my desire actually want?'; or, more precisely: 'what can I give this person to satisfy her desire to know what I want?' Thus, the child's desire materializes out of the other's desire (690, 3). And the point is that only through this somewhat perverse loop does the subject manage to join the path of his/her desire.

What is certain is that desire will continue to frustrate the subject, since no ultimate answer to the question *Chè vuoi?* can ever be given. In fantasy, the child attempts to find this answer, but what resonates in every such fantasy (until the end of one's life) is nothing other than its own inadequacy, its impossibility to fill the gap opened by desire. Fantasy then seeks to establish a degree of determinacy for the utterly enigmatic character of desire as the other's desire. This is undoubtedly a radical Lacanian contribution to the definition of subjectivity, since it posits the latter as a field whose inconsistency is to be conceived in strict dialectical correlation with the socio-symbolic universe it inhabits. Desire as such does not lead us to assert the singularity of our subjective position vis-à-vis the world; quite on the contrary, it tells us that the world we inhabit, and attribute meanings to, possesses the key to our subjectivity. This awareness should bring the ego to confront its own constitutive dislocation – the fact that the significations it purports are not unique and exclusive, but are instead caught in a mechanism that defines what the Other already is/wants.

There is also a third way of conceptualizing the subjective meaning of Lacan's maxim on desire, one that branches off from the second and leads us to the later 'Lacan of the Real', effectively returning us to the initial 'objective determination' of desire. According to this third reading, desiring the other's desire also means being fascinated not so much by the elusiveness of the other (my first interpretation of Lacan's maxim) but by the other's *jouissance*. The objective component here is preserved alongside the subjective, since we have an object of desire (*jouissance*, an enigmatic libidinal tension that attracts us) which is at the same time the substance of the other's desire, the "stuff" of his/her subjectivity. We can, therefore, list four readings of Lacan's motto:

1. I desire the other (insofar as it embodies otherness to me).
2. I desire to be desired (recognized) by the other.
3. I desire what the other desires.
4. I desire the very fascinating/disturbing desirousness (*jouissance*) that I detect in the other.

In each of these definitions the other can be written with either a lower case 'o' (e.g. another person) and with the capital 'O' (the big Other, the network of unwritten significations that sustains our being in the world). What of course should be taken into consideration is that 'o' is always contained within 'O': the otherness of our counterparts in the world is by definition, when desire is at stake, included in the big Other.

The third graph of desire

Lacan's further developed graph of desire (Graph 3), then, culminates with the question "Chè vuoi?", which comes from the Other and leads to the formula of fantasy that sustains the precarious consistency of subjectivity: $\$\Diamond a$ (Figure 7.3). As underscored by Lacan (690, 4), the very curvature of the upper part of the graph, emerging from the place of the Other, deliberately recalls the shape of a question mark.

Fantasy ($\$\Diamond a$), as we have seen, is the answer to the (unconscious) desire of the Other – the answer the subject formulates when faced by the lack experienced through the other's desire (the "chè vuoi?" intended as "what does he/she want from me?"). In this sense, as Lacan will put it in his unpublished *Seminar XIV* (*The Logic of Fantasy*, 1966–1967, session 16 November 1966), fantasy is an *axiom*, that is to say, a self-evident and uncontestable formation whose role is to attempt to fill such lack. It is in relation to fantasy that Lacan elaborates on the constitutive ambiguity of what we desire. True, the subject is

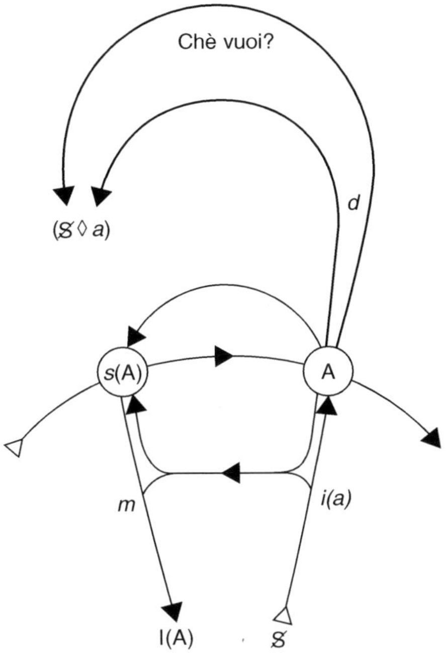

Figure 7.3 Lacan's Graph 3

left in an alienated position, but has a chance "to butt up against the question of his essence" (690, 6). This means that if misrecognition is the bread and butter of subjectivity, at the same time the subject "may not misrecognise that what he desires presents itself to him as what he does not want" (690, 6–691, 1). If Lacan tells us that, in its essence, the subject desires what he/she does not want, this is not only because the desired object is always-already what the Other wants, but because, to put it plainly, the object-cause of desire is ultimately a lack; or, to use Lacan's words, "a form assumed by negation in which misrecognition is inserted in a very odd way, the misrecognition, of which he himself is unaware, by which he transfers the permanence of his desire to an ego that is nevertheless obviously intermittent, and inversely, protects himself from his desire by attributing to it these very intermittences" (691, 1). To an attentive reading, this convoluted sentence summarizes the undecidable nature of the relation between subject and desire, insofar as it is qualified by the presence/absence of *object a* (rendered simply as *a* in Lacan's algebra). The object-cause of desire is precisely the "form assumed by negation" of which Lacan speaks. As a materialization of lack, this object embodies "in a very odd way" the misrecognition that sustains desire and, by the same token, the ego – despite the fact that, owing to the negativity lurking within such object, the ego itself is constantly negotiating the "intermittences" (the inconsistencies or contradictions) that characterize the functioning of desire.

The subversion of the subject

We can now appreciate how, in finalizing his graph of desire, Lacan introduces the possibility of the *subversion of the subject*. This possibility has to do with situating within the formula of fantasy, which is at the cusp of the graph of desire, "the moment of a fading or eclipse of the subject – which is closely tied to the *Spaltung* or splitting he undergoes due to his subordination to the signifier – to the condition of an object" (691, 3). Here we have a chance to grasp the Lacanian lesson concerning the meaning of subversion: the whole trajectory that charts the subject's necessary "subordination to the signifier" (691, 3) ends up with a formula that, if on the one hand confirms that the subject is alienated in the Other's desire (and fantasy is nothing but a coping mechanism, an axiomatic way to deal with such alienation), it also suggests that it is only by radicalizing alienation that subversion might ensue. Paradoxically, then, the only way for the subject to subvert its own alienation is by giving in completely to it, that is, by grasping itself as a metonymy of lack, as *object a* in its most radical meaning (a "form assumed by negation"). The "fading of the subject" – its collapsing into *object a* – of which Lacan speaks in relation to subversion, then, is predicated upon the subject's full submission to the signifier, inasmuch as such operation conveys to the subject that it has no content of its own. Subjective subversion, for Lacan, consists of this radicalization of alienation, and not in its overcoming through a supposedly dis-alienating process of subjective identification. All this, Lacan adds, is symbolized by the algorithm of fantasy: "The graph shows that desire adjusts to fantasy [...] but the graph also shows the inversion of the misrecognitions on which the one and the other are based, respectively" (691, 6), which confirms that fantasy also leads us to the subject of the unconscious qua *object a* (where misrecognition is inverted). Having established a link with the subject of the unconscious, Lacan can now fully engage with it by calling the drive into question.

The complete graph of desire

Lacan therefore completes his graph by adding the drive and its formula, $◊D (Figure 7.4). Significantly, the drive is defined in relation to demand (D) in a formula highlighting the fading of the subject ($) in relation to a demand that also gives way, "except that the cut remains [...] in what distinguishes the drive from the organic function it inhabits" (692, 2). The drive is, in other words, a demand where the subject fades, and in so doing makes room for a 'different demand', one characterized only by the cut as represented in Freud's erogenous zones. Through the drive, then, we can make sense of the subject of the unconscious inasmuch as it is designated by a statement the subject knows nothing about:

> Hence the concept of the drive, in which the subject is designated on the basis of a pinpointing that is organic, oral, anal, and so on, which satisfies the requirement that the more he speaks, the further he is from speaking.
>
> (692, 1)

Freud had already established that the drive, which is partial, belongs to the body and seeks satisfaction by way of connecting with its various objects (the breast for the oral drive, faeces for the anal drive, and so on). More precisely, the drive captures a limit-position situated between the psychic and the somatic. Starting from the Freudian drive, Lacan maintains that the drive's dependence on an organic function does not make it less symbolic, less tied to linguistic structures. In fact, drives isolate the erogenous zones by subtracting them from their sheer metabolic function and investing them with symbolic significations. For example, it is abundantly clear that, apart from providing an immediately pleasurable experience to the child who sucks a dummy or his thumb, the mouth is also associated by the infant with a regulatory relation with the other which involves nourishment, making certain noises, speech, etc. In other words, Lacan claims that the significance of the erogenous zones where the drives are situated derives from the subject's link with the Other, insofar as this Other is constituted by signifiers. Hence the intrinsic relation of drive and demand: "The drive is what becomes of demand when the subject vanishes from it. It goes without saying that demand also disappears, except that the cut remains" (692, 2). It is not surprising, then, that in the graph's final version the drive qua signifying chain giving shape to the unconscious desire of the subject is located right above, and connected with, the Other as the "treasure trove" of signifiers. Significantly, this connection is provided by desire, which is now doubly articulated since it also leads, as we have seen, to the fantasy.

There is, therefore, a homology between the body's erogenous zones and the Other's signifiers, one which is instituted on the notion of 'cut': on the one hand, all the erogenous zones present themselves with "the anatomical characteristic of a margin or border: the lips, 'the enclosure of the teeth', the rim of the anus, the penile groove, the vagina, and the slit formed by the eyelids, not to mention the hollow of the ear" (692, 3); on the other hand, the signifier cuts into the body so as to extract the drives from their privileged places of anatomical inscription.[20] The encounter between the signifier and the body is inevitably one that makes meaning emerge from a foundational lack of meaning. The subject 'lost' among signifiers, that is, irredeemably split by them ($), ultimately coincides with the missing cause of desire insofar as this corresponds to *object a*, which concretely represents lack in the psychic economy.

As we have seen, the two terms (subject and *object a*) are mediated by fantasy, which, precisely by providing a filling connection between the two lacks, confirms its status as a precarious and fragile, and yet axiomatic, psychic formation. To give an example, words fail us when we try to describe the reason for our passionate attachment to a given person or cause: we are, literally, lost between two or more signifiers, which never fully render the reason for our attachment. At the same time, the cause of such attachment materializes through concrete elements in the other/object, which have a hold on us beyond our awareness. Thus, while our love cannot be fully expressed in words (*\$*), at the same time it is inexplicably embodied by seemingly irrelevant 'objective' features (*a*) in the other – such as the specific way of looking, smiling, certain meaningless gestures, and so on. Crucially, the two lacks (subjective and objective) find a way of connecting through fantasy, which fills their radical elusiveness with a plethora of plausible and in principle reassuring imaginary contents. Thus, when I fantasize about a person I do so by providing an imaginary answer to the lack that triggers my affect in the first place – which is why the vector of desire that reaches the fantasy while avoiding the drive leads us back downward toward s(A) and eventually I(A). In other words, it provides a symbolic meaning, whereas by moving upward it encounters the impossibility of providing a meaning. Whatever the direction taken by the vector of desire, Lacan makes it clear that the fantasy as such always effects a substantial

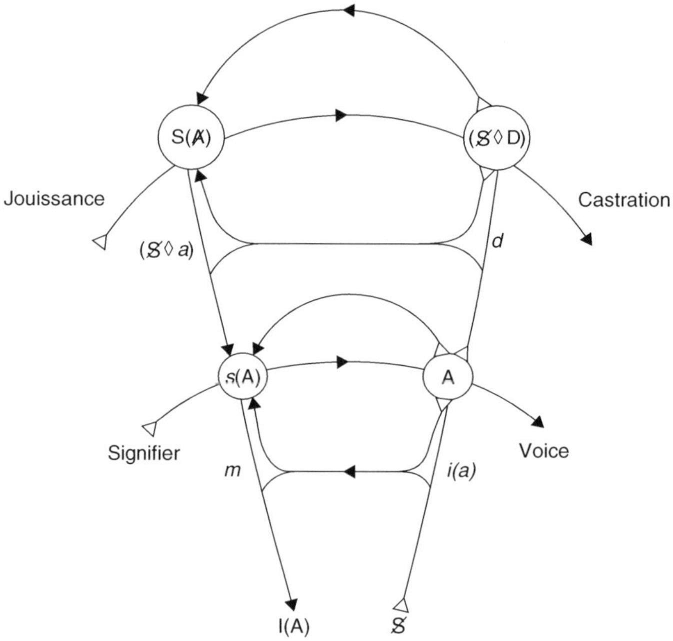

Figure 7.4 Lacan's complete graph

gentrification of the missing cause of desire, thereby obfuscating the subject's inability to justify it, while *a* should be thought of as the 'vanishing mediator' between fantasy and lack. As the fishhook vector of subjectivity indicates, *a* materializes as a remainder of the failed process of signification through the Other, which allows one to desire and consequently achieve subjective status.

The subject as object of the drive

Insofar as *a* ultimately captures the inconsistency of the desiring subject, Lacan's point here is that the subject encounters itself qua *$* precisely as the meaningless leftover (*a*) of the process of subjectivation.[21] In drive, then, the conscious subject vanishes, and in this vanishing we are given evidence of the fact that the drive has mobilized the signifier. This is confirmed if we consider that the various objects of the drive, such as the gaze (which in Lacan enjoys a privileged status)

> have no specular image, in other words, no alterity. This is what allows them to be the 'stuff' or, better put, the lining – without, nevertheless, being the flipside – of the very subject people take to be the subject of consciousness.
>
> (693, 2)

Fantasy, then, connects with *a* precisely by 'imaginizing' what is by definition not of the imaginary order, since *object a*, despite being an object, has no specular image. Think, for instance, of the dialectics inaugurated by the Lacanian gaze as the proverbially invisible pair of eyes which, despite being unlocatable, are always-already 'on us', potentially looking at us. Through this dialectic Lacan claims that we see things, and are thus able to establish meaningful relations with them, precisely because there is always a point in our visual field that we cannot see, which, for this very reason, embodies the gaze as object of the scopic drive. Thus, the subject caught in scopic drive is simultaneously the object of the gaze. Since the subject of the unconscious materializes in the drive, it comes to coincide with the (impossible) drive is exposed to the threat of anxiety. Lacan recurs to a vivid exemplification of such correspondence: "Ask someone with writer's block about the anxiety he experiences and he will tell you who the turd *is* in his fantasy" (693, 2). The anxiety that seizes someone with writer's block has to do with perceiving oneself as, literally, the (turd-like) object of the Other's whim. Put differently, it is rooted in the neurotic's belief in the existence of the Other, whose invisible gaze, and associated enjoyment, makes writing impossible insofar as, vis-à-vis such gaze, any written word becomes the source of an unbearable sense of guilt. Anxiety, however, does not lie, since the subject is nothing other than the partial object of the drive inasmuch as it "cannot be grasped in the mirror" (693, 3): a negative formation that defies representation. For this reason Lacan claims that the subject of the unconscious is not "the flip side" (693, 2) of the subject of consciousness: it is, rather, radically eccentric with regard to consciousness, a non-subsumable point of indeterminacy which at once sets up and disrupts consciousness.

To simplify things a little: what Lacan effectively tells us in the final part of his text is that the drive addresses the same deadlock inherent to desire; yet, differently from desire, it has a chance to bring about the object which is the subject of the unconscious – it is capable, in other words, to cause the subversion of the subject. As Fink (2004: 124) puts it, in the upper part of the complete graph Lacan attempts to figure out "what there is that goes beyond structure in human beings, what goes beyond the automatic functioning of the signifying order." While desire is mediated by the ambiguity of *chè vuoi?*, which signals an impasse at least partially recuperated by fantasy, drive goes a step further by taking us directly to S(Ⱥ), the "signifier of a lack in the Other" (693, 4) that simultaneously captures the subject of the unconscious and is situated next to *jouissance* as precisely that which disrupts the automatic functioning of the signifying order. While it is true, if we look at Lacan's graph, that desire coupled with fantasy might encroach upon S(Ⱥ), Lacan's topology makes it clear that desire can also join the path of the drive thereby directly leading the subject to S(Ⱥ). Just like with desire, then, with drive the Other is called upon to answer for the value of the meanings it holds (the "treasure trove of signifiers"); the difference, however, is that it has to do so "with the signifiers constitutive of the upper chain – in other words, in terms of the drive" (693, 4). Desire and drive offer two significantly different pathways concerning the outcome of the neurotic connection between subject and Other. While with desire the Other is generally able to safeguard its consistency vis-à-vis the neurotic, under the heavy blows of drive it is more likely to reveal its foundational lack, which is aptly defined by Lacan with the maxim "there is no Other of the Other" (693, 5).

From S(Ⱥ) to jouissance…

The key signifier S(Ⱥ) – the signifier of what is lacking in the Other – potentially annuls signification while at the same time grounding it, since, as Bruce Fink (2004: 125) has it, "what is *not* included in the Other as the collection or set of all signifiers is that which grounds the very functioning of signifiers." As such, it represents the decisive element in Lacanian psychoanalysis. So much so that Lacan assigns to it a position homologous to that of "the dead Father in the Freudian myth" – that is to say, of what he had renamed the Name-of-the-Father. To emphasize the foundational role of S(Ⱥ), Lacan adds: "No doubt a corpse is a signifier, but Moses' tomb is as empty for Freud as Christ's was for Hegel" (693, 7). The implication here is that for both Freud and Hegel the founding signifiers of religion are signifiers of lack rather than fullness. It is for this reason, however, that S(Ⱥ), although "a characteristic of truth's Faithfulness", is not "the last word worth giving in answer to the question,

'What does the Other want from me?'" (693, 5). Rather, as the completed graph specifies, S(Ⱥ) announces castration to be intended as the impossibility of full / absolute *jouissance*, in turn represented by the phallus.

To help us orient ourselves in the jungle of homologies embodied by S(Ⱥ), Lacan specifies that the signifier at stake in this matheme is rendered by the following maxim: "a signifier is what represents the subject to another signifier" (694, 1). This maxim conjoins signifier and subject by suggesting that the latter has no way of being represented by a signifier alone, since its existence is dependent on the endless metonymical displacement of one signifier by another. The subject is located 'in between signifiers', and in this respect S(Ⱥ) stands for the indeterminacy of the subject who has to pass through the Other. No signifier in the Other can establish once and for all the meaning of the subject; for this reason the subject is defined by a lack of meaning which corresponds to the endless shifting of its desire from one signifier to the next. As anticipated in the above quotation from Fink, the paradox of the emergence of an ever-shifting chain of signification from the lack in the Other – the ever-deferred space in between signifiers – is rendered by Lacan when he points out that one of the signifiers in the Other must be excluded for meaning to arise:

> This [a given signifier] can be symbolized by the inherence of a (-1) in the set of signifiers. It is, as such, unpronounceable, but its operation is not, for the latter is what occurs whenever a proper name is pronounced.
>
> (694, 2–3)

As Lacan exemplifies in the following formula (Figure 7.5), a statement is always the result of the signifier's priority over the signified, where the signifier (S) is to be understood precisely as (-1), the excluded signifier, while the signified equals the imaginary number, the square root of minus one (694, 4), insofar as signification is 'plagued' by the impossibility of symbolizing the signifier. If this is what takes place within every statement, then this impossibility is "what the subject is missing in thinking he is exhaustively accounted for by his cogito – he is missing what is unthinkable about him" (694, 5). Put differently: it is by relating to what it lacks that the subject is able to refer to itself as cogito.

$$\frac{\text{S (signifier)}}{\text{s (signified)}} = \text{s (the statement)},$$

with S = (–1), we find: $s = \sqrt{-1}$

Figure 7.5 Lacan's formula of the statement

But, Lacan asks (694,5), where does the signifier of lack come from? Certainly the subject of the enunciated, the 'I', is unable to account for it (694, 6). At most, this 'I' can "prove to the Other that he exists [...] by loving him, a solution introduced by the Christian kerygma" (694, 7). Through the reference to the Greek term *kerygma*, meaning 'to preach' or 'proclaim', Lacan is suggesting that Christianity (and religions in general) has found a solution to the inherent deadlock of signification by positing the existence of the Other (e.g. God), which does not necessarily depend on knowledge ("the proofs of the existence of God with which the centuries have killed him", 694, 7), but on love, or faith, of which *kerygma* is evidence. Lacan immediately adds, however, that this solution is "too precarious" and will not help to "circumvent our problem, namely: What am *I*?" (694, 8).

Through the following enigmatic claim, Lacan effectively proposes that the signifier of lack is none other than the subject: "*I* am in the place from which 'the universe is a flaw in the purity of Non-Being' is vociferated" (694, 9). The 'I' qua subject of the enunciation (the subject of the unconscious) occupies the place of the lack in the Other, the very flaw that represents the 'less than nothing' about which Žižek (2012) has written in relation to Hegel. Here Lacan plays his trump card: in his schema, this less than nothing, this flaw within nothingness itself, goes by the name of *jouissance*: "This place is called Jouissance, and it is Jouissance whose absence would render this universe vain" (694, 10). The paradox of the less than nothing is rendered very clearly: without unconscious enjoyment qua flaw that the 'I' cannot account for – that is, without the signifier in its unpronounceable and undetectable guise – the universe would lose its elementary consistency for the subject, who would therefore also vanish. This is indeed of fundamental dialectical importance: the signifier of lack – the disturbing insistence in our lives of a dimension that cannot be grasped – is precisely what keeps our universe together by 'forcing' the signifier to connect with the signified. This must be borne in mind whenever any simplistic equation between *jouissance* and subversion is put forward: in itself, *jouissance* is the indispensable ingredient of our world insofar as it guarantees that we must keep trying to make sense of it. Furthermore, Lacan adds that although *jouissance* is forbidden to me – I can never fully reach it – I am nevertheless responsible for it (694, 11). Why? Quite simply because the Other – whom I tend to blame for the disturbances generated by *jouissance* – does not exist. Which, in turn, explains why we tend to put the blame back on the 'I' via the myth of the original sin (695, 2) – also in Freud's version of the latter, namely the Oedipus myth (695, 2).

... and castration

In order to render the proper significance of the subversion of the subject, Lacan leaves *jouissance* aside and turns to the wound called castration, which is ushered in precisely by S(Ⱥ). Castration provides the key with which to grasp the meaning of the subversion of the subject as the ultimate aim of Lacan's psychoanalytic method: "In the castration complex we find the mainspring of the very subversion I am trying to articulate here by means of its dialectic" (695, 3). By embodying the ontological cut that *is* the subject, castration provides the coordinates of its subversion – although this has generally been avoided in psychoanalysis, which has resulted in "providing grist for the mill of the Philistines of general psychology" (695, 4). Castration "essentially constitutes in the subject the gap that all thought has avoided, skipped over, circumvented, or stopped up whenever thought apparently succeeds in sustaining itself circularly, whether the thought be dialectical or mathematical" (695, 5). More precisely, it designates the place "where logic is disconcerted by the disjunction that breaks through from the imaginary to the symbolic" (695, 6). This disconcertment results from the fact that castration effectively captures the lack of the imaginary phallus (ϕ), which is why in Lacanian algebra castration is expressed as $-\phi$. It is, furthermore, "the phantom known as the cause" intended as "the purest symbolization of the imaginary" (695, 7), inasmuch as it correlates with the signifier of the lack in the Other, S(Ⱥ), which Lacan, disagreeing with Claude Lévi-Strauss, refuses to describe as 'mana', since it is not a "zero symbol" but "the signifier of the lack of this zero symbol" (695, 9). This reliance on the signifier is what justifies Lacan's distortion of mathematical algorithms as symbols, inasmuch as these symbols – like $\sqrt{-1}$ – cannot "be used automatically in subsequent operations" (696, 1); in other words, as signifiers they are withdrawn from symbolic signification.

Here Lacan makes visible the connection between *jouissance* and castration:

> We must keep in mind that jouissance is prohibited [*interdite*] to whoever speaks, as such – or, put differently, it can only be said [*dite*] between the lines by whoever is a subject of the Law, since the Law is founded on that very prohibition.
>
> (696, 2)

Castration qua law therefore tells the subject that the imaginary phallus is lacking; as such, it comes before *jouissance*, to the extent that *jouissance* can only be predicated on the prohibition instated by the law; hence Lacan's pun about the law's order to enjoy ("Jouis!") and the subject's only possible reply as "J'ouïs" (I hear), "in which the jouissance would no longer be anything but understood" (696, 3). However, Lacan specifies that "it is not the Law itself that bars the subject's access to jouissance – it simply makes a barred subject out of an almost natural barrier" (696, 4). The law then mobilizes the "almost natural barrier" that Freud had discovered and named 'pleasure principle': "For it is pleasure that sets limits to jouissance, pleasure as what binds incoherent life together" (696, 4). Note here the differentiation between pleasure and *jouissance*: the latter is a consequence of the former's "almost natural" protection against chaos, incoherent life – namely the pre-symbolic

Real. But the deadlock between pleasure and its beyond (*jouissance*) depends on the castration complex: "The latter is the sole indication of this jouissance in its infinitude, which brings with it the mark of its prohibition, and which requires a sacrifice in order to constitute this mark: the sacrifice implied in the same act as that of choosing its symbol, the phallus" (696, 6).

Insofar as it stands for "the image of the penis" – the penis imagined as a detachable object – the imaginary phallus for Lacan "is negativized where it is situated in the specular image" (696, 7). The implication here is that the phallic function symbolizing potency (ϕ) can only function against the background of the impotence of its imaginary dimension ($-\phi$), that is, against the background of castration (696, 6). In this sense there is no difference (at least in *Subversion*) between $S(\not{A})$ and the symbolic phallus, since the latter is synonymous with the signifier that, on account of its 'exceptional' status as signifier of the lack in the Other, makes the articulation of meaning possible. Lacan elaborates upon Freud's theory of castration thus: the child's submission to the law represented by the Name-of-the-Father is the outcome of the child's failed attempt to construct its own identity by completing the (m)other's lack, that is, by offering itself up as the imaginary phallus (which is what defines the structure of perversion). In castration, then, the child realizes that desire can only be (partially) satisfied by the signifier qua Name-of-the-Father, which implies the endless dissatisfaction associated with the sliding of the signifier itself. Lacan's name for the intervention of the symbolic law is 'paternal metaphor', which highlights precisely how the symbolic ('metaphor') substitutes the imaginary deadlock embodied by the phallus in the child's relation to the first other (the mother). Only at this stage, after the intervention of the paternal metaphor qua castration, does the phallus illuminate the meaning of $S(\not{A})$, since the signifier of the lack in the Other now speaks for the impossible fulfillment of desire. Prior to the intervention of the signifier, then, for the child the phallus functioned at the level of the imaginary, as an object potentially endowed with the 'magical' power to satisfy the other's desire, thus being potentially conducive to complete fulfillment. In contrast to imaginary castration, which still relied on the possibility of restoring what was lost, in symbolic castration the signifier establishes the impossibility of desire reaching its complete satisfaction. As such, the endorsement of symbolic castration qua $S(\not{A})$ is the ultimate goal of psychoanalysis.

Both Freud and Lacan tell us that the specular image is fundamental for object cathexis, which governs narcissism. But the phallus, Lacan claims, complicates things substantially inasmuch as it is not merely an imaginary object, but is instead the missing point in the specular image which embodies "the most intimate aspect of autoeroticism" (696, 8). With the intervention of the paternal metaphor, this lack is mediated by the signifier, thus potentially becoming the lack that signifies the non-existence of the Other, and therefore the radical finitude and contingency of the subject. By saying that there is no specular image of the phallus qua image of the penis, Lacan therefore introduces the theme of the necessity of symbolic castration, which brings into contention the fact that there is 'no other of the Other': the Other is radically inconsistent since it can only rely upon the signifier. "The fantasy of it falling off", says Lacan about the imaginary phallus, is equivalent to the lack that constitutes the "world of objects" (696, 8–697, 1). And, by the same token, the phallus works in creating signification precisely on condition that its constitutive lack is veiled, hidden, repressed.

Lacan can now establish the link between the phallus and *jouissance* as predicated upon the lack in the Other, which in turn will lead him to introduce the issue of sexuation.

> It is thus that the erectile organ – not as itself, or even as an image, but as a part that is missing in the desired image – comes to symbolize the place of jouissance; this is why the erectile organ can be equated with the $\sqrt{-1}$, the symbol of the signification produced above, of the jouissance it restores – by the coefficient of its statement – to the function of a missing signifier (-1).
>
> (697, 2)

The square root of minus 1 is here called into question as an 'impossible' number that stands for the missing signifier and parallels the function of the phallus in structuring meaning. Insofar as it is an imaginary number, $\sqrt{-1}$ does not exist, that is to say, it is only imagined, and it is precisely through this imaginary function that "it can be equated" with the meaning of the phallus. The point Lacan is trying to make is that through its non-existence, or imaginary status, the phallus elevates *jouissance* to the place of the missing signifier. Just like an impossible/imaginary number, the phallus is therefore pure semblance devoid of any content, and as such it structures meaning.[22] Lacan adds that the volatility of the imaginary phallus is also what "reduces all coveted jouissance to the brevity of autoeroticism" (697, 3): the subject's attempt at gaining jouissance, in other words, is to be understood first and foremost in autoerotic (narcissistic, masturbatory) terms, since the first presentation of the phallus is the specular one. Lacan here briefly mentions the connection between anatomy and autoeroticism by referring to "the further perfected hand of the monkey", linking this to Mauss' reading of Freud as belonging to "the tradition of 'bodily techniques'" (697, 3). However, he suggests that, rather than lending themselves to be interpreted in terms of cynicism, these autoerotic techniques should rather be linked with the emergence of guilt, insofar as the latter "is related to the reminder of the jouissance that is not found in the service rendered to the real organ" (697, 4). In other words, guilt appears with the subject's experience of the prohibition of jouissance introduced by castration, that is, the "consecration of the signifier's imaginary function of prohibiting objects" (697, 4). This instance of prohibition also ties in with other ways of interpreting the role of the phallus, which can be seen, for example, in the traumatic "sanctification of the organ" represented by "circumcision" (697, 5).

After this passage on the connection between autoeroticism and castration, Lacan states that the symbolic equivalent of the imaginary phallus is ϕ. The fact that the imaginary phallus is located in the specular image of the male erectile organ as its lacking part leads the subject to assume that the jouissance associated with the phallus belongs to the Other; we can therefore once again see the correlation between ϕ (imaginary phallus) and Φ (symbolic phallus). The symbolic dimension of phallic function, Lacan continues, "explains both the particularities of women's approach to sexuality, and what makes the male sex the weaker sex with regard to perversion" (697, 6). Here he hints at two important issues relating to the function of the phallus as symbol of power: its sustaining feminine desire, and its embodying the masculine tendency toward perversion (since, as we have seen, the pervert fills the lack in the Other, aiming to create the illusion of a fully consistent and all-powerful Other).

An important difference between Freud and Lacan concerns precisely the issue of sexuation. If, for Freud, sexual difference is still very much developed on biological grounds, for it relies on the conundrum of the imaginary phallus, in Lacan it is clearly an outcome of the encounter with the paternal metaphor, which, as we have seen, assigns the phallus a signifying role. For Lacan, masculinity and femininity are ultimately the result of how the subject positions itself vis-à-vis the phallus qua signifier of an impossible signified. This thesis, however – at least in *Subversion*, as it can be evinced from the above reference to perversion – does not do away with sexual anatomy per se, since Lacan, like Freud, here seems to believe that the initial question concerning the imaginary phallus is inevitably based on the presence / absence of the penis.[23]

The psychopathological positions of the subject of the unconscious

Lacan's mention of perversion is brief but highly pertinent. He says that in sexuality the masculine position is by definition very close, indeed dangerously close, to perversion: "[perversion] barely accentuates the function of desire in man, insofar as desire institutes the dominance – in the privileged place of jouissance – of object *a* in fantasy, which desire substitutes for $\not{A}$" (697, 7). Instead of being aimed at the inexistence of the Other, masculine fantasy stops too short of such ontological lack, namely at the 'little other' (*a*), the at least minimally objectified and singularized detail in the Other, thus running the risk, as in perversion, of becoming "the instrument of the Other's jouissance" (697, 7). We have seen that, faced by the enigmatic presence of the Other, the subject ends up asking the following question: 'What do you want (from me)?' At this stage, that question can be reformulated self-reflexively as such: 'What am I in relation to the *jouissance* of the Other?'; or: 'What position am I expected to occupy vis-à-vis such *jouissance*?' By answering these questions, the subject of the unconscious effectively assumes a certain psychopathological position, which, structurally, can be catalogued as either that of psychosis, neurosis or perversion.

In the case of psychosis, we witness the failure or rather the foreclosure of the paternal metaphor, which means that the subject remains at the mercy of the Other's *jouissance*. Because of the lack of distance between the subject and the Other, in psychosis (e.g. paranoid or schizophrenic) meanings do not slide as they do after the intervention of the Name-of-the-Father, but instead retain a fixation which translates into the absolute certainty about what one says or does. Differently from psychosis, in both neurosis and perversion the gap between subject and Other has been inscribed by the paternal metaphor, which means that the subject is constantly grappling with lack – the lack introduced by the signifier qua law. Both the neurotic and the pervert, in other words, have relinquished themselves from the grip of an omnipotent Other, and yet – this is the common source of their different psychopathologies – they are not free from their belief in the existence of this Other and, specifically, of its *jouissance*. In brief, differently from psychotics they are not prisoners of the Other, and yet they remain subjected to its threatening presence.

How, then, do they react? More precisely: what sort of defenses do they set up against the encumbering *jouissance* of the Other? According to Lacan, the pervert does not foreclose the Name-of-the-Father, he disavows it. Rather than accepting the alienating role of the paternal metaphor, the pervert tries to deny the incidence of that role, believing instead that he can occupy the place of the phallus for the (m)other in a bid to achieve full *jouissance*. He effectively attempts to safeguard the 'dream of wholeness' concerning enjoyment. Masochism in this respect offers the clearest perverse scenario, with the masochist subject conceiving of himself as the instrument of the Other's *jouissance*. Similarly, the sadist believes himself to be the Other and as such capable of limitless *jouissance*. As Lacan puts it: "the pervert imagines he is the Other in order to ensure his own jouissance" (699). The pervert, then, thinks he knows what it is that triggers desire; his position is characterized by his presumed knowledge and control of libido as such.

With neurosis, on the other hand, perversion is generally avoided, since "one identifies the Other's lack with the Other's demand, Φ with D" (698, 2), which leads directly to the catalogue of the neurotic's drives qua $\$\lozenge D$ (698, 3). The neurotic's drives, in other words, are the consequence of his fantasies about the demands made by the Other on him/her. This predominance of the Other's demand in neurosis is, Lacan adds, a strategy to hide the Other's desire qua lack, which, however, "cannot be misrecognized when it is covered by the phobic object alone" (698, 4). The implication is that, "whether hysteric, obsessive, or, more radically, phobic" (698, 2),[24] the neurotic tends to maintain, though in a skewed and deeply problematic manner, the Other as its interlocutor. For the neurotic, castration has indeed taken place (700, 3), but the lack that castration has brought in is not fully accepted, since the neurotic continues to believe that it can be overcome. While the lack is there, inscribed in the domain of the symbolic, it causes problems for the neurotic precisely because he/she secretly holds on to the possibility of overcoming it. As Lacan puts it at the end of *Subversion*, beneath his strong ego "the neurotic hides the castration he denies" (700, 4). In other words, the neurotic represses castration, secretly continuing to believe in the possibility of a relationship with the Other that might *not* be over-determined by lack – one where the Other actually exists in an autonomous capacity. While symbolic castration has definitely taken place for the neurotic, his problem is that he relates to it in imaginary terms, as a problem that could be resolved.[25] In this respect, the neurotic's "strong ego" is a reaction against the threat of anxiety (the Other's *jouissance*) that originates in symbolic castration (700, 6). The object of the neurotic's fantasy is still the Other's demand – what does the Other want from me? – which in turn activates his/her drives. Yet, the neurotic tends to perceive himself/herself as the object of the Other's desire. In this respect the real problem of the neurotic is that, unconsciously, he/she imagines that the Other is after his/her [the neurotic's] castration in order to realize its own *jouissance*. This unbearable *jouissance* of the Other, in which he/she would vanish, is what the neurotic, whether obsessive or hysterical, is constantly struggling with. Ultimately, "although, deep down, he feels he is the most vain thing in existence", the neurotic refuses to "sacrifice his difference (anything but that) to the jouissance of an Other" (700, 7).

Lacan's argument can be summarized as follows: when confronted by the prospect of anxiety, the neurotic defends himself/herself by concealing his/her castration ($) either via identification with the 'ideal father' and consequent assumption of the imaginary phallus (ϕ); or by direct identification with the imaginary phallus itself, which is expected to fill the lack in the Other. The first position describes the obsessional neurotic's fantasmatic scenario, the second the hysteric's (698, 4). Both these positions can therefore be seen as defence mechanisms against the threatening desire of the Other, which registers in their psychic economies but is simultaneously repressed.

With the obsessional neurotic, the Other's desire is constantly negated in a bid to avoid, in fantasy, the vanishing of the subject. The obsessional neurotic is apparently in control of everything because, as anticipated, he/she identifies with the ideal father and the mastery therein embodied (698, 6). This accounts for the slavish dimension typical of his/her position: without the imaginary 'backing' of the ideal father, he/she is lost. At the same time, however, the obsessive tends to represent the Other as the 'dead father', a father who occupies a purely symbolic role, and therefore cannot enjoy (698, 7). In this manner the obsessive attempts to control the threat of *jouissance*, which would compromise his/her presumed control over reality. With the hysteric, on the other hand, the relation to the Other's enjoyment is more subtle, for the aim of this type of neurosis is to sustain one's fantasy by constantly "slipping away" (698, 4) from the position of object of the Other's desire – and yet at the same time, in fantasy, positing oneself as filling the lack in the Other, which is perceived as temporary. The hysteric, for instance, tends to experience sexuality as a threat to his/her own subjectivity, fearing that he/she will disappear in the *jouissance* of the Other, turning into a passive object of the Other's desire. At the same time, however, he/she believes the Other can only be completed by him/her.

The elementary subjective position as constituted in fantasy, in all three psychopathological cases, remains that of object of the Other's desire. Take the obvious connection between what is normally known as 'stage fright' (anxiety in relation to performances in front of an audience) and neurosis. Here are the three possible neurotic outcomes: (1) The speaker cannot perform because anxiety (perceiving oneself as the object of the audience's desire, especially through their gaze) is unbearable (phobic). (2) The speaker assumes a domineering position and tries not to interact with the audience (for instance, speaking incessantly, or avoiding eye contact) in order to keep their desire at bay (obsessive). (3) The speaker deliberately frustrates the audience so as to avoid 'congealing' into the object of their desire/jouissance (hysteric). With regard to the last two positions, Lacan says: "These features are confirmed by the obsessive's fundamental need to be the Other's guarantor, and by the Faithlessness of hysterical intrigue" (698, 5). More generally, "the image of the ideal Father is a neurotic's fantasy", inasmuch as "the true function of the Father [...] is fundamentally to unite (and not to oppose) a desire to the Law". The neurotic wishes the Mother ("demand's real Other") would "tone down" his/her desire, while the Father he/she idealizes is, ultimately, "the dead Father" (698, 6–7) – since the dead Father is symbolically active (in the role designated by Lacan as the 'Name-of-the-father') to master the excessive dimension of the subject's desire. As Lacan notes, this is "one of the stumbling blocks the analyst must avoid", which by implication means that it is also "the crux of the interminable aspect of transference" (698, 8). Lacan here warns the analyst against the risk of turning into the father qua master of the neurotic's desire, a "stumbling block" with obvious consequences for transference. More precisely, he adds that "the analyst must safeguard the imaginary dimension of his nonmastery and necessary imperfection for the other", insofar as this represents

> as important a matter to deal with as the deliberate reinforcement in the analyst of his nescience regarding each subject who comes to him for analysis, of an ever renewed ignorance so that no one is considered a typical case.
>
> (699, 1)

This means that the analyst must make every effort to preserve, for the patient, the image of his own (the analyst's) fallibility – a point that is as important as preserving the analyst's ignorance as the appropriate starting point of any session.

At this stage Lacan turns to perversion in more detail. Freud's claim that neurosis is the inverse of perversion is endorsed by Lacan: what the neurotic represses is the unconscious fantasy of being the object of the Other's *jouissance*, which, as we have seen, is precisely what qualifies the position of the pervert. The unconscious fantasies of the neurotic, then, have a perverse content:

> let us say that the pervert imagines he is the Other in order to ensure his own jouissance, and that this is what the neurotic reveals when he imagines he is a pervert – in his case, to ensure control over the Other. This explains the supposed perversion at the crux of neurosis. Perversion is in the neurotic's unconscious in the guise of the Other's fantasy.
>
> (699, 2–3)

In perversion, on the other hand, the fantasy of being the object of the Other's *jouissance* is openly endorsed because it fulfils the opposite function with regard to neurosis: while in the latter it stands for the threat of the disappearance of the subject overwhelmed by *jouissance*, against which neurosis is a defense, in perversion it strengthens the ego by creating the scenario of a fulfilled, harmonious relation to the Other, that is to say a relation governed by a law and therefore guarded from the incursions of *jouissance*. Since it is the Other that holds the key to desire and *jouissance*, the pervert identifies directly with this Other, attempting to annul the difference and complexity of his/her subjective position.

The link between neurosis and perversion, Lacan insists, is an important one to stress. A neurotic is always in danger of becoming a pervert, for the pervert's position, as anticipated, is implicit in the neurotic's. Rather than maintaining the gap between subject and Other (neurosis), the pervert enters directly the domain of the Other by imagining himself/herself as the object of the Other's jouissance. This is how he/she enjoys. Nevertheless, Lacan quickly remarks that the pervert's unconscious is not "out in the open" as in psychosis; this suggests that the pervert's structure is far from subversive since he aims at setting a limit against boundless and deadly *jouissance*: "He, too, defends himself in his desire in his own way. For desire is a defense, a defense against going beyond a certain limit in jouissance" (699, 3).[26]

The above statement about the protective function of desire is crucial if we are to understand Lacan's position vis-à-vis subversion. By hooking *object a*, desire effectively operates through a lure, namely that the Other, in its radical openness, can be replaced by *object a*. Such operation secures the fantasy in its comforting modality, thus making sure the subject keeps at a safe distance from the lack in the Other qua *jouissance*. Lacan elaborates on how this operation is based on the avoidance of the phallus as signifier of lack, a point he relates to Plato's *Symposium* and, specifically, to the figures of Socrates (qua analyst) and Alcibiades (qua analysand):

> Included in object *a* is *agalma*, the inestimable treasure that Alcibiades declares is contained in the rustic box the figure of Socrates is to him. But let us note that a minus sign (-) is attributed to it. It is because Alcibiades has not seen Socrates' prick – permit me to follow Plato here, who does not spare us the details – that Alcibiades the seducer exalts in Socrates the *agalma*, the marvel that he would have liked Socrates to cede to him by avoiding his desire.
>
> (699, 5)

It is "the absence of the penis" (699, 6) that is responsible for the circulation of desire (as Alcibiades' fascination with Socrates' *agalma* is sustained by the fact that he "has not seen his prick"),[27] since such absence is what represents the phallus (negativized specular image of the penis) as object of desire. The phallus, then, is what the fascinating appearance of *object a* ultimately hides, and as such it captures the position of women in relation to masculine sexuality: "it is the absence of the penis that makes her the phallus, the object of desire" (699, 6). Lacan then continues to link this logic – the dialectic of desire as sustained by *object a* – to transference in analysis. He does so by returning to Plato's *Symposium*, where Socrates, "the precursor of psychoanalysis" (699, 7), eventually shows his young adulator Alcibiades that his feelings are caused by his mistaken supposition that Socrates possesses the *agalma*; by contrast, Socrates demonstrates that Alcibiades' real object of desire was not himself but "Agathon the transferential object" (699, 7). In other words, the analyst sets up a strategy whereby he/she directs the analysand's desire toward himself/herself only to show the analysand how wrong that direction is, since it is based on the assumption that the analyst possesses what is in fact ontologically absent – *agalma* is only a veil over lack. This strategy allows castration (the impossibility to achieve full *jouissance*) to take place, thus opening up the way to the dialectic of desire incarnated by Alcibiades' relation to the transferential object, Agathon.

Now, the neurotic's fantasy is not only sustained by the gap between himself/herself and the Other, but more precisely by the relationship with *object a*. In fact, the very presence of *object a* in the neurotic's fantasy, quite literally as its anchoring point, reveals that "the neurotic underwent castration at the outset", which is functional to developing

> the strong ego that he is, so strong, one might say, that his proper name bothers him, so strong that deep down the neurotic is Nameless. Yet, it is behind this ego, which certain analysts choose to strengthen still more, that the neurotic hides the castration he denies. But, contrary to appearances, he cleaves to this castration.
>
> (700, 3–5)

The neurotic opposes the Other in the ways we have discussed because he fears "that the Other demands his castration" – a castration that he wants to preserve, while denying it, because "[w]hat analytic experience attests is that castration is what regulates desire, in both normal and abnormal cases" (700, 7–8). How? Precisely by guaranteeing the connection between the subject and *object a*:

> Providing it oscillates by alternating between $ and *a* in fantasy, castration makes of fantasy a chain that is both supple and inextensible by which the fixation of object cathexis, which can hardly go beyond certain natural limits, takes on the transcendental function of ensuring the jouissance of the Other that passes this chain on to me in the Law.
>
> (700, 9)

As a buffer between the barred subject and the lack contained in the object-cause of desire, fantasy makes sure that the subject's fixation on a given object against the background of lack effectively determines the necessity of the law's intervention to regulate the Other's *jouissance*. As Lacan explains at the end of his piece, desire, fantasy and the law are inextricably linked in dialectical terms. Before turning to his final statement, let us notice that Lacan offers two possible subjective strategies in relation to the Other. First, one starts by experiencing the Other's will rather than its demand – one must, in other words, break the dependency on demand. From there, it is a matter of either facing this will "as an object, turning into the mummy of some Buddhist initiation", which constitutes the pervert's position in as much as it is constituted through the subject's self-instrumentalisation; or "satisfy the will to castrate inscribed in the Other, which leads to the supreme narcissism of the Lost Cause", in turn associated by Lacan with Greek tragedy and Claudel's acceptance of a "Christianity of despair" (700, 10). This latter position defines the structure of neurosis, where castration has firmly installed lack (the "lost cause" and the "Christianity of despair") within the structure of the subject.

The inverse scale of the law of desire

The conclusive assertion of the paper is one of the most-often cited: "Castration means that jouissance has to be refused in order to be attained on the inverse scale of the Law of desire" (700, 11). By interiorizing symbolic castration, which alienates us in/through the Other while turning full or limitless *jouissance* into a mythical and deadly entity, we bring in the law that, in turn, reopens for us the possibility of *jouissance*, though this time as co-terminus with lack and represented by the ineffable object-cause of desire. Without a doubt, one of the central themes of the latter part of *Subversion* is the dialectic of language and *jouissance*. As already mentioned, for Lacan "jouissance is forbidden [*interdite*] to him who speaks, as such – or, put differently, it can only be said [*dite*] between the lines by whoever is a subject of the Law, since the Law is grounded in this very prohibition" (696, 2). The pun is truly dialectical: what is *interdite* (i.e. *jouissance* itself in its full/deadly constitution) is *dite* between the lines, that is to say as the surplus-*jouissance* (*plus-de-jouir*) generated by the intrinsic inconsistency of language, such as expressed in the formations of the unconscious. And language sustains itself precisely through the *plus-de-jouir* it generates, which by definition cannot be said. In this sense, the lack represented by surplus-*jouissance* is at the heart of Lacan's subversion of the subject, since it stands for the ontological impossibility that, on the one hand, through its gentrification (*object a*), lends a minimum of consistency to both subject and Other, while on the other hand it also confronts the subject with the possibility of the radical reconfiguration of his/her desire. Thus the impossibility of *jouissance* qua ontologically lacking surplus also stands, in a dialectical manner, for the possibility of subverting one's mode of enjoyment.

Conclusion

Having reached this final stage, two significant perspectives need to be highlighted. First, the idea that the swipe of symbolic castration, via the law of the signifier, is the necessary passage through which the subject learns to avoid being swamped by *jouissance* – which in this sense, as Lacan reiterates in *Subversion*, should be thought of as the *jouissance* of the Other, since the subject disappears in it. Think, for instance, of the aforementioned inescapability of demand, where the child has to gain a distance from the intrinsically overbearing demand that qualifies its relation to its first other (the mother). Avoiding the *jouissance* of the Other, then, leads to the formation of fantasy and desire, both of which depend on the mediation of language, that is, of the paternal metaphor. And the ego owes its existence precisely to the subject's capacity to desire, that is, to protect itself from being inundated with the maelstrom of *jouissance*, which in its final configuration coincides with death.

In Lacan, then, the intervention of the paternal metaphor can be compared to a sort of 'pulling the brakes' in respect of the subject's initial and constitutive tendency to be drawn into the Other's *jouissance*, which is by definition destructive. Thus, it would seem that the law of castration in Lacan effectively accomplishes the same 'job' of the pleasure principle in Freud: it prevents the subject of the signifier to be flooded with *jouissance*. Here, however, we must register an important change in the constitution of *jouissance* as conceptualized by Lacan. What happens to it after symbolic castration is that it appears for what it truly is, namely a meaningless surplus of sense which as such forces every desire to experience its frustration and incessant iteration. This means that, after castration, *jouissance* becomes, in actual fact, the *jouissance* of the Other. Via this emphasis on the centrality of castration we get to Lacan's 'ethics of desire', a theme that no doubt characterized his work until *Seminar VII* and can be summed up with the well-known motto from that seminar: 'do not give up on your desire'.

There is, however, a more radical way of grasping Lacan's theorization of *jouissance* in *Subversion*, which, I claim, is what makes this famous *Écrit* a veritable turning point in Lacan's oeuvre. As anticipated, it is a matter of conceiving of the passage from demand to desire and *jouissance* as a trajectory which, ultimately, does not stop at the regulatory function of castration and the concurrent ethics of desire, but takes us further to an understanding of subversion built upon the connection of drive and *jouissance* rather than desire and *jouissance*. While *jouissance* retains here its crucial convergence with lack, as instituted by the signifier, at the same time it leads the subject to confront S(Ⱥ), namely the signifier of the non-existence of the Other, which implies the possibility of the reconfiguration of one's subjective content insofar as it is dialectically connected with this Other. If we look at the final version of Lacan's graph in *Subversion*, we note that the upper chain is constituted by two vectors. The first goes from *jouissance* to castration, from left to right, following the familiar trajectory whereby the drives are, as it were, tamed and forced back into the path of desire and fantasy. However, this is certainly not Lacan's last word on *jouissance*, since he adds a second vector that moves back from castration to *jouissance* through drive, eventually encroaching upon S(Ⱥ). My conclusive point is that the importance of *Subversion* should be associated with this last and highest of vectors that does not stop at castration but, after the latter's necessary intervention, reactivates the drive in such a way as to bring about the destabilizing lack in the Other.

Notes

1 *Seminar VII* (see Lacan 1959–1960) ended on 6 July 1960, just over two months before the Royaumont conference, so inevitably there are overlaps between the content of that seminar and *Subversion*. *Seminar VII* is itself generally regarded as marking a very significant shift in Lacan's thinking – namely a shift toward the Real. While in the years immediately prior to *Seminar VII* Lacan had tirelessly emphasized the central function of the register of the Symbolic in the structuring of the unconscious and subjectivity, the end of the 1950s sees the rise of the register of the Real as a new focus of Lacan's thought. From this point on, phenomena resisting or thwarting the signifying powers of the socio-symbolic order, such as especially *jouissance*, became increasingly central to Lacan's seminars and thought in general. However, it seems clear to me that *Subversion* supplements the key theme of *Seminar VII*, namely the ethics of pure desire as that which we should not compromise or give up on, with a new focus on the drive. As Alenka Zupančič (2000: 239) has put it apropos the passage from *Seminar VII* to *Subversion*: "In order to arrive at the drive, one must pass through desire and insist on it until the very end."

2 "The thesis that being a philosopher means being interested in what everyone is interested in without knowing it has the interesting peculiarity that its relevance

does not imply that it can be settled either way" (671, 2); "Now this subject who must know what he is doing, or so we presume, does not know what is already, in fact, of interest to everyone regarding the effects of science" (672, 2).

3 "*Aufhebung* is one of philosophy's pretty little dreams" (S20, 1972–1973: 86).

4 Slavoj Žižek has successfully repoliticized the notion of ideological belief precisely by incorporating the Lacanian insight. He warns us that it is when the explicit ideological injunction begins losing its grip on its subjects that we should be most vigilant against ideological manipulation.

5 In passing, Lacan remarks that "the pilot science of structuralism in the West has its roots in Russia, where formalism first flourished. Geneva 1910 and Petrograd 1920 suffice to explain why Freud did not have this particular instrument at his disposal" (676, 6). The point, then, is that the Freudian unconscious is implicitly informed by linguistic notions that Freud himself could not fully develop.

6 "The world about which we speak and in which we live is no 'brute' reality; it is itself already mediated and structured by the signifiers of language, which allow it to appear as a meaningful and differentiated environment (*Umwelt*)" (Van Haute 2002: 10–11).

7 See also Lacan's references to Parmenides and Heraclitus in *Seminar XX* (Lacan, 1972–1973: 114).

8 This statement recalls Lacan's famous proposition, in his text "Seminar on the 'Purloined Letter'", about intersubjective communication: "the sender [...] receives from the receiver his own message in an inverted form" (30, 2).

9 Lacan (678, 8–679, 5) refers to Freud's 1911 article "Formulations on the Two Principles of Mental Functioning", which ends with Freud commenting on the dream of one of his neurotic patients concerning a father who was talking to him without being aware of his being already dead. While Freud uses this dream to expose his understanding of the unconscious death-wish against the father in neurosis, Lacan gives it a further spin by linking the 'dead father' with the 'symbolically dead' status of the signifier.

10 In this seminar, Lacan (S17, 1969–1970: 42) admonishes the subversive students involved in the 1968 upheavals that they should "sound the depth of their commitments" vis-à-vis the idea of revolution as the radical emptying of one's subjective / pathological content.

11 Literally 'the upholstery button', this expression has been translated in different ways ('quilting point', 'anchoring point'), with Fink opting for "button tie", (681, 5) in a bid to conjure up Lacan's intention to capture the idea of a given signifier that unifies a field of meaning.

12 The dialectical figure of the "negation of negation" is central to the entire *Science of Logic* (1916/2010: 89–90, 108–19, 144–45, 360, 530–32, 566).

13 If, taking the cue from Lacan's mention of the figure of the witness, we think of a crime story, we could argue that the locus of the Other encompasses both the figure of the criminal (language in its performative function; the fact that 'the letter kills') and that of the innocent bystander who witnesses the crime. It is thanks to the innocent Other as bystander that crime is sublated into a higher truth; that is to say, the Other turns language into the ultimate horizon of our being. In fact, crime and its witnessing are two sides of the same coin, and the coin is the price we pay, in terms of deception, for the acceptance of language as the untranscendable feature of our being. This is to say that the deceptiveness of the big Other is

nothing other than the deceptiveness of language itself, but, as it were, shifted to the background and given the status of the *empty framework* of language.

14 As Žižek (2012: 46) puts it, the "human language proper only functions when fiction counts for more than reality, when there is more truth in a mask than in the stupid reality beneath the mask".

15
> But an animal does not feign feigning. It does not make tracks whose deceptiveness lies in getting them to be taken as false, when in fact they are true – that is, tracks that indicate the right trail. No more than it effaces its tracks, which would already be tantamount to making itself the subject of the signifier.
>
> (683, 6)

In short, animals are unable to pretend to pretend, which is precisely the function of the Other in respect of language.

16 As claimed by Fink (2004: 116–17):

> The subject comes into being here insofar as she identifies with the Other's view of her (replete as it is with the Other's ideals and values); in other words, she internalizes the ideal for her that the Other has, what she would have to be in order to be ideal in the Other's eyes: the ego-ideal. [...] the ego-ideal is essentially a point outside the ego from which one observes and evaluates one's own ego as a whole or totality, just as one's parent observes and evaluates it.

17 Lacan acerbically asserts that such belief corresponded to

> a phenomenon of mental abdication tied to the aging of the psychoanalytic group in the Diaspora owing to the war, and the reduction of an eminent practice to a *Good Housekeeping* seal of approval attesting to its suitability to the 'American way of life'.
>
> (685, 1)

The target of Lacan's invective here are those psychologists who fled Europe during the war and, once in America, began to assert the idea that, at some point in its core, the ego must present itself as free of the conflicts between the drives and the demands of reality. From this perspective, they promoted the idea that treatment must consist in recuperating a strong and autonomous ego which is able to mediate between the activity of the drives and the social context. For Lacan this construction of the ego commits the crucial mistake of closing off none other than the unconscious.

18 Crucially, Lacan is keen to emphasize the historical implications for missing the opacity of the ego:

> The promotion of consciousness as essential to the subject in the historical aftermath of the Cartesian cogito is indicative, to my mind, of a misleading emphasis on the transparency of the *I* in action at the expense of the opacity of the signifier that determines it.
>
> (685, 5)

One should note here how the opacity of the ego is nothing but the opacity of the signifier that determines it – in other words, of the "unconscious structured like a language".

19 "For it is clear that man's continued nescience of his desire is not so much nescience of what he demands, which may after all be isolated, as nescience of whence he desires" (689, 9).

20 As Van Haute (2002: 144) comments:

> It is precisely this homology that makes it possible for the signifier to inscribe itself in the body, and conversely, for the body to be taken up in the order of signifiers and thereby in the economy of the unconscious.

21 In cinema, a perfect rendition of this logic is given in Michelangelo Antonioni's cult film *Blow-up* (1966), where the desiring subject (the photographer played by David Hemmings) eventually encounters itself in the meaningless remainder of the process of signification of reality in which he is engaged (the blurred, abstract enlargement of the photograph of a dead body). What is shocking about any such encounter is precisely the fading of the fantasy that sustains subjectivity: the entire content of the subject's self is annihilated, reduced to an inexplicable drive that insists in its path regardless of any conscious motivation.

22 Slavoj Žižek's comment on the meaning of the phallus helps us to clarify the above (infamous) passage:

> Lacan's claim that the 'imaginary' number (the square root of -1) is the 'meaning of the phallus,' its signified, is often invoked as an outstanding example of his intellectual imposture—so what does he mean by it? The paradox of the square root of -1 is that it is an 'impossible' number whose value can never be positivized, but which nonetheless 'functions.' What does this have to do with the phallus? Precisely insofar as it is the signifier of the impossible fullness of meaning, the phallus is a 'signifier without a signified'—the 'minus 1,' the supplementary feature which sticks out from the series of 'normal' signifiers, the element in which excess and lack coincide. The impossible fullness at the level of meaning (of the signified) is sustained by the void (the castrating dimension) at the level of the signifier—we encounter the 'meaning of the phallus' when, apropos some notion, we enthusiastically sense that 'this is *it*, the true thing, the true meaning,' although we are never able to explicate *what*, precisely, this meaning *is*.
>
> (2012: 846)

23 See Van Haute's criticism (2002: 211–16) of this aspect of Lacan's theory as presented in *Subversion*.

24 The place of phobia within Lacan's theory is not clarified here, and is notoriously difficult to define in his work as a whole. In *Seminar IV* (1956–1957), Lacan updates Freud's conceptualization of phobia by commenting on the case of Little Hans and claiming that phobia is a defensive mechanism against anxiety. This reading is confirmed and updated in *Seminar X* (1962–1963). In *Seminar VIII* (1960–1961), he argues, in line with what is mentioned in *Subversion*, that phobia is the most radical form of neurosis. Eventually, in *Seminar XVI* (1968–1969), Lacan claims that phobia is not a structure like neurosis or perversion, but is rather placed in between them, holding the potential to lead to either one or the other.

25 *Mutatis mutandi*, we could say that the peculiar position of the neurotic is characterized by the fact that, despite his ambivalent attachment to it, ultimately "he

cleaves to this castration" (700, 5), that is, he refuses to sacrifice it to the altar of the Other's *jouissance*.

26 In Seminar 1962–1963, session 13 March 1963, Lacan will state, for example, that the ultimate aim of the masochist is to draw out of the Other so much *jouissance* that it becomes unbearable, thus forcing this Other to evoke a law that might limit *jouissance*. The whole point is that, by making the Other anxious, the masochist subject succeeds in finding a defense against his own potentially unlimited perverse enjoyment. Ultimately, as Lacan indeed underlined in later texts, perversion is a *père-version*, in other words a desperate and disavowed attempt at establishing the law of the father.

27 In Plato's *Symposium*, Alcibiades contrasts Socrates' ugly appearance with the preciousness of his interior, comparing him to those boxes that, on the exterior, present figures of ugly satyrs, while hiding the *agalma*, that is, jewels of incommensurable beauty.

Bibliography

Choi, W. (2012) 'From or Toward the Symbolic? A Critique of Žižek's The Sublime Object of Ideology', *Décalages* 1(2), available at: http://scholar.oxy.edu/decalages/vol1/iss2/2.

Dolar, M. (2006) 'Hegel as the Other Side of Psychoanalysis', in J. Clemens, J and R. Grigg (Eds.), *Reflections on Seminar XVII: Jacques Lacan and the Other Side of Psychoanalysis*. Durham/London: Duke University Press.

Evans, D. (1997) *An Introductory Dictionary of Lacanian Psychoanalysis*. London: Routledge.

Fink, B. (2004) *Lacan to the Letter. Reading Écrits Closely*. Minneapolis, MN/London: University of Minnesota Press.

Hegel, G. W. F (1916/2010) *The Science of Logic*. Translated and edited by George di Giovanni. Cambridge: Cambridge University Press.

Lacan, J. (1961–1962) *Le Séminaire. L'identification* (1961–1962), unpublished.

Lacan, J. (1975/1998). *Book XX: Encore, On Femininity, Love and the Limits of Knowledge* (1972–1973), trans. B. Fink, ed. J.-A. Miller. London: W. W. Norton & Company.

Lacan, J. (1986/1992) *The Seminar. Book VII: The Ethics of Psychoanalysis* (1959–1960), trans. D. Porter, ed. J.-A. Miller. New York/London: W. W. Norton & Company.

Lacan, J. (1991/2007) *The Seminar. Book XVII: The Other Side of Psychoanalysis* (1969–1970), trans. R. Grigg, ed. J.-A. Miller. New York/London: W. W. Norton & Company.

Lacan, J. (2004/2014) *The Seminar. Book X: Anxiety* (1962–1963), trans. A. R. Price, ed. J.-A. Miller. Cambridge: Polity.

Lacan, J. (2005/2008) *My Teaching*. London/New York: Verso.

Pluth, E. (2007) *Signifiers and Acts. Freedom in Lacan's Theory of the Signifier*. Albany, NY: SUNY Press.

Roudinesco, É. (1993/1997) *Jacques Lacan*, trans. B. Bray. New York/London: Columbia University Press.

Sartre, J.-P. (1943/1992) *Being and Nothingness: A Phenomenological Essay on Ontology*. New York/London/Toronto/Sydney/Singapore: Washington Square Press.

Van Haute, P. (2001) *Against Adaptation. Lacan's Subversion of the Subject*. New York: Other Press.

Žižek, S. (2012) *Less than Nothing. Hegel and the Shadow of Dialectical Materialism*. London/New York: Verso.

8

POSITION OF THE UNCONSCIOUS

Paul Verhaeghe

The Unconscious is between the subject and the Other, their cut in action (712).

Context

As usually is the case with Lacan, we have to address the historical circumstances if we want to understand the importance of his article on '*Position of the Unconscious*.' The bibliographical reference in the *Écrits* (867) tells us that it summarizes his remarks made at the Bonneval Colloquium, held from October 30 to November 2, 1960. Henri Ey, who organized the colloquium, wanted to confront philosophers, analysts and psychiatrists with regard to the question of the unconscious. Lacan did not present a paper himself, but took active part in the discussions and made numerous remarks. This happened especially during the workshop 'Language and the Unconscious' ('Language et inconscient') where two of his pupils, Laplanche and Leclaire, gave a joint paper. Their presentation, '*L'inconscient, une étude psychanalytique*,' with the individual contributions clearly delineated, provoked much discussion. The fact that their reading of the unconscious was different – to say the least of it – prefigured the departure of Laplanche from the Lacanian movement.

Four years later, Henri Ey asked the participants for their papers, giving them the opportunity to rewrite them. Pontalis was asked to summarize the interventions made by Merleau-Ponty (who died unexpectedly in 1961) and Lacan was invited to do likewise with his remarks. He wrote them down in March 1964. It took another two years before the proceedings were actually published, with the title *L'inconscient* (Ey, 1966). It is my thesis that the resulting paper does not summarize Lacan's 1960 interventions. On the contrary, '*Position de l'inconscient*' is the start of the Lacanian Lacan, going beyond his return to Freud.

From the 'Rome Discourse' (1953) to 'Position de l'inconscient' (1966)

Both the year of the colloquium (1960) and the one of the actual writing (1964) are important. We have to go back to 1953 for a better understanding.

At the beginning of that year, Lacan was the President of the SPP, the *Société Psychanalytique de Paris*, itself part of the IPA. In June, he was asked to resign, because of the unorthodoxy of his praxis, as he did not follow the standard rules with regard to the fixed duration of a session. This was not an isolated incident, since it was well-known that he challenged the training programme in many other respects as well and did not agree with the direction in which psychoanalysis was moving. As a reaction to this imposed resignation, Daniel Lagache, the Vice-President of the same organization, refused to take the President's place (i.e. Lacan) and resigned too. Lagache started a new institute, the SFP, the *Société française de psychanalyse*; more than twenty members of the previous organization followed – Lacan being one of them.

Long before these developments, a congress of psychoanalysts coming from the Romance-speaking countries was already planned to take place in Rome, in September of the same year. The SPP remained the official French delegation; as a reaction, the new institute held a shadow conference alongside the official one. It is during this conference that Lacan presented what became known as his '*Discours de Rome*.'

In this paper, he propounded his views on three fundamental issues for psychoanalysis: theory, clinical practice and the consequent implications for the training or formation of analysts. He criticized the turn towards Ego Psychology and Object Relations theory, and put forward what would be coined afterwards as his 'return to Freud.' In this return, he accentuates the importance of language, hence the title of the '*Discours de Rome*,' when it was published in the *Écrits*: '*The Function and Field of Speech and Language in Psychoanalysis*.'

After the Rome conference, the SPP and the SFP went their separate ways, and in 1959 the SFP asked the IPA for affiliation. It took the IPA two years to answer, and in 1961, the SFP was granted the status of Study Group. Basically, this meant that their training procedures would be carefully watched. The next year, it became clear that the IPA would only consider a full affiliation on condition that both Lacan and Françoise Dolto were excluded. This became an official statement in 1963 and was accepted by a majority of the SFP in November. As a result, in Autumn 1963, Lacan was officially expelled from the IPA and had to start his own school. Consequently, in the fall of 1963, he terminated his annual seminar series after one session. It is no coincidence that the seminar he intended to give was entitled, *The Names of the Fathers*. No coincidence, because he questions the foundation of the Oedipal authority (Verhaeghe, 2009).

At the beginning of the following year, 1964, he started his seminar anew, and for the first time free from any institutional restraints whatsoever. The subject of his introductory lesson (January 15) of what became known as *Seminar XI*, is his excommunication.[1] Two weeks later, he puts forward his own programme starting with a question about the status of the unconscious. It is no coincidence that upon the actual publication of the seminar (1973), this particular chapter will be entitled as '*The freudian Unconscious and ours*' ('*L'Inconscient freudien et le nôtre*'). Meaning that they are different.

It is obvious that 1960 (the colloquium) and 1964 (the redaction of the paper) presented Lacan with a totally different situation. In those four years, the tensions and discords had gradually built up to the point of a final split, both on the personal (most members of the SFP voted for Lacan's exclusion), the conceptual (Lacan develops his own view on the unconscious) and the organizational level (this is the starting point of a psychoanalytic institution, independent of the IPA). In 1960, he might still have had the hope that the IPA would accept the SFP, meaning that he could develop his theory within 'official' psychoanalysis. In 1963, this is no longer the case, and from January 1964, Lacan follows his own path. *Seminar XI* is a landmark in that respect, and those early months of 1964 is exactly the time when he writes '*Position de l'inconscient*.'

It is a landmark in another respect as well. In the last sentence of the last note to the paper, appearing at the end of the very last phrase, Lacan coins it as "this sequel to my Rome discourse" (721, note 4). 'Sequel' is an understatement – with this paper, Lacan opens a new line of thought, with at its center the notion of the subject. Consequently, the paper puts forward a number of new ideas without really elaborating them, whilst at the same time it is supposed to address a number of issues raised during the Bonneval Colloquium. This results in a hybrid paper that needs much clarification. This is probably the reason why Muller and Richardson (1982) did not include it in their reader's guide to the *Écrits*. In my experience, '*Position de l'Inconscient*' can best be studied together with seminar eleven. References to this seminar are indicated as S11, followed by the pagenumber based on the original French edition. In case I refer to the English edition, this is indicated by (Sheridan, pagenumber).

The Bonneval Colloquium

Back in 1960, Lacan wanted to endorse his return to Freud via the thesis that the unconscious is structured as a language. This is a central point of discussion at Bonneval, not only with the philosophers, the psychiatrists and the IPA-analysts, but between the two 'Lacanian' speakers as well.

Leclaire followed Lacan's idea about the unconscious being structured as a language literally to the letter. He presented a case study, where the interpretation of a dream resulted in the reconstruction of a signifying chain. This reconstruction is considered to be the nucleus of the patient's unconscious and can be summarized in a formula: Poordjeli, condensing all the unconscious signifiers, even letters, that determined the obsessional neurosis of his patient. Eight years later, he published the case study in his first book (Leclaire, 1968).

Laplanche addressed Lacan's return to Freud and the linguistic structure of the unconscious from a conceptual and metapsychological point of view.

He explained Freud's double perspective, the topological and the dynamic. Topologically, the Freudian unconscious differs from the conscious because the latter contains '*Wortvorstellungen*,' whilst the unconscious operates with '*Sachvorstellungen*'. Dynamically, the difference has to do with the nature of the cathexis: free floating for the unconscious, fixed for the conscious by the association with signifiers. The conclusion based on Freud's metapsychological papers is clear (Freud, 1915/1978 a, b and c). Primal repression is the precondition for both the conscious and the unconscious. There is no language as such in the unconscious: its nucleus is preverbal.

Laplanche's rigorous reading of Freud went against Lacan's conception of the unconscious, as put forward by Leclaire. If language is identified with the verbal, then the unconscious is not structured as a language. As a matter of fact, it is the other way around. The very first association of the drive with a (non-verbal) presentation, that is, a *Sachvorstellung*, will provide the base for the further associations with word presentations. Meaning that the Freudian unconscious is the condition for language.[2]

As far as we know, during the actual colloquium, Lacan did not react to these different readings. There is only one paragraph where we find an explicit rendering of a remark made by him during the Bonneval Colloquium, in defense of Serge Leclaire (714, 5). In his presentation, Leclaire demonstrated how a dream of one of his patients was determined by a signifying chain, and – by extension – how the unconscious is structured as a language. This dream became known as the unicorn dream ('*rêve à la licorne*'). The objection made to Leclaire during the colloquium – that the unicorn sequence is not unconscious, as Leclaire himself is conscious of it – is futile, says Lacan, because the unconscious has only meaning in the Other, that is, in this case, in the analyst.

As the published papers are largely rewritten, it is difficult to have an accurate image of what was actually said. Lacan explicitly deplores this, accusing implicitly Pontalis of not having rendered accurately the interventions by Merleau-Ponty (707, 2). It is obvious that his theory from 1964 onwards is very different from the one he presented in the Rome Discourse. Ironically enough, Lacan's later theory is closer to Laplanche's presentation of 1960, although he will go much further than Laplanche. Nevertheless, he will never acknowledge this affinity, even on the contrary. In 1969, at the occasion of an interview with A. Rifflet, published in her book, he will vehemently criticize Laplanche: language is the condition of the unconscious, and not the other way around. In that book, Rifflet (1970) herself accuses Laplanche of stealing Lacan's ideas.

Studying the history of psychoanalysis is not a very comforting business. In the rest of my paper I will concentrate on the shift in Lacanian theory, as presented in his '*Position de l'inconscient*.' Lacan's text contains a number of repetitions and abrupt shifts that necessarily reappear in the close reading as well. In order to make certain parts more comprehensible, I have added explanatory paragraphs. In a final part, I will present the reader with a more comprehensive rendering of what I consider the gist of Lacan's reasoning.

Commentaries on the text

The text starts with an introductory note, written in 1966. Lacan refers to Laplanche and Pontalis as his "students" and to their presentation as a definitive conception of his work, "despite the divergence between their positions" (703, 2). He also mentions the fact that the papers have been thoroughly rewritten in the interval.

The paper itself contains five different sections, separated by a double entry. There are no subtitles. The first one is the longest, running from page 703 to the middle of page 712. This first section treats different topics, meaning that it is hard to find an apt title. It brings a delineation of the Freudian unconscious; subject and time; the teaching of psychoanalysis; the importance of the lack; temporality and topology. The second section starts in the middle of page 712 till almost the end of page 714. It explains alienation, that is, the first process in the advent of the subject. The third section focuses on the second process, separation; it starts at the end of page 714 and runs till halfway page 719. Section four runs from page 719 to the beginning of page 721 and introduces the reader to Lacan's interpretation of the drive. The final section is very small; it consists of four paragraphs (721).

First section (703–712)

The unfreudian Unconscious (703–708, 2)

How thoroughly innovating this paper is, appears from the first section, where he starts with a new idea: "The Unconscious *is* a concept founded on the trail left by that which operates to constitute the subject" (703, 10). Note: 'to constitute *the subject*' (my italics). The very same innovation appears also in the title of the 1966 introduction to the '*discours de Rome*': '*On the subject who is finally in question*' ('*Du sujet enfin en question*,' 189). The 'finally' is very telling – revealing that Lacan himself was convinced of the necessity of this notion, and that it was lacking in his previous conceptualizations.

With the exception of one sentence ("The importance I attribute to language as the cause of the subject (…)" (704, 2)), we have to wait until the next section before Lacan will expand on this enigmatic thesis. A number of things are already obvious: the unconscious is not a thing, it is a concept (704, 2); hence, it is our way of understanding a certain operation. Which operation? The one *that constitutes* the subject. We have to keep this in mind for the next sections.

The enigmatic sentence is followed by a larger explanation of what the unconscious is not. It does not indicate a part of psychological reality that lacks the qualification of consciousness (703, 11). Of course, there are such parts, but they have nothing to do with the psychoanalytic conception of the unconscious, in spite of the homonymous denomination (704, 1). Even more so, the unconscious as psychoanalysis knows it, did not exist in pre-freudian times: in that period, the un-conscious had no more consistency than the 'un-black,' meaning the union of all the things that are not black, or not conscious (704, 5–6).

Lacan enumerates different examples of this not conscious, referring to an old book by Dwelshauvers (the sensory unconscious, the automatic unconscious developed by habit, etc.) to point out to the reader that these have nothing in common (704, 7). They can only be grouped together based on a totally wrong understanding of the unconscious as something primitive and instinctual (704, 8).

At that point, he formulates a first fundamental critique on psychology. This chaotic enumeration reflects the central error of psychology, that is, the assumption that consciousness is by itself a unitary phenomenon, operating its supposedly synthetic function in the same way as in "the dialectic of judgment, and in ordinary daydreaming" amongst others (705, 1). The irony is that this error is based on an experience that marks the break with assurance based on intuition (705, 4). This experience is Descartes' *Cogito*, indicating in its double movement precisely the rareness of the moment. Extrapolating this experience to all conscious phenomena is an error (705, 2). Consciousness is heterotopically distributed (705, 6), and the only homogeneous function of consciousness resides in the 'That's me' imaginary capture of the I by its mirror image: "The only homogeneous function of consciousness is found in the ego's imaginary capture by its specular reflection, and in the function of misrecognition that remains tied to it" (705, 7). It is obvious that Lacan takes his distance from a Hegelian idea about self-consciousness and the presupposition of absolute knowledge (705, 5)

Note that Lacan associates psychology with misrecognition. This brings him to the formulation of a second criticism: psychology promotes ideals and is at the servitude of society, meaning today (i.e. 1960!): market research. This explains why it receives so much credit (705, 9–11). And he adds that this psychology has enrolled Freud as well. By way of example, he refers to the discourse of consumption, which convinces women that they can only become a 'true woman' if they buy the right products to realize their potential (706, 1). Consequently, psychology is by and large an ideological enterprise, serving the powers that be. As the refusal of any ideology is the basic ethical stance of science (706, 2), psychology is both unethical and unscientific.

At that point of his reasoning (706, 3), Lacan turns to the colloquium where, he says, remarkably enough, the Freudian conception of the unconscious took a central stance. Remarkably, because many analysts, also those at the Bonneval Colloquium, are hoping to join the psychologists, who are not very fond of Freud (706, 4). This trend has been reversed at that colloquium because of his own teachings, which obliges him to account for the path that he follows (706, 5). Instead of sustaining the primitive mentality and the kind of interest general psychology serves, psychoanalysis needs to expose what is at stake (706, 6); meaning the economic interests psychology submits to. This explains the justified prejudice towards psychoanalysis in Eastern Europe (706, 8).

Instead of attempting to join general psychology, psychoanalysis should focus on its ethics and take the responsibility for the presence of the unconscious in the field of science (706, 9). This is what Laplanche and Leclaire, "my students" (706, 10), have done during the Bonneval Colloquium, whilst he himself situated them in their respective positions towards the unconscious. At this point in the paper, Lacan deplores the lack of genuine transcripts, and blames the organization for the lack of them (707, 2). In a footnote Bruce Fink tells us that Lacan is here criticizing Lagache; yet, as Lacan mentions no name, it might be directed against H. Ey as well. In the next paragraph, Fink recognizes a sneer to Lagache in a pun ('l'occasion là gâchée' [Lagache] – 'the opportunity that was missed,' 707, 3).

Lacan concludes that this has given him the opportunity to rewrite his interventions and to present the reader his updated ('à ce jour') theory of the unconscious (707, 3). This is all the more important since, during the colloqium, he could not express himself freely because of what he coins as "the resistances of a peculiar allocation of roles" (707, 3). This is what I referred to in my introduction, concerning the split between the SFP and the SPP and Lacan's hope, at that time, that the new group would be accepted by the IPA. When he writes '*Position of the Unconscious*,' this hope has proven to be idle, and Lacan knows that he has to go his own way.

The circumstances are political, but the paper is not merely a matter of politics. Lacan takes care to tell the reader that his doctrine is above all technical. Analysts are part of the concept of the unconscious, not only because we forged it to understand a number of things, but especially because the unconscious is addressed to us, as analysts. As Lacan situates the unconscious in the Other, it has to be found in its enunciation (707, 4). And he who sustains its presence – the analyst – must be called into question and has to experience "his own splitting by the signifier" (707, 5).

The next paragraph testifies to the evolution in Lacan's thinking, compared to 1960. During the colloquium, he was very much in favor of Leclaire's reading, and afterwards took his distances from Laplanche. Now, he refers to "the sense of an arrested spiral" one has in reading their work. Meaning of course the sense *he* has, in reading their work. They limited the testing of his (Lacan's) theory to a "spare part" (707, 6). By implication, what Lacan is elaborating here, goes way further. As we will see later, in our close reading of the paper, this way further was already announced in one of the opening sentences: "The unconscious *is* a concept founded on the trail left by that which operates to constitute the subject" (703, 10).

This unconscious has nothing to do with the instinctual; it has everything to do with language. Writing down the analytical experience demonstrates what is operational, that is, the "metaphorical and metonymical effects" (708, 2), which constitute the mechanisms of the unconscious, as described by Freud.

Subject and time (708, 3–709, 3)

Starting from the idea that the mechanisms of the unconscious as described by Freud come down to metaphor and metonymy, Lacan wonders whether these belong to language or to speech ("[...] are they effects of language or or of speech?" (708, 3)). This apparently simple question is not simple at all, as it entails the question of temporality. For de Saussure, the founding father of structural linguistics, language as such is there, in a timeless synchrony, whilst speech functions in a linear diachrony. The interpretation made by Jacobson (1956/1995) – well-known by Lacan – links language, synchrony and metaphor, whilst speech combines diachrony and metonymy. Let us not forget that both concepts took a central stance in Lacan's Rome discourse, as made obvious by its very title: *Function and Field of Speech and Language*.

The importance of this disjunction – either synchrony or diachrony – has everything to do with clinical practice and the possibility for change. If we are determined by our past – determined by language, as it exists in a timeless now – then nothing can change, and the Other (as language) is the determining factor. If language-in-action, that is, speech, is related to causality, then there is a possibility for change. This is beautifully expressed in *Function and Field of Speech and Language*: "What is realized in my history is neither the past definite as what was, since it is no more, nor even the perfect as what has been in what I am, but the future anterior as what I will have been, given what I am in the process of becoming" (247, 7).

In my interpretation, this explains why Lacan needed the notion of the subject and its 'advent,' together with a new theory on causality and determination. The difficulty resides in the way temporality is understood in relation to who we are. As Lacan explains, it is not a matter of either synchronicity or diachronicity, it is both. The subject is caused by langage ("language as cause of the subject" (704, 2); "The effect of language is to introduce the cause into the subject" (708, 5); "For his [i.e. the subject's] cause is the signifier" (708, 5) and produced by speech, albeit in such a way that it is never realized and keeps disappearing ('fading') during its actual production. The subject is what the signifier represents to another signifier, and yet to another, etcetera. In this paper, the differentiation between determination and causality is not fully elaborated. As with many other ideas in it, the elaboration takes place in the months to follow, that is, in *Seminar XI*.

Indeed, synchrony and diachrony are intertwined. Synchrony expresses a determinative effect, that is, the divided subject as a production of the Other: "As an effect of language, in that he is born of this early split, the subject translates a signifying synchrony into the primordial temporal pulsation that is the constitutive fading of his identification" (708, 7). As we will learn later, this pulsation contains an opening and a closing moment, with a gap in between. It is in this gap that appears the desire of the Other (709, 3). Desire means lack, that is, something that is not determined. What does the Other want from me? Precisely this opening opens the possibility for change via separation. Its effect is that "the subject of desire" is not allowed "to realize that he is an effect of speech"; that he merely is an effect of the desire of the Other (709, 3).

Teaching psychoanalysis against identification (709, 4–710, 7)

This theory is not just a theory, as it has consequences for the analytic practice, the teaching of psychoanalysis included. If the desire of the Other plays such a central role, the teacher of psychoanalysis – he who transfers signifiers to his pupils – must be aware of his responsibility (709, 4). Lacan claims to do so in his seminars, and this is all the more the case, because those who attend his teaching, are not rookies (709, 5–6).

Generally speaking, students are badly educated in matters of philosophy (709, 7) and taught an ideal of authority that gives them a false sense of certainty. This finds an expression in "a koinè of subjectivation" (709, 12), a common supposedly cultivated language and knowledge, giving them a false sense of mastery – "the false evidence of the ego" (709, 12). This reminds the reader of the Freudian idea about the ego not being the master of its own house (Freud, 1917/1978: 143).

Teaching psychoanalysis has to go against such a 'koinè,' otherwise the experience of being in analysis will be distorted, especially if it has to be expressed in the terms of this koinè (710, 1). Notice that Lacan here ascribes the same function to the teaching – his teaching – of psychoanalyis as to the analytic experience itself: the sublation of certainties based on imaginary identifications. In his Rome Discourse he had made this very clear:

> For in the work he does to reconstruct it for another, he [the analysand] encounters anew the fundamental alienation that made him construct it like another, and that has always destined it to be taken away from him by another.
>
> (208, 1)

In the present paper, he links it to the "scientific spirit" (710, 2). This expresses Lacan's hope at that time to introduce psychoanalysis into positivist science, based on cybernetics.

As mentioned above, the theme of teaching psychoanalysis and the very idea of a training analysis took a central stance in Lacan's conflict with the IPA. Earlier in the paper (707, 4), he stated already what he repeats here as well: this is not only a 'political' issue; the ideas about training have everything to do "with the affirmation of the unconscious" (710, 4).

In the paragraphs that follow, he explains that his use of Hegel does not mean that he joins the Hegelian idea about a progress towards a final synthesis and the end of history. On the contrary, what Lacan loves about Hegel is the *Aufhebung*, the sublation of certainties and the occasion to point out "the avatars of a lack" (710, 7).

"To confirm the function of this point of lack" (710, 8–711, 1)

One of the novelties in the Lacanian Lacan is the idea of an original loss and its function in the advent of the subject. In that respect, Freudian theory does not suffice, although it provides a path towards it. Plato's dialogue on love – *the Symposium* – provides a better entry. At that point in the text, Lacan mixes his references, because he switches from the *Symposium* to the *Politeia* with Platon's famous allegory of the cave. The reference to the *Symposium* will be elaborated much later, in the section of separation (716, 9 and 717, 1–2). There, it becomes obvious that his reference to the *Symposium* concerns the parable told by Aristophanes, because it is in that story that we find an explanation for the loss operating as a continuous cause.

According to the fable, the original human being was round, his back and sides forming a circle; he had four hands and four feet, one head with two faces, looking opposite ways, set on a round neck and precisely alike; also four ears, two privy members, and the remainder to correspond. These original humans did not suffer any lack whatsoever; they were complete. They were even so complete that the Gods became jealous of them. Zeus decided to punish them for their pride, by cutting them in two and thus diminishing their strength. This had a terrible effect. After the division the two parts of man, each desiring to be whole again, went madly looking for the other half. And when they had found it, they threw their arms around one another, entwined in mutual embraces. Longing to grow into one, they were on the point of dying from hunger and self-neglect, because they could not do anything apart. As a result, mankind was being destroyed, and Zeus had to invent a new plan. He turned their sexual organs round to the front. After the transposition the male generated in the female in order that by the mutual embraces of man and woman they might breed, and the human race might continue. This explains how the desire of one another became implanted in humans. Ever since, this becoming whole again is the basic need of men. The loss of completude and the installation of a lack cause a never-ending need to mend it.

This is the brief summary of the larger story that one can find in Plato's dialogue on love. The message in Aristophanes' fable is clear: love is our longing to be made whole again by joining the other. But we should hear the other message as well: sexuality is a *secondary* attempt to reach this original wholeness. What was lost, precedes sexuality as we know it. Lacan will take up this reasoning further in the paper, and in *Seminar X*. In order to explain the origin of desire and the lack of a final answer, he constructs a myth, about what he calls a 'lamelle' – the part of ourselves that we lose at birth, setting into motion a never-ending circular but nonreciprocal articulation between subject and Other. This loss functions as a basic cause, that is in itself not determined; the articulation determines the subject via the signifiers – this is the unconscious as an ever failing process. It fails, because it can never provide an answer to what was lost. As a result, the determination is not total, and via the repetitive attempts to find an answer, the subject has a possibility for change.

Topology of the Unconscious: "An entrance one can only reach just as it closes" (711, 2–711, 7)

In opposition to a received wisdom – the koinè Lacan referred to earlier – the unconscious should not be considered as an 'inside' (711, 7). Topologically speaking, it is an opening and a closing at the same time, an "edge" or 'rim,' and as analysts, we have to account for the gap. Lacan calls the cut 'irreducible' (711, 6). Especially the way it closes should be examined by the analyst. This echoes the "temporal pulsation" mentioned earlier in the paper (708, 7). Again, these ideas will receive a larger elaboration in the early lessons of *Seminar XI*, where Lacan talks about the status of the unconscious. There, he describes it as an ever failing attempt to realize something.

On January 22, 1964, he starts his seminar with a surprising question: what is the unconscious? The title of that part – *The Freudian Unconscious and Ours* – warns us that his audience is in for something new. Indeed, he questions the very status of the unconscious; his answer elaborates the always-difficult tandem of cause and effect. The unconscious – that is, the Lacanian unconscious – enters the scene between cause and effect, precisely at the point where something goes wrong and fails in its very realization. The locus is an inbetween, hence the idea of an opening, a gap, a crevice; hence, the accompanying metaphors: the unborn, the limbo, the larval state. No wonder that Lacan considers the status of the unconscious as something precarious, obliging the analyst to an ethical stance: we have to go for it, lest it disappears (S11, 1964: 34). Its productions (the symptoms) share a typical quality: they are all failures; disappearing the very moment we see or hear them.

A classic reading supposes a solid background to this process, says Lacan, but for him, it is exactly the opposite. We have to take the 'un' of unconscious very seriously, meaning that something is fundamentally lacking. The unconscious does not have any ontological status whatsoever. In this respect, he puts forward an essential difference between Freud and Descartes. The latter finds his existential certainty in a supposed being, an '*être*,' a 'res extensa,' whilst Freud finds his certainty in an absence. The unconscious is not ontological, it is pre-ontological, as it concerns a border process, a movement of opening and closing within the chain of signifiers where something that has to do with desire, is time and again not realized. He talks about the pulsating function of the unconscious, thus anticipating on the fourth fundamental concept of *Seminar XI*, the drive ('pulsion'). In '*Position of the Unconscious*,' he had already put forward this idea of a temporal pulsation. Topology meets time.

Temporality of the unconscious: 'a circular, albeit nonreciprocal articulation' (711, 8–712, 7)

The first thing that comes to mind with respect to Lacan's view on the temporality of the unconscious is his unearthing of the Freudian idea of *Nachträglichkeit*. Based on Saussurean linguistics this is easy to understand: it is only at an interpunction in the chain of signifiers that an effect of meaning may be produced and this necessarily in a retroactive and always provisional way. The concept itself is difficult to translate into English, the traditionally used 'deferred action' being a poor equivalent. Literally, it means to carry (German: *tragen*) something afterwards (German: *nach*). Something that was produced earlier, receives only later a certain weight and meaning, in view of an interpunction in the signifying chain. When the chain continues, that weight and meaning will be changed again. Freud used this reasoning to explain a peculiar characteristic of a trauma: it might have its meaningful effect much later, at a time when its signification has changed because of new signifiers.

Although Lacan refers here to this idea of *Nachträglichkeit*, at the same time he evokes the idea of "a temporal structure of a higher order" (711, 9). This higher order is indeed higher, as it obliges Lacan to introduce us to the idea of causality as something different from "the retroaction of the signifier in its efficiency" (712, 1). In that respect, he turns implicitly to Aristotelian theory on causality, and especially to the difference between the *causa finalis* and the *causa efficiens*. This needs some explanation.

According to Aristotle, nature – *physis* – is goal-directed and contains right from the start an end goal that causes and directs each particular change. This is the final cause: everything carries an ultimate goal within itself, and everything that happens, has to be considered as mere steps towards that goal. He interprets this as the *entelechie*: the aim of each change is the realization of being. A seed, for example, contains certain characteristics causing a number of things to happen, with a particular tree as the final goal, the tree being the *entelechie* of the seed. The changes during this process go back to the *causa efficiens*, the one that set things into movement. The example give by Aristotle is quite Lacanian avant la lettre: the father causes the child (Aristotle, *Physics*, book II, 3).

In '*Position of the Unconscious*,' it is the Aristotelian final cause that introduces "the functioning relationship" between overdetermined forms, that is, a "circular, albeit nonreciprocal articulation" (712, 3). Lacan gives the reader an inkling of what will follow with his indication that this relationship operates between the subject and the Other. As it has to do with the final cause, this relationship implies a teleology, a final aim. Later in the paper, it will become obvious that this cause is a loss at the very start of our life, the aim being to restore it. This aim will never be reached, thus causing an endless thrust forward.

This something is the subject, the Lacanian subject that is, as a *hypokeimenon*, a supposed being that is never fully there. The pre-ontological status of the unconcious, as put forward in the first lesson of January 22, 1964 against the Cartesian certainty, reads here: "The subject, the Cartesian subject, is what is presupposed by the unconscious" (712, 5). The production of the subject happens via the signifiers that represent the subject for other signifiers. This is the *causa efficiens* in action, the determination, with the Other as a production machine.

The next two sections of '*Position of the Unconscious*' elaborate this "circular, albeit nonreciprocal articulation" (712, 3). The advent of the subject is caused by a primordial lack at the start of life, the loss of something that will never be recovered. In the never-ending attempt to recover this loss, two processes continue in a flywheel motion: alienation and separation.

Before commenting on these two sections, I think it might be useful to explain how new these ideas are, compared to the earlier Lacan. Before 1964, the idea of alienation already occupied a very prominent place in his theory. His paper on the mirror stage demonstrates that alienation is a necessary operation, which cannot be restricted to the process of socialization, for it is precisely what determines this process.[3] With his further elaboration of the mirror stage, alienation was introduced into the structural relation between the imaginary and the symbolic, that is, the imaginary alienation is determined by the symbolic one, which relies on the Other.[4] The subject wants to be loved/desired by the Other and models/alienates her or himself on the image of what s/he thinks is desirable for this Other. At that time, the goal of psychoanalysis was to recognize this Other and its influence. Separation is understood as a major operation, installed through the paternal metaphor and – if need be – via the analytic process. It is the function of the father to separate the child and the first (m)Other.

In '*Position of the Unconscious*' and in *Seminar XI* all this is considerably changed. There is a pre-ontological causality at work, that is, an original loss on the level of being. Alienation is part of the process to restore this loss, but it takes the subject away from its being, in the direction of the Other. As a process, it comes down to a necessary choice, the alternative being death. Separation is the opposite process, inasmuch as it redirects the subject towards its being, thus opening a possibility of escape from the determining alienation coming from the Other. The net result is that there is no reciprocal relationship between subject and Other, only a circular one.

Second section. The causation of the subject: alienation (712, 8–714, 5)

The previous section ended with what Lacan called two domains (the subject and the Other) and their conjunction, with the unconscious between the two of them, as their "cut in action" (712, 4 and 7). This action – this is the unconscious – consists of two operations ordered in that circular, nonreciprocal relationship upon which Lacan keeps insisting (712, 8). "The first, alienation, constitutes the subject as such" (712, 9).

We learn that only the relationship with the signifier may engender alienation and that the signifier has priority over the subject, as demonstrated by Freud's experience. For example, a *Witz* lights up "the subject's division from himself" (712, 10). This division is not only made clear by the signifier, it is also because of the signifier, and not because of signs. A sign represents something to someone, even to the universe, as long as this 'someone' concerns a center where information can be totalized (713, 2). This does not apply for the subject, as the idea of totalization goes against the notion of the divided subject. A signifier represents a subject for another signifier, and this explains the division of the subject. Starting from a being that cannot speak, the signifier produces something (the subject) by making disappear what was there (the being) in its very attempt to put it on the scene. "[...] it disappears, no longer being anything but a signifier." (713, 3). Here, again, Lacan draws our attention to the temporal structure, using both senses of the French imperfect "*il y avait*." Something was there, but it is no longer where we thought it was; and yet, it does not make its appearance where we expect it to appear, the only thing appearing is a signifier, shifting to another signifier (713, 3). This is the unconscious in action – the cut in action – that Lacan describes in *Seminar XI* as a failure; time and again, something is not realized and remains unborn, unconscious.

In what resides alienation then? Not in the fact that this operation starts in the Other; this starting point does explain why a subject can never be its own cause (712, 4). Alienation lies in the division of the subject. Its logical structure has to be understood by a new reading of the either/or alternative (Latin: *vel*) (713, 5). Normally, this presents the idea of a choice: you choose either this or that. The new 'vel' imposes a choice because one of the two terms between which we are supposed to make a choice, is eliminated beforehand (713, 6). Consequently, the choice is limited: you can choose the remaining term or refuse it, *sic aut non*, yes or no (713, 8).

This mysterious description becomes clear when Lacan presents his examples: "your money or your life"; "liberty or death." In both examples, the only choice you can make is whether you want to live or not (713, 7, 8), knowing that this life will be impaired: you have lost your money, your freedom. In the long run, this means that the 'yes *or* no' becomes a 'yes *and* no' ("*sic et non*"); at the end of the day, we will lose our life anyway (714, 2).

Applied to the subject, he can choose for an imposed meaning (the signifiers coming from the Other) or for petrification (being without meaning). If he sticks with the meaning, he will have to face the absence of meaning that follows from his change into signifiers, and hence with a precarious identity. This nonmeaning arises from the field of the Other, but is produced as an eclipse, a fading of the subject (714, 3). In *Seminar XI*, Lacan describes this as follows:

> Alienation consists in this *vel*, which – if you do not object to the word *condemned*, I will use it – condemns the subject to appearing only in that division which, it seems to me, I have just articulated sufficiently by saying that, if it appears on one side as meaning, produced by the signifier, it appears on the other as *aphanisis*.
>
> (Sheridan: 210; S11, 1964: 191).

Lacan continues with this idea of nonmeaning arising from the Other, because it gives him the opportunity to relate this to clinical praxis and to his view on interpretation. Earlier in this paper (706, 9), he had already made clear that the analyst is responsible for the unconscious, that it is his ethical duty. Here, we learn that the unconscious has to take a seat in the armchair of the analyst, not to provide a meaning to it (although the unconscious has only meaning in the Other). Even on the contrary: in *Seminar XI*, where he elaborates alienation more extensively in his lesson of May 27, 1964, he states that "Interpretation is directed not so much at the meaning as towards reducing the signifiers to their non-meaning, so that we may rediscover the determinants of the subject's entire behaviour" (Sheridan, 212).[5] Here, in this final paragraph on alienation, we find the same idea: interpretation is not operative because of an effect of meaning. On the contrary, it is operative because of the articulation in signifiers, without any meaning at all (714, 5).

To conclude: alienation takes place between subject and Other and concerns the mythical point of origin in which being (*l'être*) as such has to make its appearance in the field of the Other. The effects are quite dramatic: when being makes its appearance at the level of language, it disappears under that language. The element lost in the process of becoming a human being is being itself, the pure being, the Real, leaving us with a basic lack as a condition for our becoming, which Lacan (S11, 1964: 31) calls the '*manque-à-être*' (want-to-be, or lack-of-being). Thus, right from the start, the subject is divided between the necessary loss of its being on the one hand and the signifiers coming from the Other on the other hand.

What is less clear in Lacan's description is the motive, the driving force of this process. He had already put forward the idea of causality earlier in the text; in the next two sections, he will present a further elaboration of the *causa finalis* and the ensuing 'circular but nonreciprocal movement.'

Third section. The causation of the subject: separation (714, 6–719, 6)

The second process in the causation of the subject, separation, also takes place between subject and Other, during what Lacan had already called "the cut in action" (712, 4 and 7), that is, the opening and closing of the unconscious. Separation has to do with the closing of this causation. The division of the subject, as a result of the signifier, is here joined by a division of the object. In this respect, Lacan refers to one of Freud's very last papers, without giving much explanation (714, 6): *Splitting of the Ego in the Process of Defence*. In this unfinished paper, Freud (1940b/1978) discusses the splitting of the Ego based on the disavowal of castration. I will return to Lacan's reference later.

Separation is situated in the intersection between subject and Other (714, 7). The schematic representation in *Seminar XI* by two overlapping circles makes this easier to understand (S11, 1964: 192). Normally, in such an intersection we would expect something substantial, that is, the common part belonging to the two circles. In this case, it is exactly the opposite. The intersection contains two lacks and their interaction. The first one belongs to the subject. During the advent of the subject, he loses his being, resulting in the lack of being ('*manque-à-être*') because of the alienation, that is, the identification with the signifiers coming from the Other. At that point, the subject with his own '*manque-à-être*' is confronted with the desire of the Other and hence with the lack of the Other: what does s/he want from me?

The paradoxical result of these combined lacks is that it permits the subject to realize oneself (715, 2; Bruce Fink translates '*le sujet se réalise*' as 'the subject is actualized,' thus losing the active modus as present in the original French). This explains why separation opens a possibility for change, that is, a possibility to escape from the determining impact of the Other. What this 'oneself' might be, is not clear, but based on Lacan's reasoning, it is obvious that it is not an original being. Surprisingly enough, he links it to Freud's death drive (715, 2). This association with Thanatos becomes clear in the next paragraph (715, 3). As Freud (1940a/1978: 148) described, the aim of Thanatos is to undo connections. Here, death drive means separation from the larger whole, from the Other; to separate oneself from the Other (Latin: *separare*) means to engender oneself (Latin: *se parere*), as a separate part (Latin: *pars*).

Lacan takes care to warn us about the illusion of a whole, as this might be evoked by the idea of a part. There is no whole, on the contrary. Playing on the homonymy between partition and parturition, he accentuates that the subject realizes itself only via its division (715, 4). This realization has nothing to do with giving birth to oneself, even on the contrary; it is the juridical and social meaning that counts.[6]

At this point in the text, Lacan refers to the chain of signifiers, and – even more importantly – to the gap between them. The interval between the first signifier, S_1, and the second signifier, S_2, repeats itself through the chain and this is where desire appears in a metonymical way (715, 5). There, in this gap, the subject meets something different than the effects of meaning, as put forward by the alienation; he meets the desire of the Other, albeit without being able to grasp the concrete object of this desire (715, 6). Even on the contrary, the desire of the Other remains an enigma.

The answer produced by the subject to the desire, and hence, to the lack of the Other, may come as a surprise. The subject presents itself in its absence: 'can the Other afford to lose me?' (716, 1). Strange as this may seem, this is a common fantasy, even in the psychopathology of everyday life. Fantasies about our own death – even about our suicide – depict more often than not the reactions of those left behind: will they miss me, do they feel guilty? Understand: how important am I for them, can they afford to lose me? How much do they desire me?

Previously in his paper, Lacan had evoked a "circular, albeit nonreciprocal" articulation; refering to a "functioning relationship between these forms" (712, 3). This nonreciprocal circularity is what appears when the subject presents its own disappearance as an answer to the lack of the Other. Instead of answering the lack of the Other, the subject returns to his point of departure, where he lost his being. "Therein lies the twist whereby separation represents the return of alienation" (716, 2).

Again, this theory on the unconscious as 'cut in action' has repercussions for clinical praxis. The intervention of the analyst operates on the pulsating process, the opening and closing of the unconscious, via which the being of the analysand has to arise, being that resides beyond this border process (716, 4). In the next paragraph, Lacan gives us a precious insight about transference: the expectation of this being of the analysand in relation to the desire of the analyst constitutes the true mainspring of transference (716, 5). In my reading, this echoes what Lacan writes elswhere: "The analyst too must pay [...] with his person" (490, 10) and, much later, about the necessary 'subjective destitution' of the analyst at the end of the treatment (Lacan, 1968: 23). During the advent of the subject, being is lost and the Other dominates the scene. As a result of the analytical process, via transference, the loss of being shifts to the side of the analyst, making it possible for the analysand to create something new, a *sinthome*, independently of the alienation arising from the Other (for a more extensive discussion, see Verhaeghe and Declerq, 2003).

The obvious question – obvious in the light of Lacan taking his distance from the idea of a substantial original identity – is what this being is about (716, 6). In his answer, Lacan plays with Plato's allegory of the cave: the cave's walls (displaying the projected shadows of the objects, taken for reality by the chained humans) have to "come alive with a palpitation whose movement of life [*le mouvement de vie*] must be grasped now" (716, 6). Now meaning: "after we have articulated function and field of language and speech in their conditioning."

Here, Lacan turns to sexuality, adding that he wants to present something new, reminding us that psychoanalysis has not put forward that much new in this field, by making use of a myth (716, 8). He takes up the reference earlier made (710, 8) to Aristophanes and his parable, as told in the *Symposium* (see above). It is no coincidence that this reference appears during Lacan's presentation on separation. Aristophanes' double-backed creatures are cut in two by Zeus, each one looking for their lost half ever since. The original sphericity of the primordial double man is compared by Lacan to a Magdeburg sphere whilst the organic aspect reminds him of an egg (717, 2). He refers to the development of the embryo, where in the very early stage, the differentiation in layers ('membranes') results in the placenta, as half of an original whole that will feed the other half, meaning the embryo as such. When the umbilical cord is cut at birth, the baby does not lose its mother, it loses its own anatomical complement, called "after-birth" by the midwives (717, 3). Later in the text, Lacan will refer to an even earlier process, that is, the special cell division (meiosis) that takes place during sexual reproduction (718, 10). During that process, one half is also lost, and death becomes a structural necessity.

Here, Lacan inserts his own myth. Imagine, he says, that when the membranes burst, a phantom flies away. A phantom that is a far more primal form of life (717, 4) compared to the newly born. The breaking of the egg gives birth to man (French: *l'homme*) as well as to Manlet (French: *l'hommelette*; wordplay on omelette) (717, 5).

The description that follows in the next paragraphs is not very reassuring (717, 6–718, 3). The Manlet, later called lamelle, is omniscient and immortal. A fight between man and Manlet is lost on beforehand for man, as this lamelle is guided by the pure Real (and not by sensory-based reality as is the case for man): its attacks are unpredictable, it knows no obstacles, it cannot be educated, and it is impossible to trap. Trying to destroy it results in its multiplication, the only solution being to lock it up in a Magdeburg sphere, taking care that the whole of it is put in there, preferably by itself, because it is not wise to touch it.

The next paragraph brings a surprise. This Manlet/lamelle is what Lacan understands by libido (718, 3), meaning that man can never win the battle with 'his' libido, as it is not 'his.' For Lacan, libido is closer to an organ than to a force field, as one might have expected. It is as a surface that it commands this force field. He refers the reader to Freud's conception of the drive as a montage – meaning not something along the lines of an instinct. In *Seminar XI*, he compares it to a surrealist collage and presents a vivid description: "[…] the resulting image would show the working of a dynamo connected up to a gas-tap, a peacock's feather emerges, and tickles the belly of a pretty woman, who is just lying there looking beautiful" (Sheridan: 169; S11, 1964: 154). The same lesson of May 6, 1964 links this idea of a surface, more explicitly to the idea of '*leur structure de bord*,' translated by Sheridan as 'their rimlike structure' (ibid.). In '*Position of the Unconscious*' (718, 5) Lacan talks about a "closed rim, which is the erogenous zone." Notice that the lamelle/libido operates on erogenous zones, presenting a border structure, just as the unconscious does.

Lacan reminds the reader of a certain aspect of Freud's drive theory: the constancy of the drive pressure, meaning that the flow (German: *Schub*) of the drive is not to be mistaken for its discharge; a better description is the back and forth evagination of the libido as an organ (718, 5–6). Stoke's theorem from electromagnetic theory explains the reason for this constancy. Lacan adds an explanatory footnote, which is in its turn explained by a translator's note, that I reproduce here in a note as well.[7]

This organ (the libido) "must be called an unreal one," in the sense that it precedes and causes human reality, that is, "the subjective realm it conditions." With his self-constructed myth about the lamelle flying away at the time of birth, Lacan "strives to provide a symbolic articulation for [it]" (718, 7–8). Here, the implicit reference is to Lévi-Strauss and his understanding of myths as evolving stories based on an already existing symbolic system into which the subject is born, which is governed and structured by linguistically determined rules of exchange. Lacan's myth explains how the human drive works. Libido, as an irreal organ, determines human behaviour, because it is based on the 'montage' that the drive is; and this montage has nothing to do with instinct, let alone with instinctual discharge, it operates continuously as a force field. Its cause is an original loss; the goal is to restore a lost completude, but the aim (i.e. the effect of the goal) is the traject, the circling around the (ever missing) object (S11, 1964: 163; Sheridan: 178).

In the next paragraphs, Lacan changes his description, moving from the differentiaton between placenta and embryo to the even earlier expulsion of half of the chromosomes during the meiosis (718, 9–719, 1). In both cases, half of an original whole is lost (the part of the fertilized egg that becomes the placenta; half of the chromosomes) and that lost part flies away (717, 4). This lost part is eternal life as we have to lose it because of sexual reproduction (718, 9).

Lacan does not give much information, but it is plausible that he refers here to the major difference between sexual and non-sexual reproduction. The latter happens by mitosis, which produces two perfect copies of the original cell; the former happens by meiosis, thus losing half of the original two cells, creating something new but thereby introducing death for the individual, as a structural necessity. The things that are important for Lacan in this reasoning are that one loses half of oneself right at the start (see placenta, see half of the chromosomes), that this creates something new (see separation) but that we lose the possibility of eternal life.

These ideas of partition and losing part of oneself permit Lacan to give a new meaning to the psychoanalytic notion of partial object. The function of such an object is determined by the type of anatomical cut (719, 2). Readers who are acquainted with classic Greek will recognize Lacan's remark between brackets – *ana temnein*, to cut apart. A new meaning, because, for example, the partial object par excellence, the breast, is usually interpreted as part of the mother's body, standing for warmth and tender loving care, something that is lost and hence longed for. This does not explain its erotic value, which is better rendered by Sint Agatha in the painting by Tiepolo, presenting us her breasts on a plate (719, 3).

Here, breast has nothing to do with womb (the French *sein*, breast, means also womb) but has to be understood as something that can be taken away and hence, as a prefiguration of castration (719, 4). Ever since Kleinian investigations, weaning is situated far too much in the fantasy of the partition from the mother's body. As a result, we are not aware any longer of the fact that the separation takes place between the mother and the breast (and not between the child and the mother), thus turning the lost object into one of erotic desire (719, 5). This explains Lacan's reference, at the start of this section (714, 6), to Freud's paper on the splitting of the ego (1940b/1978). The division of the subject implies a division of the object as well, as something that can be cut off and separated from the own body, as a prefiguration of castration.

This reasoning permits Lacan to put the breast on the same plan as the placenta. In both cases, mammalian organization installs a parasitical relation, first between embryo and placenta, second, between infans and breast. Placenta and breast function as an ectopia of one individual (the child) on the other (the mother). In this description, the major characteristic put forward by Lacan appears in the last words: "a certain type of organism *which remains specified by this intersection*" (my italics, 719, 6). The intersection where something is lost forever, that keeps operating as a force field.

Fourth section. Sexuality between the two sides of the gap (719, 7–721, 2)

It is no coincidence that Lacan ends his conceptual innovation in '*Position of the Unconscious*' by presenting his ideas about the drive (every drive is a partial drive) and about sexuality (there is no such a thing as a sexual relationship). The Lacan of the signifier is here moving towards the Lacan of object *a*. He makes a differentiation between body and organism on the one hand, and the subject in its dialectical exchange with the Other on the other hand. Between them, we find the libido as "organ" (719, 8), operating as a force field and based on the loss of half of the original organism.

The libido/lamella pushes the organism's being to its limit, beyond the body; conversion symptoms in hysteria testify to this extreme elasticity (719, 8). Because of our relation to the signifier, we have learnt about death. Consequently, the speaking being understands the "deadly meaning" of the libido and its link with sexuality; every drive comes down to the death drive (719, 9).

What is the part of the original organism in the dialectics of the subject with the Other? Before the advent of the subject, the sexed being has lost half of itself (placenta; meiosis) and hence, lost eternal life, precisely because of becoming a sexed organism. This loss is materialized in an immaterial organ, the libido, operating as a constant force. During its advent, the subject puts forward his loss, that is, this uncorporal organ, at the time of separation. In that way, the subject presents his own death, his own disappearance as the object of desire of the Other (720,1).

Following that presentation, the subject can present the object that he loses by nature: excrements, and the props he finds in the desire of the Other, that is, his gaze and his voice (720, 2). This is what Lacan understands as 'drive': dealing with these objects in order to restore the original loss (720, 3). Later, in *Seminar XI*, Lacan puts a different accent: the aim of the drive is the traject, the circling around the (ever missing) object (S11, 1964: 178) Here, Lacan joins Freud in his reading of Platon: the aim of the drive is to return to an original state (Freud, 1920/1978, 57–58). The way this return is attempted runs via partial objects, meaning that the drive is always a partial drive. This points to an essential lack in our functioning: "the absence of anything that could represent in the subject the mode of what is male or female in his being" (720, 4). Doubts about masculinity or femininity have nothing to do with our supposed biological bisexuality. These doubts are much better explained by the absence of a sexual bipolarity in the dialectics between subject and Other (720, 5).

This brings us to the conclusion of Lacan's paper: sexuality is distributed between the two sides "of our *rim*" – this rim being the threshold of the unconscious (720, 6). At the side of the living, the subject is looking for an object that might give him back the eternal life that he lost in becoming a sexed being; this search operates via partial objects, meaning that the subject will never meet the other sex (720, 7). At the side of the Other, that is, the exchange of signifiers, order and norms must be installed, telling the subject what he has to do as a man or as a woman (720, 8). We were not made man or woman, as some people think, based on the bible (720, 9). And a reference to Lilith doesn't make much difference (721, 2).

Lacan does not give any explanation concerning this reference to Lilith. She figures in Jewish folklore, as Adam's first wife, who was created at the same time and from the same earth as Adam. This contrasts with Eve, who was created from one of Adam's ribs. Lilith refused to obey Adam and is considered a female demon, source of evil and seduction. What is probably important for Lacan is that Eve was created from Adam's body, which is a far echo of the loss of half of oneself (see Aristophanes; see placenta/embryo; see meiosis). Lilith is created independently of Adam and stands on her own.

Fifth section. Leaving Bonneval (721, 3–6)

In these final paragraphs, Lacan takes his leave from the debates at the Bonneval Colloquium because they invited 'irresponsible interventions' coming from a certain side (721, 3). The fact that someone from that side has in the meantime studied the Oedipus complex from a hermeneutic point of view, is for Lacan a confirmation of what was already happening back in 1960 (721, 5). Here, he is implicitly referring to Paul Ricoeur (1965/1970), one of the speakers at the colloquium, who published afterwards his hermeneutic reading of Freud.

It is obvious that this final section refers to the historical circumstances that I mentioned in my introduction. The result of these 'irresponsible interventions,' Lacan says, was exactly the opposite: instead of silencing him, the whole situation obliged him to come into the open (721, 4). *Seminar XI* proves his point, as it is the first one that has an open access policy. The irony is that this is a direct result of the prohibition by the IPA of his teaching.

Lacan's seminar will go much further than a mere return to Freud. The final footnote gives us an inkling of what is to follow (721, note 4). The message in that footnote is clear: forget about the post-freudian partial object, think 'object *a*,' what Lacan considered as his only invention. This object *a* has nothing to do with regression, that is, with the usual post-freudian reading of partial objects. It has to be understood structurally, and in relation to minus phi, "as 'cause' of the castration complex." In that respect, Lacan refers the reader to the next paper in the *Écrits, On Freud's 'Trieb' and the Psychoanalyst's Desire.*

Between Signifier and Drive: Position of the Unconscious

Between the Bonneval Colloquium (1960) and the actual writing of the paper (1964) Lacan is facing two problems. With his return to Freud he had explained how unconscious processes function as linguistic mechanisms governed by inherent rules. He taught his pupils not to be seduced by the meaning of words – on the contrary; it is the material aspect of the signifier that appears prominently in this linguistic determination. Free association is anything but free; it operates according to an inner determination. The question then is: how can we ever escape the unconscious of the Other and its determinative effect, or to rephrase it clinically: what are the possibilities for change, based on a psychoanalytic treatment?

The second problem seems unrelated to the first one. Freud's major discovery concerns the impact of sexuality in the causation of neurosis. If the object *a* is Lacan's invention, then 'drive' might very well be called Freud's. But what is the place of the Freudian drive in Lacan's linguistically determined unconscious? Or of the body, for that matter?

'*Position of the Unconscious*' treats both problems, but we need to study *Seminar XI* to understand the new answers.

Conclusion

(1): The Unconscious as an ever-failing border process

Lacan starts *Seminar XI* by questioning the very status of the unconscious. In the second lesson (January 22, 1964) we learn that the unconscious enters the scene between the 'cause' and its 'effect,' precisely at the point where something goes wrong and fails in its very realization. The locus is an inbetween, hence the returning idea of the unconscious as an opening, a gap, a crevice and the accompanying metaphors: the unborn, the limbo, a larval state, functioning as a pulsating movement where something is opened at the same moment that it is closed. No wonder that Lacan considers the status of the unconscious as something precarious, obliging the analyst to an ethical stance: we have to go for it, lest it disappears. Its productions share a typical quality; they are all failures, disappearing the very moment we see or hear them. This reminds us of an all too easily forgotten fact: the reason why we know about the unconscious is that it tends to repeat itself, albeit in its own failure. Precisely the results of this repeated failure – from neurotic symptoms to dream formation – provided Freud with the material ground for his discoveries.

A classic reading supposes a solid background to this process, but for Lacan it is exactly the opposite. We have to take the 'un' of unconscious very seriously, meaning that something is fundamentally lacking. The unconscious does not have any ontological status whatsoever. On the contrary, it is pre-ontological, as it concerns a border process, a movement of opening and closing within the chain of signifiers where something that has to do with desire, is time and again not realized. Lacan talks about the pulsating function of the unconscious, thus anticipating his fourth fundamental concept in *Seminar XI*, that is, the drive. In this respect, he puts forward an essential difference between Freud and Descartes. The latter finds his existential certainty in a supposed being, a *res extensa*, whilst Freud finds his certainty in an absence and in a failure. These failures are what Lacan coins as the 'productions of the unconscious,' that is, the symptoms.

The material context of this production is the network of signifiers. In these early lessons we learn that the network has to do with a primary classificatory function that is operational before the actual formation of the subject.[8] Lacan refers to the Freudian metapsychology, more particularly the letters 48 and 52 to Fliess, the last chapter of *Die Traumdeutung* and the papers of the 1915s. The chain of signifiers contains an ordering that includes gaps in which the unconscious operates in such a way that something fails to be realized. It has to do with causality and determination. What is not clear is the causal factor.

(2): Causality and determination

Seminar XI introduces us to a radical new perspective on causality, echoing presocratic ideas. From Plato onwards, science has been confronted with the question of the primary cause, Aristotle's 'Unmoved Mover,' within a linear determination (a determines b determines c, etcetera). This leads to a typical deadlock: what determines 'a'? In his answer, Lacan makes a differentiation between law and cause. The first one determines a series, thus permitting predictions. The second one belongs to a different register that is literally unthinkable; hence its typical appearance as a failure, a gap. The latter is interpreted via Aristotle's idea of *tuché*, the former as an illustration of its counterpart, the *automaton*. Both of them permit Lacan to elaborate his theory on the pre-ontological status of the unconscious and its relation to the 'productions of the unconscious.'

A classic critique of psychoanalysis concerns its determinism. In its caricatural version: everything is determined from the age of five, the human being is driven by dark forces arising from an almighty unconscious, there is no such a thing as chance, everything is written beforehand in an unknown handwriting. The early Lacan elaborated this determinism in a scientific way, by interpreting this dark unconscious as a linguistic system, governed by laws and thus predictable. The later Lacan concentrates on the drive and the Real, thus making room for unpredictability and causality as such.

Seminar XI contains both. On the one hand, Lacan elaborates the determinism he finds in the human psyche, which leads to a deterministic part in psychoanalytic practice as well; on the other hand, he confronts us with causality beyond determinism, entailing an opening for change. *Automaton* stands for the deterministic part. *Tuché* resides beyond the *automaton* and is the name for the ever-missed meeting with a new order that becomes more and more prominent in Lacan's thinking: the Real.

The *automaton* concerns the 'network,' the 'chain,' the 'procession' of signifiers. These denominations as well as Lacan's elaboration accentuate the linear ordering of the signifiers, based on two kinds of laws.

The first kind comes down to the linguistic mechanisms of metaphor and metonymy, whose elaboration goes back to an older paper (1957), *The Instance of the Letter in the Unconscious or Reason since Freud*. The second kind has everything to do with mathematical laws. Their elaboration can be found in *Seminar II* and the accompanying paper (1957), *Seminar on The Purloined Letter*, especially in its addendum. Lacan's decision to put this paper at the beginning of his *Écrits* (and thus breaking the otherwise chronological order) says a lot about the importance he attributed to it at that time. More specifically, it expresses his hope for a clinical praxis based on these lawful determinations. It is the period where Lacan believes in the possibility of a complete analysis (finding, constructing the last signifier) and a predictable subject (computation).

If we study these mathematical laws, there is one thing that stands out right from the start: they concern solely the formal aspect of the signifier, independently of the signified. Hence the possibility for Lacan to replace the chain of signifiers by a series of pluses and minuses obtained by pure chance (coin flipping). He designates this formal aspect as the materiality of the signifier, the letter – a term which figures prominently in the title of the two papers already referred to. This material chain of signifiers, obtained by a chance sequence of pluses and minuses, is governed by laws which determine the possibilities of circulation and production of these signifiers. In the addendum to *Seminar on The Purloined Letter*, he demonstrates that a chance series of pluses and minuses contains predictable sequences, on condition that one groups them by three. Again, this concerns a purely formal elaboration. In the actual paper itself he presents us with a meaningful elaboration focusing on Poe's story, *The Purloined Letter*. A signifier, 'letter,' deviates in a certain way from its path and determines thereby a number of effects on those who hold it. The meaningful content of the letter is supposed but never exposed, thus reducing this letter to its material character.[9]

Mathematical laws explain the deterministic effect in which the original chance event (coin flipping) is surpassed; the chain produces 'spontaneously' its own determination. This is the *automaton*, literally something that moves by itself. This idea tallies perfectly with the process of free association, which is here exposed as an automatic association. Such an inherent determinism of the chain of signifiers does not only open the possibility of interpretation, it makes this interpretation predictable.

Clinically, this mathematical determination must be linked to the linguistic mechanisms. Their combination presents us with the divided subject as a determined effect of the chain of signifiers. It is this combination that explains the well-known sayings: 'The unconscious is structured like a language' and 'The signifier represents the subject for another signifier'. Lacanian reinterpretations of a number of Freudian analyses in this respect are very instructive. In the case of the Rat Man, for example, the chain of signifiers produces the signifier 'rat' in a very determined way: *Rat*, *heiraten*, *Hofrat*, *Rate* ... With the Wolf man, the same goes for 'Wolf' and for the letter 'V'. Probably the most instructive case is to be found with Anna O who, under hypnosis, had to reproduce the entire chain of signifiers between symptom and cause, in order to make this symptom disappear. The determinism inherent in this chain is so obvious for Freud, that he keeps referring to it in his last chapter of the *Studies on Hysteria*.[10]

Hence, the *automaton* contains no chance event. On the contrary, it displays a systematic, lawful determination. This supposedly complete determinism opens up the possibility of a supposedly complete analysis, meaning that the last signifier representing the subject can either be found or constructed. If this is the case, psychoanalysis would join hard science. For a certain period, Lacan had high hopes in this direction. For had he not discovered a scientific determinism underlying Freud's 'free' association? This explains his enthusiasm for S. Leclaire's contribution at the Bonneval Colloquium. As mentioned above, Leclaire presented a case study in which the final signifier – a combination of letters summarizing the core of that particular analysand's determination – could be constructed.

This brings us to the second concept, *tuché*. The automatically functioning chain of signifiers does not only determine the sequence of signifiers. From time to time it meets with an impossibility, with something that cannot appear in the chain itself. In Lacan's first theory, this idea of a lack was already present, but at that time the impression was that this lack was nothing but a lacking signifier, that is, something that could be found or constructed through the very process of analysis itself. This changes when Lacan interprets this lack as the *tuché*.

This idea is one of the cornerstones on which *Seminar XI* is built. As a matter of fact, it goes back to Freud's cornerstone as well, that is, repression and the real nature of the trauma. Already for Freud, the trauma came down to something where normal representation failed: the traumatic experience could never find an appropriate symbolic expression. Freud would discover an analogous process at the base of neurosis. He described this as the primal repression, meaning that something remains fixated at a non-verbal level, making it forever impossible to turn it into words, and thus constituting the kernel of the System Unconscious. This is the Freudian metapsychology where Laplanche referred to, during his contribution at Bonneval. In *Seminar XI*, Lacan coins this as an ever-missed encounter with the Real and links it to the drive. Freud's so-called secondary repression (usually abbreviated as 'repression') concerns the later psychological derivatives of the trauma and determines a lack that can be filled in during the analytic treatment. Freud elaborated especially this secondary repression, whilst his theory on primal repression remained rather vague.

With *tuché*, Lacan concentrates on this primal process and tries to understand causality. Whilst automaton explains a systematic determination coming from the symbolic, causality has to be looked for in something undetermined coming from the Real. "In short, there is cause only in something that doesn't work" (S11, 1964: 25; Sheridan: 22). Three weeks later (session of 12 February 1964), Lacan introduces his audience to a number of ideas whose importance will only grow: the body, the drive, the Real; object *a*. This is not the body from the mirror stage, hence Lacan's use of the word 'organism'. As cause it calls for "an appointment with a real that eludes us" (S11, 1964: 53; Sheridan 53). This Real lies beyond the *automaton*, is not determined and cannot be represented. This explains why the idea of cause implies for Lacan the idea of failure. The symbolic fails to represent something of the Real; a certain process does not happen, thus causing something else to fill the scene.

Much later in *Seminar XI*, we will learn that this Real comes down to a crucial feature of the sexed organism, more particularly to a primal loss at the birth of life. This loss has a causal impact: it causes the organism to an endless attempt to regain what is lost forever. These ever failing attempts happen unconsciously. "For what the unconscious does, is to show us the gap through which neurosis associates with a Real – a Real that may well not be determined."[11] The in itself non-determined Real, operating as a cause, drives the organism and later, the subject. The net result is a failure, indicated by Lacan's negative denominations: 'the not-realised,' 'the un-born,' thus permitting him to make explicit a direct connection with the 'un' of the Un-conscious (S11, 1964: 25–26; Sheridan: 22–23).

The very same idea of failure reappears in his description of the becoming of the subject. This brings Lacan to an important conclusion: there is a structural homology at work on several levels, in which a primal lack asks for an answer without ever finding one. "At the level of the unconscious there is something at all points homologous with what occurs at the level of the subject" (S11, 1964: 27; Sheridan: 24).

This theory on causality changes considerably the ideas about determination. Previously, Lacan considered the determination by the symbolic as omnipresent; now, a different causality enters the game, arising from the Real of the body.[12] From this point onwards in his theory, it is the interaction between those two orders that has to be studied. *Tuché* puts the accent on the unconscious as a cause, *automaton* on the productions and the effects of the unconscious – the symptoms – which are determined in a systematic way. Moreover, both of them are structurally interwoven and determine each other in a mutual interdependence, which is circular but not reciprocal.

As stated above, Lacan's theory about the *automaton* in *Seminar XI* is not new. In his second seminar, he had already demonstrated that the appearance of any signifier is determined by 'law,' that is, there is a system determining which signifier can appear at a given point in the chain of signifiers and which cannot. This is important, because it provides us with the scientific base of Freud's free association. During the analytic treatment, free association is governed by an underlying determination, resulting in a kind of automatic memory. A number of lost signifiers can be retrieved and worked through during the treatment. Nevertheless, clinical practice demonstrates that this process of rememoration succeeds only up to a point, after which the chain stalls and stops.

It is there where the second line starts: this 'full stop' of the symbolic, the point of causality 'where it doesn't work' concerns the not-realized, the unborn in the chain of signifiers, the non-verbal remainder, even when desire has been expressed in the words of a demand. At that point, Freud had already met repetition compulsion rather than rememoration. The point where the chain stalls, is the very point where the Real makes its appearance. The 'meeting' with the Real is an ever-missed meeting, because there is no appropriate signifier. Lacan formulates this idea by paraphrasing Spinoza: "Cogitatio adaequata semper vitat eamdem rem": an adequate thought avoids always the same thing (S11, 1964: 49; Sheridan: 49).

As a consequence, there is no final analysis possible, nor a definite computation of the subject. Repressed signifiers are determined, and can be found back up to a certain point. Beyond that, we meet with something different, where the signifier is lacking and the Real insists, acting as a *primal cause* for the chain of signifiers and for the subject. On the positive side, this means that the subject escapes total determinism. On the negative side, this means that talking is not enough and that psychoanalysis as a practice has to redefine its goal. It will take Lacan another ten years to come up with a new answer: identification with the *sinthome* (S23, 1975–1976: 70; Verhaeghe & Declercq, 2003).

This reasoning explains why Lacan considers the subject as a *hypokeimenon* with a pre-ontological status. Here, we can see the differences with Aristotle's ontology. For Aristotle, the *causa finalis* directs every being at the full realization of its being, whilst the *causa efficiens* determines all the intermediate changes. For Lacan, the *causa finalis* is a loss in the heart of being at the start of life, causing the ever failing attempts to remediate it. The attempts at remedial take place in and via the chain of signifiers; but the introduction of mankind into the symbolic order caused the primal loss. Consequently, these attempts are structurally doomed to fail, and there will never be a final realization of being. The net result is the ever-continuing process that Lacan calls 'the advent of the subject'. During that process, the *causa efficiens* is at work, meaning the determination that is inherent to the chain of signifiers.

In the later parts of *Seminar XI*, the whole question as put forward by *tuché* and *automaton* reappears, although this time with a focus on the accompanying structure. The concepts as such are not used any more. This structure can be understood as follows: it amounts to an attempt at answering a loss from a previous level by installing something that concerns the lack or loss of the next level, as a result of which the original loss is endorsed, giving rise thereby to a never-ending flywheel movement. A pulsating movement of opening and closing in a circular but non-reciprocal way.

(3): A circular but non-reciprocal dialectic

The Real of the organism functions as cause, in the sense that it contains a primal loss. Which loss? The loss of eternal life, which paradoxically enough is lost at the moment of birth, that is, birth as a sexed being (S11, 1964: 187; Sheridan: 205). In order to explain this, Lacan constructs the myth of the lamella flying away at birth. This lamella stands for the life instinct, the primordial form of the libido, object *a* in its pure form.[13] The myth goes back to a biological fact: non-sexual reproduction implies in principle the possibility of eternal life (cf. single-celled organisms and clones), sexual reproduction implies in principle the death of the individual. In the latter case, each sexed organism tries to undo this loss, and wants to return to the former state of being. This was already with Freud the basic characteristic of the drive, here to be read as Eros and Thanatos, the life and death drive. At this stage, we are talking about the drive, which precedes any form of sexuation and the accompanying reversal into component or partial drives, meaning phallic drives.

Thus considered, the first level in the movement of opening and closing concerns the both mythical and real appearance of individual life, 'the advent of the living' and the simultaneous loss of eternal life. The opening of the sexually differentiated forms of life takes place through the closure of eternal life as such. The attempt to return takes place through sexual reproduction, which means that as a return to eternal life, it is a failure. From that moment onwards, this non-reciprocal although circular relationship will continue on different levels, each time with the same effect. That is to say: the process doesn't manage to mend the loss; on the contrary, it endorses the loss. This is the start of the structural homology between drive, unconscious and subject.

The next level in the attempt to regain what is lost, brings the formation of the I via the primary identification of the mirror stage. The living being acquires an initial identity through the unified image of his body coming to him from the mirror Other; at the same time this 'I' loses the Real of its body, on top of the preceding loss of eternal life. Consequently, this 'I' will try to join its body again (see Descartes' 'Je pense, donc je suis'), this time via the symbolic Other.

This leads to the next level, that of the advent of the subject. The 'I' attempts to fuse with the (m)Other, in order to recapture it's body and to be *m'être/maître à moi-même*, to belong to myself, to be master of myself (S17, 1969–1970: 178). Instead of regaining its body, the I disappears and the subject enters the scene as a divided product of the signifiers that cannot meet the desire of the Other.

If we continue this series, we arrive at a fourth level wherein the divided subject tries to become whole again by joining the other sex. This is what the Oedipus complex does, in its own peculiar way – that is, by interpreting the original loss in terms of castration. This phallic interpretation will be applied retroactively to all preceding levels, meaning that each loss is read in a phallic way.[14] Gender identity is the final stage of this circular but non-reciprocal relationship. The original gap between life and death, between the body and the I, between the subject and the Other is reproduced and worked over in the gap between man and woman. Moreover, this repetition produces the same effect: if the aim of the relationship is to become whole again, then failure is inevitable.

The negativity of this conclusion – 'There is no such a thing as a sexual relationship' – hinders us in seeing the positive side to it: "It is always about the subject as indeterminated" (S11, 1964: 28; Sheridan: 26). The core of the subject is symbolically undetermined. This opens a possibility for choice and change, beyond the determination coming from the Other. A possibility for separation. For Lacan, this delineates the difference between science and psychoanalysis.

(4): Science and psychoanalysis

The subject's need for a final answer coming from the Other leaves us with a faulty impression: it seems as if the subject wants to gather knowledge. This is the meeting ground between the subject of science and the subject entering analysis: both want to know. Freud's case study on Dora is a standard illustration and demonstrates immediately the particular character of this knowledge (Freud, 1905b/1978). Through her dreams and symptoms, she continually asks what it means to be a woman and a daughter in relation to the desire of a man. It is the same field of interest that haunts the child, more particulary on three specific points: what is the difference between boys and girls? where do babies (where do I) come from? what is it that connects my father to my mother? The child, says Freud, proceeds like a scientist and will forge genuinely explanatory theories. That is why Freud calls them infantile sexual researches and infantile sexual theories (Freud, 1905a/1978: 194–197).

Lacan interprets these ideas from a structural point of view. The subject wants to know, but at the same time, this wanting to know covers the passion of not wanting to know about our division. The goal of science is described by Lacan (1966) in his *La science et la vérité* as 'la suture du sujet,' the suturing or stitching of the subject (731, 6).[15] This is what drives every subject right from the start: the desire for a complete Other, a finally closed symbolic system which has retrieved the lost object *a* and solved – 'sutured' – the division of the subject.

This process is endless, interminable as Freud said, because every new signifier endorses the original loss. That's why the subject in analysis has to keep producing new signifiers, that's why the subject of science has to keep secreting new knowledge. The subject of science believes that nature will reveal to him the final meaning. In this respect, he is the same subject as the analysand believing that psychoanalysis will present him with the final meaning of his symptom.

Lacanian psychoanalysis has the ambition of confronting this division in its very causality, thus betting on the subjectivation of an originally alienating process. Lacan's attempts in that respect – the Sinthome, the 'passe,' the act – share one denominator: the belief in creativity *ex nihilo*.

Notes

1 *Seminar XI* was published in 1973. Alan Sheridan translated it in English and *The Four Fundamental Concepts of Psycho-Analysis* were published as soon as 1977 by the Hogarth Press and the Institute of Psycho-Analysis – the same editor of Freud's complete works in English.

2 The nature of the unconscious was the subject of my master's thesis back in 1978, focusing on Freud's metapsychological papers and the different interpretations made by Leclaire and Laplanche at Bonneval (Verhaeghe, 1978). The historical circumstances as well as the discussion between Leclaire, Laplanche and Lacan are summarized by Roudinesco (1986: 317–328).

3 See *The Mirror Stage as Formative of the Function of the I as Revealed in Psychoanalytic Experience.*

4 See *Remarks on Daniel Lagache's Presentation: "Pychoanalysis and Personality Structure".*

5 "L'interprétation ne vise pas tellement le sens que de réduire les signifiants dans leur non-sens pour que nous puissions retrouver les déterminants de toute la conduite du sujet" (S11, 1964: 192). The next paragraph in *Seminar XI* refers to Leclaire, just as is the case in *Position of the Unconscious.*

6 Let us not forget that the title of the first part of the Rome Discours talks about the "psychoanalytic realization of the subject" (206).

7 This is Bruce Fink's note:

> 'Curl flux' is perhaps more commonly known as 'the flux integral of the curl of a vector field,' 'the surface integral of the normal component of the curl of a vector field,' or 'the collective measure of rotational tendency taken over the entire surface.' Stokes' theorem says that the flux integral of the curl of a vector field over a surface is equal to the line integral of the vector field around its boundary curve. Thus, for a given closed curve, the 'curl flux' over any surface whose boundary is exactly this closed curve is the same. The theorem gives the conditions for which the flux remains constant.
>
> (843 [847, fn 1])

8 The same idea can be found in Lacan's paper on the mirror stage, where he situates the birth of the *je* "prior to being objectified in the dialectic of identification with the other" (*Mirror Stage*, 76, 4).

9 The background of these ideas is probably to be found in Shannon's theory, although Lacan does not refer to it. In collaboration with Weaver, Shannon elaborated in 1949 a mathematical theory in the field of informatics. Their theory presents a formula expressing the probability of the appearance of a certain sign at a certain place in the message, and this without taking into account the content or meaning of the message. This probability is then used in a second formula which calculates how much information the said sign contains. The greater the probability of appearance of that sign in a particular place, the smaller its information value, and vice versa: the smaller its probability of appearance at a particular place, the greater its information value. This theory had an enormous impact not only in the field of informatics but also in the wider field of communication and discourse theory.

10 All these consequences of the pressure give one a deceptive impression that there is a superior intelligence outside the patient's consciousness which keeps a large amount of psychical material arranged for particular purposes and has fixed a planned order for its return to consciousness.

(Freud, 1895/1978: 272; see also 275–76, 286–87)

11 S11: 25, my translation. Sheridan (p. 22) translates the French "la béance par où la névrose se raccorde à un réel" as "the gap through which neurosis recreates a harmony with the real." The whole point of *Seminar XI* comes down to the demonstration that any harmony with the real is lost forever.

12 If one studies Lacan's work in this respect, it becomes obvious that he struggles with this new idea of causality, and that he has great difficulty in abandoning the previous unidimensional determination by the symbolic. This struggle can very well be illustrated with one lesson of *Seminar X* (session of 9 January 1963). He starts with repeating the reason why the subject is first of all and originally unconscious: "qu'il nous faut d'abord tenir pour antérieure à cette constitution [du sujet] une certaine incidence qui est celle du signifiant" (my translation: "that we need first of all to consider a certain incidence, the one of the signifier, as anterior to this constitution [of the subject]"). Based on this, one could infer that the signifier can be interpreted as primal. The next sentence offers a different story: "Le problème est de l'entrée du signifiant dans le réel et de voir comment de ceci naît le sujet" (my translation: "The problem concerns the entry of the signifier into the

real and the way in which the subject is born from this"). In this, the real acquires greater eloquence and the relation with the body is clear from the very beginning. Indeed, the signifiers do not appear out of thin air, on the contrary: "Ce qui permet justement à ce signifiant de s'incarner, c'est bien entendu ce que nous avons là pour nous présentifier les uns aux autres notre corps" (my translation: "What precisely permits this signifier to incarnate itself, is of course that what we have to present one to another, that is, our body"). This was already acknowledged in *Seminar II*:

> Les premiers symboles, les symboles naturels, sont issus d'un certain nombre d'images prévalentes – l'image du corps humain, l'image d'un certain nombre d'objets évidents comme le soleil, la lune et quelques autres.
> (Lacan, S2, 1954–1955: 352)

(My translation:

The first symbols, the natural symbols have come forward from a certain number of prevalent images – the image of the human body, the image of a certain number of evident objects, such as the sun, the moon and some other.)

This introduces us to a second theme, that is, causality arising from the real of the body. Previously, Lacan used expressions such as "signifiers furnished by nature". This is a very strange expression in the light of his theory concerning the supremacy of the symbolic. There are a number of analogous expressions, which prepared the field for his new theory on the body and the real as cause. I have quoted a few of them below:

- "Le Es dont il s'agit dans l'analyse, c'est du signifiant qui est là déjà dans le réel, du signifiant incompris" (Lacan, S4, 1956–1957: 49); my translation: "The Id which is what analysis is about, concerns the signifier, the incomprehensible signifier which is already there in the real";
- "Quand nous abordons le sujet, nous savons qu'il y a déjà dans la nature quelque chose qui est son Es, et qui est structuré selon le mode d'une articulation signifiante marquant tout de ce qui s'exerce chez ce sujet de ses empreintes, de ses contradictions, de sa profonde différence d'avec les coaptations naturelles" (Lacan, S4, 1956–1957: 50); my translation: "When we start with the subject, we know that there is already in nature something which is his Id, and which is structured following the way of a signifying articulation that marks everything of this subject by its imprints, by its contradictions, by its profound difference with natural cooptation".

A more extensive elaboration can be found in the opening chapter of *Seminar XI*: "Nature provides signifiers, and these signifiers organize inaugurally human relations in a creative way, providing them with structures and shaping them" (Lacan, S11, 1964: 20). In this quote, the signifiers precede the subject, but nature furnishes them. A few months later, this "primary classificatory function" will be associated with the biological difference between male and female around which the "combinatory" comes into being and is developed. The conclusion of this reasoning is: "What would make it legitimate to maintain that it is through sexual reality that the signifier came into the world" (Lacan, S11, 1964: 151). In the next paragraph, Lacan combines this "combinatory" with the one at work in genetics, including the loss in the process of meiosis. Eventually in *Seminar XI*, it becomes clear that, according to Lacan, nature saddles us with an essential loss, that of eternal life in itself, and subjectivity is an effect of this loss.

13 Lacan links the idea of object *a* and the libido as an organ that is lost in an answer to a question by Safouan.

> The *objet a* is something from which the subject, in order to constitute itself, has separated itself off as organ. This serves as a symbol of the lack, that is to say, of the phallus, not as such, but in so far as it is lacking. It must, therefore, be an object that is, firstly, separable and, secondly, that has some relation to the lack
>
> (Sheridan: 103; S11, 1964: 95)

See also Sheridan: 197–198 (S11, 1964: 179–180), where Lacan explicitly refers to the Bonneval Colloquium.

14 "there is no access to the opposite sex as Other except via the so-called partial drives wherein the subject seeks an object to take the place of the loss of life he has sustained due to the fact that he is sexed" (720, 7).

15 See also *Seminar XII*, session of 16 December 1964 and *Seminar XXIII*, session of 13 January 1976.

References

de Saussure, F. (1976) *Cours de linguistique générale*, Paris: Payot.

Ey, H. (1966) *L'inconscient (VIe Colloque de Bonneval)*, Paris: Desclée de Brouwer.

Freud, S. (1905a/1987) 'Three Essays on the Theory of Sexuality,' in J. Strachey (Ed.), *The Standard Edition of the Complete Psychological Works of Sigmund Freud*, Vol. 2, London: The Hogarth Press and the Institute of Psycho-Analysis, pp. 123–245.

Freud, S. (1905b/1978) 'Fragment of an Analysis of a Case of Hysteria,' in J. Strachey (Ed.), *The Standard Edition of the Complete Psychological Works of Sigmund Freud*, Vol. 2, London: The Hogarth Press and the Institute of Psycho-Analysis, pp. 1–122.

Freud, S. (1915a/1978) 'Instincts and their Vicissitudes,' in J. Strachey (Ed.), *The Standard Edition of the Complete Psychological Works of Sigmund Freud*, Vol. 2, London: The Hogarth Press and the Institute of Psycho-Analysis, pp. 109–140.

Freud, S. (1915b/1978) 'Repression,' in J. Strachey (Ed.), *The Standard Edition of the Complete Psychological Works of Sigmund Freud*, Vol. 2, London: The Hogarth Press and the Institute of Psycho-Analysis, pp. 141–158.

Freud, S. (1915c/1978) 'The Unconscious,' in J. Strachey (Ed.), *The Standard Edition of the Complete Psychological Works of Sigmund Freud*, Vol. 2, London: The Hogarth Press and the Institute of Psycho-Analysis, pp. 159–215.

Freud, S. (1917/1978) 'A Difficulty in the Path of Psycho-Analysis,' in J. Strachey (Ed.), *The Standard Edition of the Complete Psychological Works of Sigmund Freud*, Vol. 2, London: The Hogarth Press and the Institute of Psycho-Analysis, pp. 135–144.

Freud, S. (1920/1978) 'Beyond the Pleasure Principle,' in J. Strachey (Ed.), *The Standard Edition of the Complete Psychological Works of Sigmund Freud*, Vol. 2, London: The Hogarth Press and the Institute of Psycho-Analysis, pp. 7–64.

Freud, S. (1940a/1978) 'An Outline of Psycho-Analysis,' in J. Strachey (Ed.), *The Standard Edition of the Complete Psychological Works of Sigmund Freud*, Vol. 2, London: The Hogarth Press and the Institute of Psycho-Analysis, pp. 141–207.

Freud, S. (1940b/1978) 'Splitting of the Ego in the Process of Defence,' in J. Strachey (Ed.), *The Standard Edition of the Complete Psychological Works of Sigmund Freud*, Vol. 2, London: The Hogarth Press and the Institute of Psycho-Analysis, pp. 271–278.

Freud, S. and Breuer, J. (1895/1978) 'Studies on Hysteria,' in J. Strachey (Ed.), *The Standard Edition of the Complete Psychological Works of Sigmund Freud*, Vol. 2, London: The Hogarth Press and the Institute of Psycho-Analysis.

Jacobson, R. (1956/1995) 'Two Aspects of Language and Two Types of Aphasic Disturbances,' in L. Waugh and M. Monville-Burston (Eds.), *On Language*, Cambridge, MA: Harvard University Press, pp. 115–133.

Lacan, J. (1968) 'Proposition d'Octobre,' *Scilicet*, 1, pp. 14–30.

Lacan, J. (1973) *Le Séminaire, livre XI, Les quatre concepts fondamentaux de la psychanalyse* (1964), ed. J.-A. Miller, Paris: Éditions du Seuil.

Lacan, J. (1973/1994) *The Seminar. Book XI: The Four Fundamental Concepts of Psycho-Analysis* (1964), trans. A. Sheridan, ed. J.-A. Miller, Harmondsworth: Penguin.

Lacan, J. (1978) *Le Séminaire, Livre II: Le moi dans la théorie de Freud et dans la technique de la psychanalyse* (1954–1955), ed. J.-A. Miller, Paris: Éditions du Seuil.

Lacan, J. (1991) *Le Séminair, Livre XVII, L'Envers de la Psychanalyse* (1969–1970), ed. J.-A. Miller, Paris: Éditions du Seuil.

Lacan, J. (1994) *Le Séminaire. Livre IV: La relation d'objet* (1956–1957), texte établi par J.-A. Miller, Paris: Éditions du Seuil.

Lacan, J. (2005) *Le Séminaire. Livre XXIII: Le sinthome* (1975–1976), texte établi par J.-A. Miller, Paris: Éditions du Seuil.

Laplanche, J. and Leclaire, S. (1966) 'L'inconscient: une étude psychanalytique,' in H. Ey (Ed.), *L'inconscient (VIe Colloque de Bonneval)*, Paris: Desclée de Brouwer, pp. 95–130.

Leclaire, S. (1968) *Psychanalyser. Un essau sur l'ordre de l'inconscient et la pratique de la letter*, Paris: Éditions du Seuil.

Muller, J.P. and Richardson, W.J. (1982) *Lacan and Language – A Reader's Guide to Écrits*, New York: International Universities Press.

Ricoeur, P. (1965/1970) *Freud and Philosophy: An Essay on Interpretation*, New Haven, CT: Yale University Press.

Rifflet, A. (1970) *Jacques Lacan. Avec un préface de J.Lacan*, Brussels: Ed. Ch.Dessart.

Roudinesco, É. (1986) *La bataille de cent ans. Histoire de la psychanalyse en France, 2. 1925–1985*, Paris: Éditions du Seuil.

Roudinesco, É. (1993) *Jacques Lacan. Esquisse d'une vie, histoire d'un système de pensée*, Paris: Fayard.

Shannon, C.E. and Weaver, W. (1949) *The Mathematical Theory of Communication*, Urbana, IL: University of Illinois Press.

Verhaeghe, P. (1978) *Psychoanalyse: woord en beeld. Een metapsychologische studie*, Universiteit Gent: Faculteit der psychologische en pedagogische wetenschappen.

Verhaeghe, P. (1998) 'Causation and Destitution of a Pre-ontological Non-entity: On the Lacanian Subject,' in D. Nobus (Ed.), *Key Concepts of Lacanian Psychoanalysis*, London: Rebus Press, pp.164–189.
Verhaeghe, P. (2002) 'Causality in Science and Psychoanalysis,' in J. Glynos and Y. Stavrakakis (Eds.), *Lacan & Science*, London/New York: Karnac, pp. 119–145.
Verhaeghe, P. (2009) *New Studies of Old Villains. A Radical Reconsideration of the Oedipus Complex*, New York: Other Press.
Verhaeghe, P. and Declercq, F. (2003) 'Lacan's Analytical Goal: "Le Sinthome" or the Feminine Way,' in L. Thurston (Ed.), *Essays on the Final Lacan – Re-inventing the Symptom*, New York: The Other Press, pp. 59–83.

9

ON FREUD'S "TRIEB" AND THE PSYCHOANALYST'S DESIRE

Theo Reeves-Evison

Context

The short essay '*On Freud's "Trieb" and the Psychoanalyst's Desire*' started life as a series of impromptu remarks at a colloquium at the University of Rome in January 1964. The colloquium was organized by Enrico Castelli under the title '*Technique and Casuistry*', and featured presentations from high profile speakers working at the intersections of philosophy, psychoanalysis, hermeneutics and phenomenology, such as Paul Ricoeur, Antoine Vergote and Alphonse De Waelhens. While Lacan's original contribution was delivered entirely without notes, he later published a summary of his remarks both in the conference proceedings and a few years later in the Écrits (Castelli, 1964).

The historical backdrop to the essay is significant. Lacan attended the conference shortly after the *International Psychoanalytical Association* revoked his status as a training analyst in October 1963, and this decision, which Lacan descibed as an 'excommunication', was made precisely on acount of the techniques he was using at the time. Three days after Lacan had visited Rome he began his eleventh seminar on *The Four Fundamental Concepts of Psychoanalysis* (S11, 1964), which was held at the *École Normale Supérieure* at the invitation of Louis Althusser. The seminar had hitherto been held at the Saint Anne hospital in central Paris, but his 'excommunication' no longer made this possible, and the change in venue also marked a change in the audience he spoke to.[1] Alongside the loyal disciples who had followed him in the 1950s was a new generation of young philosophy students, who would lend Lacan's work a greater systematic rigor in the years to come. The decision by Lacan to present his remarks '*On Freud's "Trieb" and the Psychoanalyst's Desire*' at a philosophy conference, then marked a shift in the reception of his work and a conscious step towards addressing a broader and more philosophically aware audience.

The newly systematic approach to Lacanian theory that was being incubated at the *École Normale Supérieure* stripped away the inconsistencies and surrealist influences in Lacan's early work. Lacan actively encouraged this, and in many ways *On Freud's "Trieb"* could be said to inaugurate a kind of 'clean up operation' where certain concepts were clarified, categorized and distinguished from one another (Roudinesco, 1993/1997: 306). The major thrust of this *Écrit* is to distinguish the concept of the drive from both instinct and desire, and to think through the role of the latter in the operation of psychoanalysis. The drive is further discussed as one of the four fundamental concepts of psychoanalysis in Lacan's seminar later that year, and *On Freud's "Trieb"* could be said to lay the foundations for the epistemological clarification that the concept was to undergo (S11, 1964).

Although it is the shortest of Lacan's essays published in the Écrits, *On Freud's "Trieb"* is extremely rich, and contains ideas that were formulated at a significant juncture in Lacan's life and work. Some 'post-Lacanian' authors such as Renata Salecl and Slavoj Žižek have suggested that around this time we can see a transition from an 'early Lacan' of desire, to a 'late Lacan' of the drive (Žižek, 1997: 148). *On Freud's "Trieb"* can be seen as establishing the initial cleavage between the two concepts, and marking a transition from one stage of his work to another.

Commentaries on the text

Lacan's decision to use the German word *Trieb* in the title of the essay is given further weight in the first two paragraphs when he takes great care to distinguish it from 'instinct'. Lacan considers the wholesale substitution of the word 'instinct' for the German *Trieb* in the English translation of Freud's works (and of *instinct* for *pulsion* in the French translation) an unforgivable mistake, especially where Freud had the German word *Instinkt* at his disposal but chose *Trieb* instead (Freud, 1915/1957).

On a semantic level, the word instinct carries obvious biological connotations, whereas *Trieb* has a greater polysemic complexity, at once suggesting propulsion, stimulation, or force – all of which hint at some of the models and metaphors Freud borrowed from nineteenth-century physics. The word *Trieb* also carries the sense of an activity or motivation, as in 'what are you driving at?' [*Was triebst du da?*] whereas instinct assumes a more passive position.

For Lacan this mistranslation represents more than just the oversight of a single translator, it reflects the erroneous direction "psychologizing thought" as a whole was taking at the time. In the first paragraph, he links this direction to an assumption of "the existence of morals in nature" (722, 1). This point should be understood in the context of debates around 'genital love' and the subordination of the drives to reproductive sexuality. It is worth pointing out that at the time the Écrits was first published in French, conversion therapy aimed at 'curing' homosexuality was still widespread, and until 1973 it was classified as a mental disorder in the *Diagnostic and Statistical Manual of Mental Disorders*.[2] For Lacan, drives can be distinguished from instincts precisely on the grounds that they have no 'natural' object or outcome, least of all procreation, but rather are involved in an economy of *jouissance*.

Lacan builds on this point with a discussion of the concept of libido, which he again categorically distinguishes from 'sexual instinct'.[3] For Freud, libido is the underlying current that charges the drive. In his most extended treatment of the drives in '*Instincts and their Vicissitudes*' ['*Triebe und Triebschicksale*'], Freud puts forward an energetic theory of the libido. The problem for Lacan is that this theory does not set out a means of quantifying libido in the same way that energy might be measured in other fields, in physics for example, where energy is measured in joules. While "libido is subjected to a kind of quantification" this is "useless, since only certain *quanta* of constancy are recognized therein" (722, 4). Lacan makes this point at greater length elsewhere, when he affirms that it is unhelpful to speak of libido as a quantity of energy unless it can be fixed to a numerical value and compared with other values (Lacan, 1973/1987: 22). As Johnson points out, this distances Lacan from a vitalist strain in French thought in the 1960s that could be described as 'neo-Bergsonian', on account of its debt to the philosopher's quasi-mystical theorisation of energy (Johnson, 2005: 314–315).

As Lacan reminds us, Freud insisted on the sexual character of libido, which brought him into direct conflict with Jung, who again in a vitalist mode, characterized it as neutral life energy. But at the same time that Lacan reaffirms Freud's position, he makes a surprising claim, that the 'sexual coloring' of the libido is "the color of emptiness: suspended in the light of a gap." (722, 5) What could this poetic formulation mean?

In the first place, the 'emptiness' referred to by Lacan is linked to the fact that the object of the drive can never fully stand in for the lost libidinal satisfaction it tries to compensate for. If we think of satisfaction as being attributed to a specific object in the psychic economy, we will be disappointed, because this object is always lacking; we are confronted with an empty space, and more specifically, with a gap. In the functioning of the drive, certain objects serve as impoverished substitutes for an initial, almost mythical (insofar as it is pre-conscious) experience of satisfaction.

Second, the idea of a 'gap' [*béance*] is a frequent motif in Lacan's work, used in a variety of senses, and here it is linked to Freud's central concepts of the pleasure and reality principles. In abbreviated form, the pleasure principle is defined negatively on the basis that it aims at the avoidance or discharge of unpleasurable tension. This search for satisfaction is moderated by the 'reality' it encounters in the outside world, which complicates things by imposing conditions and detours on the route to pleasure. Lacan follows Freud (1933/1978: 223) in asserting that the pleasure and reality principles are not simply opposed to one another, as one might expect, because the reality principle still in some ways facilitates the acquisition of pleasure – just as a road diversion facilitates the movement of traffic from A to B, only via a longer route. Since this is the case, the 'gap' Lacan speaks of is not the gap between the two, but rather a gap at the far reaches of *both* the pleasure *and* the reality principle – and to extend the road metaphor, the 'destination' that neither the diversion nor the direct route allow us to reach.

Here we touch on an essential point about desire, namely, that it functions by means of a set of limits. It is precisely on account of the destination being out of reach that it is desired in the first place. Lacan writes that it is from "a field of praxis [...] that Freudianism hews a desire, the crux of which is essentially found in impossibilities" (722, 6–7). As we shall see, the object of desire is essentially a social product for Lacan, and the impossibilities of desire that the subject encounters can be understood as the translation of a structural impossibility into social prohibitions. Lacan will develop this point later in the essay.

What follows this extremely compressed set of opening remarks is a passing reference to two related Freudian concepts. The first of these is "wishful thinking" and the second "the omnipotence of thought" (723, 1). Freud discusses these concepts in Totem and Taboo, primarily in the context of a discussion about animism and magic (1913/1955). He argues that these fields "reveal in the clearest and most unmistakable way an intention to impose the laws governing mental life upon real things" (1913/1955: 91). Animism and magic, as well as certain cases of obsessional neurosis and paranoia, involve the systematic overvaluation of the power of thought, whereby one believes that it is possible to influence reality simply by thinking (or with the aid of an object such as a voodoo doll, for example). For Freud, the idea that such practices can actively shape reality amounts to wishful thinking, even though it may not be immediately clear what the unconscious wish is.

As Lacan is quick to point out, these concepts do not simply imply megalomania, "but rather the reconciliation of opposites" (723, 1). That is to say, the mechanism of projection, whereby reality is disguised or denied, can be used as a means to deal with conflicts within the psyche. Ambivalent emotional states can be projected outwards and embodied in warring spirits or demons, thus resolving conflict between two competing desires by attributing agency to outside forces (Freud, 1913/1955: 60–61). Understanding these mechanisms leads to what Lacan described as "theological decline" (723, 2). In Freud's work the heavens are depopulated, as one by one the gods are shown to be projections that result from a combination of "wishful thinking" and the "omnipotence of thought".

Nevertheless, Lacan goes on to introduce a concept with obvious religious resonance: the "Name-of-the-Father". Here and elsewhere the homophony between *le nom du père* (the name of the father) and *le non du père* (the 'no' of the father) is exploited to emphasize the dual function of the father as both the one who prohibits incest in the Oedipus complex, and the name that, according to Lacan, symbolizes the Law in Freud's myth of the primal horde. This moves the essay into a discussion of the Oedipus complex in general, and of the place of desire in its functioning.

The fact that Lacan writes Law with a capital 'L' alerts us to the fact that we are not talking about everyday legislation here, but a fundamental principle of the symbolic order itself, which presides over all social life, and creates the conditions under which desire can emerge. Drawing inspiration from Claude Lévi-Strauss and Ferdinand de Saussure, in Lacan's work 'the Symbolic' is figured as a locus of differential elements that allow for social mediation and exchange. Here and elsewhere, Lacan emphasizes that it is only through castration that one can fully accede to the symbolic order. "Psychologists" who stress the "importance of being gratified by one's mother" [*gratification maternelle*] (723, 5) are guilty, according to Lacan, of abandoning this central discovery and infantilizing adults – a criticism that he extends to psychoanalysts as well in the following paragraph. While maintaining continuity with Freud, Lacan in effect radicalizes the former's approach to castration, a move with far-reaching clinical implications. From a Lacanian perspective, the Oedipal crisis, which culminates in castration, occurs when the child realizes that it does *not* have all that the mother wants. The child cannot be the sole object of her desire – an object that Lacan labels 'the imaginary phallus'.[4] In giving up its attempt to play the role of the phallus for the mother, the child renounces a certain amount of *jouissance*, which creates the "lack on the basis of which desire is instituted" (723, 8).

In parentheses Lacan makes the point that castration applies equally to both genders. This is another point of departure from Freud, who claimed that the castration complex represented the point of entry to the Oedipus complex for girls, rather than its terminal crisis. For Lacan it is the terminal crisis for both genders, on account of the role of the phallus in the operation, which neither sex has a privileged relation to: "it is the phallus by default that constitutes the amount of symbolic debt: a debit account when one has it, a disputed credit when one does not" (723, 9). In this convoluted sentence both monetary metaphors imply dispossession. For Lacan the symbolic phallus is a signifier that has no opposite, and as he argues in *Seminar IV*, this means that while the woman can be said to lack the symbolic phallus, this lack is still in a way a form of having (S4, 1956–1957: 153). This paradoxical relationship is what is designated by the metaphor of "a disputed credit", which highlights the indeterminate status of the object of possession, without negating the act of possessing itself. For the man on the other hand, having the phallus is only possible on the precondition that he has already assumed castration, and that is why his account is in "debit".

Many of the ideas presented on the Oedipus complex are already established in Lacan's work by the time he comes to present *On Freud's "Trieb"*. So why go over them again here? The reasons seem to be twofold. First, as a means to once again critique certain strains of psychology and psychoanalysis (723, 5)[5] and second, to demonstrate that desire is fundamentally inculcated in the symbolic order, and that it is only by accession to this order through castration that desire can function. As we shall see, the drive functions in an altogether different register.

Before moving on to a discussion of the drive proper, Lacan drops in a reference to *The Symposium*, Plato's famous text set at a drinking party where the guests make speeches about love. Having already made an extended reading of *The Symposium* in *Seminar VIII* (1960–1961), Lacan stops only to make a passing remark and draw attention to the word agalma, *ἄγαλμα*, meaning a precious object, hidden within unremarkable outer 'packaging'. The character Alcibiades uses the word to pay a rather double-handed compliment to Socrates.[6] In the final discourse of the text, Alcibiades lays bare his unyielding desire for Socrates, who he calls his eron, *ἐρῶν* or beloved. Yet despite his gushing tributes, Alcibiades accuses Socrates of selfishly withholding his 'agalma'. The significance of this interchange for Lacan is that the 'agalma' is something that Socrates never had. In the context of the discussion, the example serves once again to remind us of the function of lack as it relates to desire, but also to lay the ground for a discussion of the desire of the analyst, who is aligned to Socrates in *Seminar VIII*, on account of his strategy of mobilizing Alcibiades's desire for his self-betterment. In this seminar the agalma is also related to the concept of 'object *a*'.

Returning to the subject of the drives, Lacan makes several allusions to Freud's work in quick succession. First, he writes that the "the concept of the drive represents the drive as montage" (723, 12). In *Seminar XI* this claim is illustrated with a colorful surrealist vignette whereby "a dynamo [is] connected up to a gas-tap, a peacock's feather emerges, and tickles the belly of a pretty woman" (S11, 1964: 169). Lacan then rearranges the elements of this assemblage to show that the drive essentially operates in a circuit that turns back on itself, involving the four elements that Freud isolates: pressure, aim, object, and source (Freud, 1915/1957).

Second, he repeats Freud's claim that "the drives are our myths" (723, 13). Freud made this point on account of them being "magnificent in their indefiniteness" (Freud, 1933/1978: 95). In some ways this indefiniteness is constitutive, and in underlining the problem, Lacan makes a larger point concerning the difficulty of grasping the drives independent of their psychical representatives. The drives in effect 'mythify the real' – that noumenal realm beyond the tapestry of language – and in so doing they carve up the Real in the same way Greek mythology carves up the heavens.

Third, and this is where Lacan finally spells out one of the central points of the essay, "Desire comes from the Other, and *jouissance* is located on the side of the Thing" (724, 3). We know from *Seminar VII* that this might as well be read 'the *drive* is located on the side of the Thing', for it is here that Lacan argues that the Thing is the apparent goal of the drives (S7, 1959–1960: 110). But what is 'The Thing' in the first place? In short, it is a forerunner for the concept of object *a* – simultaneously posited as a beyond-of-the-signifier, a Kantian 'thing-in-itself', and the void which emerges on the basis of a split between mother and child. Given this range of meanings, it is misleading to consider 'The Thing' an object in any straightforward sense. Lacan's argument is that desire stops short of the Thing, remaining at the level of the symbolic order. Like the lizard that looses its tail, desire drops off when it approaches the Thing, whereas the drive carries on, gaining satisfaction by perpetually encircling "the hedges of *jouissance*" (724, 2).

As Lacan begins to draw the essay to a close he turns finally to the subject of the analyst's desire.[7] After asking "what then can the analyst's desire be? What can the treatment to which the analyst devotes himself be?" (724, 6). Lacan runs through a series of negative answers. The analyst's desire should neither be to preach a certain life direction guided by moral principles, nor to embody the 'physician's privilege' (724, 8). At this point we should recall that Lacan has already rejected the moral of so-called '*gratification maternelle*' mentioned earlier in the text. Both of these paradigms involve the prescription of ends (*fins*), and ready-made road maps of how to get there. As such they ignore the singularity of the subject, and lead to 'the political segregation' of those unable to fit a certain symbolic mold. (724, 9) The analyst should take on board the message of Moliere's *The imaginary invalid* (no doubt the author Lacan has in mind when he speaks of 'the great writer of comedies') and question the socially sanctioned role of the physician with his or her ready-made solutions.

For Lacan, the analyst's desire should remain an unfathomable '*x*', only then can it serve as the driving force of the analytic session – an idea that has ramifications for the training of analysts as well. Lacan sums up this approach with the paradoxical term *fin première*. At once translatable as 'primary aim' or 'first end', *fin première* is opposed to the *fin dernière* of eschatology, and implies an initial cause, the cause of desire, which in turn sets the analysand's desire to work. Steering clear of eschatological ends can also be considered a way of avoiding fixed meanings as the outcome of an analysis, and encouraging the productive deadlocks of nonmeaning. In short, the aim of Lacanian analysis cannot be to facilitate a coherent meta-narrative at the end of the treatment, which then recodes everything that came before it, nor can it be the pursuit of ideal outcomes such as 'health', 'happiness' or 'genital oblativity'. The 'aim' of analysis has to be placed beyond (or rather before) these explicitly therapeutic aims and to put the analyst's desire to work as a desire for difference. The distinction between a therapeutic aim of psychoanalysis, and this other, altogether more radical approach Lacan is advocating comes to the fore in the analysis that trainee psychoanalysts undergo, which by definition has an aim beyond therapeutics. When it comes to training analysts (lest we forget, an activity the IPA had prohibited Lacan from doing just months before) the primary aim must also be mobilized, and as such the analyst's desire must play a crucial part.

This is the major concluding point of *on Freud's "Trieb"*, and it is somewhat tantalizing that a more explicit connection between the drive and the desire of the analyst is not made. Later the same year, in *Seminar XI*, Lacan will add flesh to the bones of this *Écrit* by further developing its themes and concepts. It is in this seminar, and not in the *Écrit* itself, that the analyst's desire is shown to have the capacity to expose the subject's relationship to the drive. Nevertheless, in its anticipation of this link, and its affirmation of productive space of indeterminacy that the analyst's desire keeps open, *On Freud's "Trieb"* remains a crucial, if condensed companion piece to *Seminar XI*, and a gateway to the later Lacan as a whole.

Notes

1 The title of Lacan's eleventh seminar was originally announced as 'On the Names of the Father', and commenced at the St. Anne Hospital on November 20, 1963. Due to Lacan's 'excommunication' from the IPA this was to be the first and only session of a seminar under this title. It was not until the January 15 the following year that Lacan took up his seminar once again, under the new title '*The Four Fundamental Concepts of Psychoanalysis*'.

2 In 1973, a vote was taken by the American Psychiatric Association to reclassify homosexuality. In the seventh printing of the DSM-II in 1974, it was labeled a "sexual orientation disturbance" instead. (American Psychiatric Association, 1973)

3 The concept of libido is exclusively (and problematically) masculine in Freud's work (Freud, 1933/1978: 131) – a point that Lacan reaffirms (*Signification*: 584) – whereas instincts cannot be attributed to either gender exclusively. This is one of the ways Lacan distinguishes drive from libido.

4 To be distinguished from both the biological penis and the symbolic phallus (*Signification*).

5 Despite their mutual respect, Lacan may have had Donald Winnicott in mind here. Winnicott claimed that the analytic environment should be a 'holding environment' (Winnicott, 1986: 119). As Luepnitz writes, 'his idea was that a person deprived of maternal provision could use the "good breast" of the analyst; offering more access thus could be reparative'. This could be seen to 'infantilize adults' (Luepnitz, 2011: 11.)

6 Agalma is difficult to translate into English, and can mean shrine, object of worship or ornament. The term appears in the Écrits in Greek.

7 It should be pointed out that the term *le désir de l'analyste* is equivocal in French. It could simultaneously mean the desire that the analyst actually has, or the desire imputed to the analyst by the analysand (Evans, 1996: 39).

References

American Psychiatric Association (1973) *Homosexuality and Sexuality Orientation Disturbance: Proposed Change in DSM-II, 6th printing, page 44*, Washington, DC: The American Psychiatric Association. APA Document Reference No. 730008.

Castelli, E. (1964) *Tecnica E Casistica*, Padova: Cedam.

Evans, D. (1996) *An Introductory Dictionary of Lacanian Psychoanalysis*, Hove: Routledge.

Freud, S. (1913/1955) 'Totem and Taboo', in J. Strachey (Ed.), *The Standard Edition of the Complete Psychological Works of Sigmund Freud*, Vol. 13, London: The Hogarth Press and the Institute of Psycho-Analysis, pp. 1–162.

Freud, S. (1915/1957) 'Instincts and their Vicissitudes', in J. Strachey (Ed.), *The Standard Edition of the Complete Psychological Works of Sigmund Freud*, Vol. 14, London: The Hogarth Press and the Institute of Psycho-Analysis, pp. 109–140.

Freud, S. (1933/1978) 'New Introductory Lectures on Psycho-Analysis', in J. Strachey (Ed.), *The Standard Edition of the Complete Psychological Works of Sigmund Freud*, Vol. 22, London: The Hogarth Press and the Institute of Psycho-Analysis.

Johnson, A. (2005) *Time Driven: Metapsychology and the Splitting of the Drive*, Evanston, IL: Northwestern University Press.

Lacan, J. (1973/1987) 'Television', *October*, 40, pp. 7–50.

Lacan, J. (1973/1994) *The Seminar. Book XI: The Four Fundamental Concepts of Psycho-Analysis* (1964), trans. A. Sheridan, ed. J.-A. Miller, Harmondsworth: Penguin.

Lacan, J. (1986/1992) *The Seminar. Book VII: The Ethics of Psychoanalysis* (1959–1960), trans. D. Porter, ed. J.-A. Miller, New York/London: W. W. Norton & Company.

Lacan, J. (1991/2007) *The Seminar. Book XVII: The Other Side of Psychoanalysis* (1969–1970), trans. R. Grigg, ed. J.-A. Miller, New York/London: W. W. Norton & Company.

Lacan, J. (1994) *Le Séminaire. Livre IV: La relation d'objet* (1956–1957), texte établi par J.-A. Miller, Paris: Éditions du Seuil.

Luepnitz, D. A. (2011) 'Thinking in the Space between Winnicott and Lacan', in *Between Winnicott and Lacan: A Clinical Engagement*, New York: Rouledge.

Roudinesco, É. (1993/1997) *Jacques Lacan*, Cambridge: Polity Press.

Winnicott, D. W. (1986) *Home is Where we Start From*, London: Penguin Books.

Žižek, S. (1997) 'Interview: Renata Salecl and Slavoj Žižek: Interviewed by Andrew Long and Tara McGann', *Journal for the Psychoanalysis of Culture and Society*, 2(2), pp. 147–151.

10

SCIENCE AND TRUTH

Ed Pluth

Context

'*Science and Truth*' is a written essay that Lacan delivered orally at the start of his thirteenth seminar in December 1965. With few exceptions (some notes and the short prefatory material such as '*On Our Antecedents*') it is the newest essay to be included in the volume, appearing in print just eleven months after its delivery. (Although it was in fact first published even earlier, in February of 1966, in the first issue of *Cahiers pour l'Analyse*.) This makes its status rather distinct. The essays included in the *Écrits* that come from the period when Lacan was teaching his seminar (after 1953) are typically working with concepts and topics that he had been developing throughout the previous year, or years. '*Science and Truth*' is not the result of a previous year's work in this sense: it does not act as a sort of resumé or ultimate doctrinal statement of a year, or more, of theoretical elaboration. Its content, while mostly drawing from what Lacan had been working on in previous seminars, is thus much more like the content of the seminars themselves: it is at times more speculative, and some of it Lacan never returns to again. Indeed, if one reads transcripts of the rest of the thirteenth seminar for more on some of the topics Lacan brings up in this essay, one is disappointed. Even in subsequent seminars Lacan does not return, for example, to the four discourses he concludes this essay with (magic, religion, science, psychoanalysis) and their connections to the four Aristotelian causes. Yet the odd thing about '*Science and Truth*' is that Lacan's sometimes speculative remarks and asides now do remain in print alongside essays whose content is relatively more fleshed out, and whose obscurities can usually be clarified by consulting the seminars in which the difficult material was developed. With this essay, that is not the case.

But there is some polished material in this essay; most notably the topics of science, psychoanalysis's relationship to it, and the notion of the 'subject of science'. '*Science and Truth*' is a significant statement of Lacan's views on all these matters at this time, and my commentary will focus on them. Lacan's position seems to be that psychoanalysis as an autonomous discourse is something that still needs to be developed, and its debts to both the natural sciences and to structuralism need to be settled in order to finish the job.

Commentary on the text

Lacan's seminar for the year prior to the delivery of '*Science and Truth*' was entitled *Crucial Problems for Psychoanalysis*. Lacan opens this year's seminar, his thirteenth, entitled *The Object of Psychoanalysis*, by asking whether last year's work puts him in a position to say that he has "established the status of the *subject* in psychoanalysis" (726, 1). The answer seems to be yes: he says that he developed in that seminar "a structure" that accounts for what he calls the splitting of the subject – and that this split subject is the one with which psychoanalysts work (726, 1).

Lacan is using the German word *Spaltung* (splitting) in this context because of its presence in the title of a late essay by Freud entitled '*Das Ichspaltung im Abwehrvorgang*' ('*Splitting of the Ego in the Defensive Process*'), written in 1938, not completed, and published after Freud's death in 1939. Lacan refers to this essay directly on the next page, and will return to it in the essay's concluding paragraphs. In it Freud discusses the circumstances in which the ego engages in a simultaneous rejection and acceptance of some aspect of reality – in the case Freud discusses, of the mother's lack of a penis. Lacan will in this essay retool Freud's discussion of the ego, split between a refusal and an acceptance, into a subject split between an (unacknowledged) truth and a (semi-delusional?) knowledge. Lacan adds that psychoanalysts detect this subject on a "more or less daily basis" in their work (726, 2). They can't avoid encountering the subject as split since they deal with the unconscious all the time, and an analyst can even be said to be submerged by its "constant" manifestations (726, 2).

While recognizing the unconscious in the clinic "suffices to ground" the split subject Lacan is talking about, he expresses worries throughout the essay that psychoanalysis is still not adequately grounded (726, 2). The fact that psychoanalysts deal with the unconscious every day does not guarantee that any of them really know what they are doing, or why what they are doing works. An analyst could well be aware of the subject's splitting, of the unconscious and its manifestations and what all that means, but beyond that exposure and experience Lacan claims that "a certain reduction" is necessary for a psychoanalyst to "know the status of his practice" and for clarity to be gained about what that practice is working on – its "object" (726, 3). Lacan links such a reductive gesture to the birth of any science. This introduces us to the topic of science, and psychoanalysis's relationship to it, obviously another one of the main themes of the essay. For now the relationship is put in terms of an analogy: psychoanalysis needs to gain clarity about the nature of the objects it works with, and this is needed for any science to take off. But whether and how psychoanalysis would count as a science Lacan leaves open at this point.

How does a "reduction" help a science to "constitute its object"? Lacan is agreeing with thinkers like the historian of science Alexandre Koyré (1892–1964) and the philosopher Alexandre Kojève (1902–1968) on the origin of the natural sciences. Grossly simplifying matters here, according to these authors the sciences emerged only when natural objects and phenomena were "reduced" to measurable quantities. With this reduction (to the mathematizable) it became clear that the objects of the natural sciences were something other than what appears to us in the richness of our lived experiences, with all its diverse qualities. Epistemology is supposed to focus on the particularity of objects of knowledge in different domains, but Lacan claims that up to now this branch of philosophy has not been "equal to the task" – presumably not equal to the task of specifying the object of psychoanalysis, and perhaps not even the object of the natural sciences, as he suggests later: "something in the status of science's object ... seems to me to have remained unelucidated since the birth of science" (733, 3; 726, 3).

What has been overlooked (by epistemologists, presumably) is a "decisive change" brought about by the natural sciences involving a "modification that has occurred in our subject position" (726, 4). What Lacan has in mind here is what will be another one of the main topics of this essay, what he'll call the 'subject of science' – a new subject position that emerged as a consequence of the scientific worldview. So on the first page of the essay alone Lacan has introduced the reader to its three main threads: the distinctness of psychoanalytic theory and practice, its relationship to science, and the subject position that has emerged as a consequence of the natural sciences.

Saying that last year he left open the question of whether psychoanalysis was a science, or could be one, he notes that what he did do involved a focus on this "moment of the subject" that he considers to be "an essential correlate of science, a historically defined moment" (727, 2). This moment is the articulation of the *cogito* in the work of René Descartes (1596–1650), which Lacan is taking to be a first indication of what the subject position of the subject of science looks like.

In the next paragraph he refers to the Cartesian *cogito* as a "correlate," a "moment" and a "defile" – a waste product or after-effect – of "the rejection of all knowledge" (727, 3). Of course, Descartes (1641/1979: 13) tells us in the *Meditations* that he was going to apply himself "earnestly and openly to the general destruction of my former opinions." What Descartes is engaging in is, indeed, a rejection of knowledge, albeit provisionally: but Lacan finds the gesture of rejection more important than the certainty Descartes ends up with. Even in the extreme hypothesis in which an evil Genius might be deceiving Descartes about the reality of his experiences and the truth of his knowledge (including mathematics), Descartes concluded that in order for him to be deceived at all ... he must at least exist. This is why Lacan writes that for Descartes the *cogito* serves as a sort of refuge from the moment of radical un-knowledge, offering an "anchoring in being," that defines "the subject of science" (727, 3). Fink's note on this passage observes that the "anchoring" could refer back to the "rejection of all knowledge" as well (844, n856, 4). Does Lacan agree that this anchoring in being found in Descartes's work really defines the subject of science, or is it not, rather, a defense, along the lines of what Lacan will discuss below as a suturing?

How does Lacan conceive of the subject of science? We've already seen that he associates the object of the natural sciences with quantification: a stripping away of a natural object's qualities. It has been argued that the Cartesian *cogito* is a similarly stripped-down subject: reduced not to the measurable, but to the mere act of thinking. Jean-Claude Milner (2000: 38) has called this a "thought without qualities," and identifies the work of the Descartes scholar Martial Gueroult (1891–1976) as Lacan's source for this reading of Descartes. The emergence of this subject without qualities – a reduced, if not quantified, subject – is the most important consequence of the rise of the sciences. It is worth quoting Milner (2000: 37–38) at length on this topic:

> Physics eliminates every quality from existents, therefore a theory of the subject that wishes to respond to such a physics must also strip the subject of every quality. [What were the qualities of a subject? Precisely thinking, reflecting, doubting, knowing, perceiving… -- EP] This subject, constituted following the characteristic determinations of science, is the subject of science … The qualitative markings of the empirical individual are not appropriate to the subject, whether they are somatic or psychic, nor are the qualitative properties of a soul. The subject is neither mortal nor immortal, neither pure nor impure, neither just nor unjust, neither sinner nor saint, neither damned nor saved. Even the properties that for a long time have been believed to constitute subjectivity as such are not appropriate: this subject has neither self, nor reflexivity, nor consciousness.

Registering a slight disagreement with it, Russell Grigg also quotes this passage in his excellent study of the subject of science (Grigg, 2008: 144). Of course, this conclusion is different from Descartes's actual position on the *cogito*, and to arrive at it Milner observes (2000: 38) that one must, as Gueroult argued, read Descartes according to "the order of reasons" – according to what his work strictly implies, regardless of where he went with it. Clearly Lacan is in pursuit of such a radically dehumanized subject as well, and this, we will see, is what he thinks is the unthought of scientism itself.

So he notes that reading Descartes the previous year "did not guide me in vain," since it led him to the insight that the split subject of psychoanalysis can be thought of in terms of "a division between knowledge and truth" (727, 4). That is, it is divided between a rejection of knowledge and a certainty about the truth of being, of existing, qua thinking thing. Although, again, it seems to me that when it comes to the subject of science Lacan is interested mainly in the fact of this division or split, which we've already seen can be found in Freud. Plus, it seems to me that Lacan will read the relationship a little differently later in this essay, when he considers the truth as the cause of the subject's division, and (unconscious) knowledge as a sort of pearl constructed around the truth's traumatic grain of sand.

Lacan used the one-sided Möbius strip as a model in the previous year's seminar for how to think of this division: knowledge and truth could be written on such a surface, and what would appear as a distinction between them (it might seem like they are on opposite sides) would be only an apparent distinction: instead there is a continuous, imperceptible shift from one to the other. Not only do the two apparent sides not really differ from each other, but each is generated from one and the same source (the twist in a ribbon or sheet that makes it a Möbius strip).

In the next paragraph Lacan shifts gears, and he will not return to his discussion of the divided subject of science until several paragraphs later. What seems to be the topic of this next section of the essay is method: Lacan's when reading Freud, but also Freud's with respect to the sciences of his own day. And so, ultimately, the point is to shed further light on the relationship of psychoanalysis to science, by way of Freud's scientism, and the structuralist turn of Lacan's own day.

In the following paragraph Lacan describes his return to Freud as one in which he "synchronically" resituates some of Freud's key concepts according to one guiding principle, namely that of "the subject – the subject caught up in a constituting division" (727, 5). A structural approach to Freudian theory, Lacan is saying, can set aside the temporal development (the diachronic aspect) of Freud's theory, and even look at it backwards chronologically ... such that Freud's latter topography of the Id, Ego, and Superego can be understood as a dialectical reworking of the first topography (the unconscious, conscious, preconscious systems) in light of the further experience gained with what analytic experience works with – "the subject caught up in a constituting division" (727, 5).

As an example of what his synchronic strategy regarding Freud accomplished, Lacan alludes to the "discordance that supposedly characterizes" the reality principle in Freud's work (727, 6). In 1911, Freud introduced the idea of a reality principle that acted as a supplement to the otherwise dominant pleasure principle: a principle that would explain why the psyche would start to represent "not what was agreeable, but what was real" (Laplanche and Pontalis, 1967/1974: 380). Left to its own devices, under the sole rule of the pleasure principle, Freud seemed to think that the psyche might hallucinate itself to death. So the idea was that the reality principle would emerge to interrupt the tendency for the psyche to obtain satisfaction in the quickest and easiest way possible (by hallucination, or fantasy). This principle was developed in the period of Freud's first topography, and it pitted the consciousness/pre-consciousness system against the wishes of the unconscious.

Consciousness and the unconscious this way became antagonistic, driven by different goals: delayed gratification versus direct satisfaction, with the reality principle ultimately putting the goal of survival above satisfaction. However, with the second topography (id, ego, superego), it would seem that the reality principle permeates both levels of the psyche, the conscious and unconscious systems. This could be taken to entail a contradiction, or a rejection of the earlier view. Also: do we need to conclude that the unconscious is opposed to its own satisfaction? Lacan's position seems to be that if we recall the importance of the divided subject, this is not a contradiction at all: discordance, in fact, does rule the psyche.

Lacan's approach, then, can lead us to see the reality principle as something that highlights an essential aspect of the experience of what he is calling the subject of science: the two principles are highlighting the kind of psychic life that emerges in the wake of the shift in the subject position associated with the subject of science (727, 7).

This leads Lacan to his next point: that psychoanalysis "as a practice" and "the *Freudian* unconscious as a discovery" could not have emerged without or before the birth of the sciences in the seventeenth century (727, 9). And the subject of this science is at the "nexus" of how the new mathematized natural sciences differ from what preceded them. Because of this "all humanist references become superfluous in science, the subject cutting them short": Lacan takes the subject of science to be this stripped-down, minimalist subject, a subject that is not much more than the site of a division (728, 2). Hence, much of what has been said and thought about the nature of the subject since the seventeenth century is going to turn out to be a misunderstanding: the subject is not deep, or full, as we shall see. It is certainly not what Descartes argued it was: a thinking substance. Lacan will be engaging in a sustained critique of what he describes as a 'humanist' view of the subject in this essay, found in disciplines ranging from hermeneutics to Marxism to psychology.

Despite the importance of the sciences for the emergence of psychoanalysis, the link between Freud and the sciences should not be misunderstood. Yes, Lacan admits that Freud's patients perhaps "came to him in the name of science" and this cultural belief undoubtedly put Freud in a position to make the discoveries he made (728, 3). Lacan's mention of a "trumped up … break on Freud's part with the scientism of his time" is probably a reference to Paul Ricoeur's *Freud and Philosophy: An Essay on Interpretation*, published the same year as this talk (1965), and by the same editor and in the same series as Lacan's own *Écrits* would be (728, 4). Roudinesco (1993/1997: 324) notes that the "publication of his book made Lacan furious: the whole text was on the subject of Freud and his disciples but made no reference to the teaching of Lacan, whose seminar Ricoeur had attended for five years". Ricoeur (1913–2005) presents Freud as a hermeneutic thinker, someone who was developing a system for interpreting human actions and beliefs from a non-naturalistic point of view: from Ricoeur's perspective, human actions and beliefs only make sense within their practical context (chemistry cannot shed light on ethics). Thus, he takes Freud to have been breaking with the dominance of the natural sciences of his day, regardless of how Freud himself thought of the status of his insights (and Freud's enthusiasm for the natural sciences is hard to overlook).

Lacan wants to affirm, however, that it was precisely Freud's "scientism," and this alone, that led him to his discoveries (728, 4). No break with scientism occurred at all, and one does not understand psychoanalysis better by replacing the naturalism that founded it with a humanism. Lacan thinks Freud's scientism is manifested in his inclination to mathematize "physiology and the mental functions considered to be included therein" – reducing the realm of the human, and the meaningful, to basic thermodynamic principles (728, 4). He names one of Freud's professors in Vienna, von Brücke, who led the charge in this direction at the time. Ernst Wilhelm Von Brücke (1819–1892) was a positivist who was skeptical of then current vitalist approaches to organisms. One of the things that displeased him about vitalism was its openness to mysticism and, in a term that will be used by Lacan later in this essay when discussing religion, obscurantism – flirting with the idea that there is some sort of life-force. Lacan also alludes to Helmholz and Du Bois-Reymond. Jean-Claude Milner (2000: 60, n18) observes that Hermann von Helmholz (1821–1894) "had explicitly raised the question of a thought without self-consciousness" and that this position shows the "historical articulation between scientism and the unconscious." (Emil Du Bois-Reymond (1818–1896) was a physiologist who explored the connections between nerves and muscle tissues and electricity.)

Lacan acknowledges that after Freud's foundation of psychoanalysis, "deviations" from scientism did occur (728, 6). The fact that Freud "opposed these deviations with timely sureness and inflexible rigor" is a testament to his commitment to the ideal of science (728, 23–24). Among these deviations, Lacan mentions the case of Jung specifically, whose work he takes as "an attempt to reinstate a subject endowed with depths": very much not how Lacan understands the subject of science (728, 7). Indeed, for Jung Lacan claims that the subject is thought to have a "relationship – said to be archetypal – to knowledge," whereas the subject of science is notable for its birth from an "erasure" of knowledge – the rejection he alluded to earlier in Descartes (728, 7). He adds that the subject of science's relation to knowledge itself is also "punctual and vanishing" (728, 7).

Because of Freud's commitment to science, because of this "indubitable origin," of psychoanalysis, "blatant in all of Freud's work," another prominent discipline, Marxism, "is unable … to attack his ideas on the basis of their historical extraction" (728, 8). Perhaps the thinking here is that a Marxism might engage in a historicizing or culturalist critique of Freud's insights – not, like Ricoeur, minimizing his scientism and naturalism, but focusing on other aspects surrounding the "historical extraction" of Freud's insights (and thus perhaps in this way calling into question their validity). Specifically Lacan mentions a number of Freud's biographical details, his "affiliations": with "the society of the dual monarchy" (the Austro-Hungarian empire), his "spiritual aversions" (which Lacan attributes to his Jewish background), and his affiliations with "the capitalist order that conditioned his political agnosticism" (728, 9). Lacan makes an aside here, asking who in his audience would be able to write an essay like Lammenais's *Essay on Indifference in Matters of Religion* (1817): Lammenais (1782–1854) was an ultramontane, arguing that the French state should not intervene in religious matters, since religious authority resided in the papacy. If Lammenais was arguing that the state should be indifferent to religion, and Freud is critiqued for his non-radicality by some Marxists, Lacan is perhaps wondering here if a psychoanalyst could write something like Lammenais wrote, arguing that psychoanalysis too should be politically indifferent.

Then finally Lacan refers to Freud's "affinity" for "bourgeois ethics" and alludes to the "dignity" of Freud's life compared to that of other "revolutionary agitators" (729, 1) (one thinks of the surrealist André Breton's disappointment at meeting Freud in Vienna in 1921). Despite all this, Freud's work should have a similar status to revolutionary works that have left their "mark on language" Lacan thinks (729, 1). The point seems to be that none of these historical or biographical details matters more for determining the status of psychoanalysis than Freud's scientism does.

Lacan then seems to be saying that he wishes he could assume that people were clear on the basics of psychoanalysis – the field within which it operates, the conditions for its emergence and continued practice – but says that he will "nevertheless have to rehash" here what he takes to be psychoanalysis's "least debatable certainties" (729, 2).

The first certainty he mentions, which should come as no surprise given what he has been saying so far, is that "the subject upon which we operate in psychoanalysis can only be the subject of science" (729, 3). Lacan considers right away how "paradoxical" this might sound: far from working with some sort of minimalistic, reduced, subject-without-qualities, isn't psychoanalysis in fact working with subjects who live, who work, who exist socially and historically with a host of real identities and desires (729, 4)? Isn't psychoanalysis working with concrete, suffering individuals? Can psychoanalysis ignore the subject's multiple contexts, its concrete life? In other words: isn't the subject of psychoanalysis what we could call the empirical, psychological individual? Lacan warns his readers that if one does not see clearly the nature of the subject psychoanalysis works with, "everything gets mixed up" and a sort of "objective" dishonesty sets in (729, 4). Regardless of their good intentions, if analysts don't recognize the mistake they have made about the nature of the subject they work with, and again, maybe no matter how good they are or effective they may well be as analysts, some serious problem is occurring in their practice: it is the duty of the analyst to maintain the position strictly implied by psychoanalysis. Fink, in his note to this passage, claims that Lacan is likely alluding to the group of psychoanalysts who, under pressure from the IPA, sided with Lacan's exclusion from the Société Française de la Pyschanalyse as a teaching analyst, leading Lacan to found his own school, the École de la Cause Freudienne, in 1964 (844–45, n859). This fairly recent event, and some of his former students involved in it, is very much on Lacan's mind in this essay, as we shall see.

Lacan adds that a psychoanalyst cannot be allowed to take on the position of a beautiful soul either – a Hegelian figure who laments the evils of the world, detaches herself from action and intervention in it, overlooking her own participation and investment in the evil world (for a good discussion of this position, from someone close to Lacan, consult Hyppolite (1946/1979, 512ff)). Psychoanalysts should not shy away from acknowledging the nature of the subject they really work with, even if it seems to them to be dehumanizing: any attempt to incarnate this subject, which is a "relapse" for psychoanalysis into something other than a science, is faulty, even if it seems fruitful in other ways (729, 6). This is especially a problem "when the subject is incarnated in man, himself nothing in such theories but a child" (729, 6).

Lacan has something specific in mind here: what Claude Lévi-Strauss (1908–2009) called "the archaic illusion" in chapter seven of his *Elementary Structures of Kinship* (1949/1969) (729, 7). The illusion in question consists in comparing the minds of children in more advanced societies to the minds of people in less advanced ones (and vice versa), such that the 'primitive' mind is taken to be frozen in a state of perpetual childhood (while contemporary perspectives in psychology and ethnography would be very careful not to argue in such a way, insofar as a distinction is still made between thinking rationally and thinking non-rationally, logically or non-logically, the same error Lacan is talking about here might still be said to occur). Lacan's point is that this (humanist) perspective misunderstands both children and 'primitives.' For Lacan's purposes in this essay its seems like the illusion involves something quite basic, and he will associate it with 'psychologizing' others – a danger intrinsic to trying to get into the mind of another (child, primitive, adult, or what have you) in order to understand how it thinks and what it knows. This is certainly a difficult trap for an analyst to avoid.

Lacan is saying that psychoanalysts are vulnerable to this error if they overlook the fact that the subject of psychoanalysis is the subject of science. It follows that psychoanalysis is not going to be a "science of man," not necessarily because it isn't a science, but because the "man" of the human sciences itself is a theoretical error: "there is no such thing as a science of man because science's man does not exist, only its subject does" (729, 9–730, 1). From the point of view of the sciences (which, remember, are based on a fundamentally reductionist gesture regarding natural objects), the "man" dealt with and conceived in a variety of disciplines (but Lacan is referring mostly to ethnography and psychology) is a colorful fiction: the subject, too, needs to be reduced somehow.

Lacan discusses what might be an exception – the "case of psychology" (730, 3). Why? Not because it is actually a science, in Lacan's consideration, or because it successfully reduces the subject, but because it has been able to persist, and thrive as a sort of science of the human by becoming a service-branch of the technocracy. The French philosopher and historian of science Georges Canguilhem (1904–1995) delivered a talk, "*What is Psychology*," in 1956 about the relationship between psychology and science, on the one hand, and psychology and philosophy on the other. Canguilhem argues there that psychology's relationship to both is problematic and not entirely thought out. Lacan seems to be agreeing with Canguilhem's perspective. At the end of his essay he presents psychology with a choice: it could work on its philosophical foundations and become more academic and rigorous, or it could continue to do what it is already doing, which is to develop a body of knowledge (or rather techniques) in the service of the state. Canguilhem (1958/2016: 213) suggests that it is a choice between an ascent to the Pantheon or a descent to the Police Department:

> It is rather vulgarly then, that philosophy poses to psychology the question: tell me what you aim for so that I may find out what you are? But a philosopher can also address himself to the psychologist in the form of offering orientation advice … and say to him: when one leaves the Sorbonne by the street Saint-Jacques, one can ascend or descend; if one ascends, one approaches the Pantheon, the conservatory of great men; but if one descends, one heads directly to the Police Department.

Notice there is no mention of a "toboggan" ride down to the Police Department, which is a flourish Lacan adds (730, 3).

Other sciences "in this class" (the alleged "human" sciences, presumably) fail to be real sciences of man also (730, 4). Lacan asks us to consider the cases of Lévy-Bruhl and Piaget and their central concepts of 'prelogical mentality' and 'egocentric thought,' respectively. The French ethnologist Lucien Lévy-Bruhl (1857–1939), in works like *How Natives Think* (1910), argued that tribal peoples engage in a non-logical, non-analytical, 'magical' way of thinking (Lacan will comment on this later), much like the children and mad of civilized societies do. Lévy-Bruhl and the Swiss psychologist Jean Piaget (1896–1980) are serving here as exemplars not only of the archaic illusion but of the humanist, psychologizing error. Their approaches are working with only "the assumed mentality, presumed thought, and actual discourse of science's subject" (730, 4). "More valuable" sciences are able to be more fecund by ruling out the "archaic illusion" altogether – an illusion which Lacan describes now explicitly as a " 'psychologization of the subject' " (730, 5).

Game theory provides Lacan with an example of a very different approach, one that he will endorse and see present in the work of Lévi-Strauss. The subject supposed, or in question, or posited, in game theory is "strictly reduced" to the formula "for a matrix of signifying combinations" (730, 6). Game theory does not psychologize the players or agents in a game because there is no attempt by this science to get into a particular individual's head and imagine what his or her thought processes might actually be like when working on a strategy, or what a player might believe or understand: game theory simply takes into account the rules and works on what an ideal strategy would be. We could describe it as a manifestation of Kantian morality outside of the moral sphere: it assumes a strict, emotionless application of the law. In chess, an example of the humanist error Lacan is describing would be like making a move you know looks strong but is actually bad, just hoping your opponent doesn't see the right reply to the flaw … whereas one should, ideally, make the best move the position dictates, regardless of what you think the other may or may not see. We can understand this as a difference between the imaginary and the symbolic, although Lacan does not bring those registers up here at all. Also relevant here is Lacan's mockery of the boy the detective Dupin tells us about in Poe's "*The Purloined Letter*," who would beat people at the game of "even or odd" by imitating their facial expressions so that their way of thinking would just come to him, and he could predict what they would do next (14, 3).

Linguistics, and Lacan probably has only structuralist linguistics in mind here, also avoids the psychologizing error, but Lacan describes its situation as "subtler" since it does have to deal with the difference between the "enunciated and the enunciation" (730, 7–731, 1). In other words, the "subject who speaks" is necessarily a factor and a presence for linguistics (731, 1). Yet linguistics can avoid getting bogged down in the empirical and psychological issues working on such a subject might involve by focusing on "something else – namely, the battery of signifiers, whose prevalence over signification effects must be ensured" (731, 1). Language is of course seen by structuralist linguistics as a system of signs responsible for the generation of meanings: Saussure, when trying to specify what linguistics studied, set aside considerations such as history, psychology, physiology, etc. Lacan concludes that a structural turn even allows linguistics to construct "a poetics" that is independent of any consideration of what was in "the mind of the poet" (731, 1).

Lacan mentions several linguists in the next few lines, and suggests that the differences "between … Jakobson, Hjelmslev, and Chomsky" can be derived from differing perspectives on the relationship between logic and grammar (731, 3). Lacan holds that "the formalization of grammar must literally circumvent this logic if it is to be successfully carried out" (731, 5). His reference to "modern logic" and the "third example" is to his forthcoming discussion of science in contrast to magic and religion, a discussion that will focus on the position of the subject in each: here he already indicates his view that in science the subject is sutured (731, 6).

Jacques-Alain Miller gave a talk with this as its title in Lacan's seminar from the previous year, and it was published in the same issue of *Cahiers pour l'analyse* that '*Science and Truth*' was first published. This concept will play a very important role in Lacan's effort to distinguish science from psychoanalysis. Suture is a word used to get at the position of the subject in a structure, and Miller's view is that structures only operate or become effective (actualized) through a misrecognition of what is missing from them.

> Suture names the relation of the subject to its discursive chain; the subject figures therein as an element that lacks, under the guise of a place-holder. Because, although it is missing from it, the subject is not purely and simply absent.
>
> (Miller, 1966/2002: 98)

The misrecognition involves this: the subject as place-holder covers up lack, but ironically indicates the very location of lack at the same time. This is a structure Lacan will bring forth a couple of times, especially at the end of '*Science and Truth*' with his discussion of phobic and fetish objects.

Here Lacan is saying that "Gödel's last theorem" can be used to demonstrate the ultimate failure of any suturing mechanism (731, 6). Lacan probably has Gödel's second incompleteness theorem in mind, which asserts the inconsistency of any formal system: within any system, statements can be generated that are not provable or disprovable by it, that are strictly undecidable as to their truth status. In a similar fashion, science is not able to rid itself of its subject-effect. The subject "remains the correlate of science," and not in a harmonious way (731, 6). The subject is an "antinomic" correlate since science is "defined by the deadlocked endeavor to suture the subject" it generates (731, 6). The errors he has been discussing are no doubt connected to the suturing of the subject. Lacan always describes the humanist subject as full, or deep, or concrete, whereas we could assume the subject of science is characterized by division, lack, etc. The suturing of the subject of science (replacing it, we could say, with one more in line with humanist ideology), is a continued failure (one thinks of Sartre's definition of humanity as a "useless passion," vainly trying to attain the status of a full being-in-itself); hence the "deadlock" Lacan refers to. Also notice how this line of reasoning is creating some separation between psychoanalysis and science, even though the latter is its precondition: if science sutures the subject, yet the subject psychoanalysis works with is the subject of science, presumably psychoanalysis does not do to the subject what science does.

Where does psychoanalysis stand with respect to structuralism, though? Compared to the natural sciences and, apparently, "modern logic," Lacan thinks contemporary structuralism is doing something rather unique by bringing the subject of science (as an object of consideration) explicitly into "every 'human science' it conquers" (731, 7). It does this by finding a way to include this subject into the structures it studies. It would seem that this is something psychoanalysis should do as well; but we will see that Lacan also takes some steps away from structuralism in what follows.

The relationship Lacan sees here between subject and structure is expressed topologically by a Möbius strip, which Lacan also throughout his seminars called an "inner eight" (731, 7). It does not seem to be the case that Möbius strips are commonly called 'inner eights,' and this designation was perhaps peculiar to Lacan. He may be calling it this because when he would draw a Möbius strip on the board for his audience, it would look like a figure eight with the top lobe folded down over the other, as it were. When he presents this figure in his ninth seminar, he does not link it to the Möbius strip, but instead presents it in the context of a discussion of Euler circles, and thinks the figure would be a way to describe the presence of an excluded group inside another group (S9: 11 April 1962). As we see here, Lacan wants to say this figure would show how the subject is "internally excluded from its object" (731, 8).

According to Lacan, Lévi-Strauss is on board with this subject in structure being the subject of science. In *The Savage Mind*, Lacan takes Lévi-Strauss to be demonstrating how the classification systems of "savages," in which knowledge of fauna and flora "surpasses our own," is arrived at through a "mathematics of the signifier" (731, 9). Lévi-Strauss even argues that some of the ways in which plants and animals are classified, that strike us as random or arbitrary, are actually governed by a series of important oppositions, just ones that are different from the Linnean classifications we are used to. In fact, Lévi-Strauss will even describe the rigor and precision of tribal classification systems as Linnean. But the most important accomplishment of structuralism is its radical separation of knowledge from the subject. Lévi-Strauss presents a coherent system of knowledge (mythologies, kinship structures, classifications) on its own terms and makes it, much like the unconscious, a knowledge that works on its own; without a knower, without a thinker. For Lacan this work effectively "extracts the subject from the combinatory in question – the subject who on the graph has no other existence than the denotation *ego*" (732, 2). The graph referred to here is not Lacan's graph of desire I think but a table – several, actually – used by Lévi-Strauss in the earlier *Elementary Structures of Kinship*. The term *Ego* is used to mark the position of one particular person in a vast network of kin, with each kin member labelled according to their relation to "ego" (Lévi-Strauss, 1949/1969: 209, 297). (Incidentally, one also finds precursors of what Lacan called "Schema L" in that book. Lévi-Strauss uses that very same diagram to illustrate exchange systems among four parties or groups (Lévi-Strauss, 1949/1969: 187, 300)). No reference to the Freudian Ego is being made here either; instead Lévi-Strauss is just using the Latin word for "I," which Lacan seems to like as a designator for the subject of science – a subject that is but a location or placeholder in a larger scheme of relationships and positions.

Another book by Lévi-Strauss, *The Raw and the Cooked* (1964), on mythemes (basic units of mythology), shows us that it is the "apparatus" constituted by the "mytheme" alone that has analytic power (732, 3). We are not being presented with any insights at all into the mind or nature of the "myth-maker" (in opposition to what would have been the goal of, say, Lévy-Bruhl and Piaget's approaches, discussed earlier), nor is the goal of Lévi-Strauss's work to ascertain the true meaning of a myth, and how it might have been understood by members of a particular culture (732, 3). Lacan observes that an ethnologist's "informer" could himself have written *The Raw and the Cooked* ... but only if the person had separated himself from his function (culturally) as a myth-maker – giving us a bit more insight into what Lacan has in mind with the subject of science, suggesting that it is closely tied to alienation (732, 3). Lacan is saying here that in order to attain the perspective of the subject of science, it would be necessary to check what makes one human, or a member of a culture, "at the cloakroom ... at the Museum of Man" (732, 3). In other words, to be able to adopt Lévi-Strauss's perspective on structures one's "assent" to the structures that shape one's life (one's participation in them, one's place in them, one's belief in them) must be kept in check (732, 3). Lacan says he is using the word "assent" here in the sense used by Cardinal John Henry Newman (1801–1890), who tried to argue that assent is a type of knowledge distinct from what we do when making inferences. The "grammar of assent" was allegedly at work in claims that were believed unconditionally (like those concerning matters of faith, he argued), whereas the category of inferences are always only probabilistic. Lacan is saying then that even this ground-level set of assumptions, the things we seem to always implicitly believe, must be set aside to attain the perspective appropriate to the subject of science. Lévi-Strauss's structuralism provides Lacan with a model: it dispenses with considerations about the mental states of myth-users and myth-creators or myth-tellers. Hence "the object of mythogeny ... is not linked to any development or stasis of the responsible subject. It is not concerned with this latter subject but rather with the subject of science" (732, 3). And the more the writer or researcher reduces her own "presence to that of the subject of science" the "more correctly is the collecting [of myth versions] carried out" (732, 3).

Should psychoanalysis be a structuralism then? Is this the way for psychoanalysis to qualify as a science? Lacan wants to say that psychoanalysis can do the same sort of thing that Lévi-Strauss is doing: the practice of psychoanalysis requires the same subject of science for its object and also the same subject's perspective on the part of the analyst. That is, a psychoanalyst must also check his beliefs at the door, and withdraw from the "grammar of assent" governing his fundamental cultural beliefs and assumptions, especially when it comes to transferential relationships. Lacan seems to think that Lévi-Strauss might not be so sure about psychoanalysis's ability to do this, since psychoanalysis works not with myths but dreams, and what are dreams without transferential relationships, especially when told in a clinical setting? It would seem difficult, in light of this, for psychoanalysis to avoid the humanistic and psychologizing errors Lacan is keen to avoid. It would also seem like some psychological dimension would persist within psychoanalysis, the very dimension that a structural analysis is supposed to set aside. But of course, we know that one of the main points Lacan is defending in this essay is that psychoanalysis only works with, and on, and in the wake of, the subject of science. Now we can add that it only works when the analyst is also taking on the perspective of this subject. But still, it is not clear if this means that psychoanalysis is a science, or a structuralism.

This is what Lacan is thinking about in the next paragraph. The subject of science is described by Lacan as a "nonsaturated but calculable" one (nonsaturated: it is without depth …), and he wonders if this subject could in fact come to dominate the conjectural (human) sciences, such that these sciences would once and for all rid themselves of their humanistic, archaic illusions (732, 6). Could this subject take pride of place in the human sciences, on the assumption that they take a structuralist turn? Lacan's answer may be a bit surprising. He writes that this is "all the less indicated" because this subject is "part of the conjuncture constituting science as a whole" (732, 7). It would be hard for this subject to be what these sciences deal with because, as Lacan has already claimed, while this subject is a by-product of the sciences, its suturing is essential to their efficacy (although it does not seem to me that we are given clear reasons as to why this must be the case, at least not in this essay). This suggests to Lacan that another perspective is needed in order to deal with this subject properly, and this is precisely what he seems to be saying psychoanalysis provides us with – beyond the sciences, and beyond structuralism.

Distinguishing between the "exact sciences and conjectural sciences" (and maybe trying to argue that the latter might be able to deal with the subject of science?) would not help matters, since Lacan finds the distinction to be "no longer sustainable" (733, 1). The fields and objects studied by the conjectural sciences (traditionally) are now "subject to exact calculation (using probability)" (733, 1). But we shouldn't be too quickly or easily satisfied with the formalism that is practiced in these sciences either. The "trappings" of formalism themselves need to be explained (733, 2). The point being, maybe, that these trappings do not surge up all at once – they are not obvious, and are the products of "crises" on science's path to more and more efficacy (733, 2).

Striking a different note, in a line I quoted earlier, Lacan observes that "something in the status of science's object … seems to me to have remained unelucidated since the birth of science" (733, 3). Lacan is perhaps reminding us here of the shift from the qualitative object of lived experience to the mathematized, merely measurable object of the sciences. He will shift now to discuss the object of psychoanalysis, a topic that returns him to a question he says he asked when he first mounted "this rostrum" – is psychoanalysis inside or outside science (733, 4)? Lacan is referring here to his seminar's presence at the École Normale Supérieure since 1963. In his eleventh seminar, in the first session, the topics of psychoanalysis, science, and religion are indeed broached, and Lacan makes some comments about the nature of science's object there: most notably, that it changes, and has changed beyond the shift from quality to quantity. For example: "We cannot say that the object of modern physics is the same now as it is at its birth, which I would date in the seventeenth century" (S11: 8). That the objects of the sciences change at all may be what he thinks has not been elucidated.

Lacan reveals next, no doubt not to anyone in his audience's surprise, that the object of psychoanalysis is what he calls object *a*. If this is what the object of psychoanalysis is, does this mean that psychoanalysis is the science of object *a*? Is psychoanalysis, if it is a science, the development of a knowledge about this object? Lacan's answers to these questions are negative, and he suggests that they may be the wrong questions to ask: equating "knowledge of object *a*" with "the science of psychoanalysis" is something that "must be avoided" (733, 5–6).

What follows next is perhaps the reason why, and we start to see how psychoanalysis is different from the sciences. When Lacan writes that "object *a* must be inserted ... into the division of the subject" I take him to be saying that we need to see object *a* as the cause of this division – a topic he'll be elaborating on in the next few pages (733, 6). Yet there is an ambiguity in the phrase, and as the next paragraphs suggest perhaps this insertion into the subject's division is something that psychoanalysis brings about practically as well. Generally speaking in the next paragraphs Lacan seems to be turning our attention toward what psychoanalysis does, as a praxis, and away from its epistemological status as a possible science: the thesis may be that psychoanalysis is less a (scientific) knowledge of object *a* than a know-how or handling of it: (re)placing it as the cause of the subject's division.

In the next paragraph he describes analytic work as a "taming" of object *a*, an object that itself is "not peaceful," it "does not leave you in peace" – especially not psychoanalysts (733, 9). Lacan says that Freud's famous "call" – '*Wo Es war, soll Ich werden*,' which he renders as 'where it was, there must I come to be as subject' – should remind us of the subject's division between truth and knowledge, or should be thought of in these terms (733, 9–734, 1). We can associate the Es/it here with object *a*, and so the call could be re-retranslated as "where object *a* was there must the subject come to be". Yet put this way, it sounds like psychoanalysis is a reconciliation, a bringing together of what was opposed (I must come to be where It was). Lacan thinks the phrase should instead be taken as a paradox. How can this "obscure being" – the It, or object *a*, "who was forever awaiting me" (there where it was) – "come to be totalized" (that is, how can it be fused together with the subject, possibly ending the division between knowledge and truth) "by a line that can only be drawn by dividing this being still more clearly from what I can know of it" (734, 2). In other words, rather than bridging the division between knowledge and truth, Lacan seems to be saying here that psychoanalysis highlights it, and perhaps exacerbates it.

To get at this another way, Lacan refers to Freud's notion of a "double inscription" in the psyche, his own understanding of it, and a dispute that emerged during a conference at Bonneval in 1960 that was dedicated to the topic of the unconscious (734, 3). Two of Lacan's students at the time, Jean Laplanche (1924–2012) and Serge Leclaire (1924–1994), presented papers from a Lacanian orientation (Lacan was at the conference but did not give a talk: the essay '*Position on the Unconscious*' is a résumé of his remarks during it), yet they held differing views about the status of language in the unconscious. Leclaire gave his famous '*Licorne*' case there, in which he demonstrates how a meaningless cluster of signifiers, linked to his analysand's proper name, were overdetermining many of his symptoms – very much showing the strengths of Lacan's key insight that the unconscious is structured like a language (see Roudinesco, 1986/1990: 310–312 for a discussion of this). Laplanche, as Roudinesco (1986/1990: 312) describes it in her section on this conference in *Jacques Lacan and Co.*, "took his distance" from Lacan's ideas on language and the unconscious, and in a sense was challenging the rigor of Lacan's return to Freud by returning to Freud himself and showing that Freud's views on language and the unconscious were quite different from Lacan's. According to Freud, Laplanche argued, language was "secondary in relation to the unconscious" (Roudinesco, 1986/1990: 313). This is because of the distinction Freud made between thing-presentations and word-presentations, the former being visual, the latter, obviously, linguistic. Furthermore, the unconscious consisted of Thing-representations in Freud's first topography, whereas word-representations were in the conscious/preconscious system. Despite taking issue with how strictly Freudian Lacan's view of the unconscious was, Laplanche developed a Lacanian take on metaphor in his paper, defending the idea that metaphor does illustrate the structure of repression.

What does this have to do with the notion of double inscription? In Freud, this idea was about representations that were both "in the unconscious, on the one hand, and in the preconscious-conscious system on the other" (Laplanche and Pontalis, 1967/1974). And the controversy is about how to understand what this means for the relationship between the two (Laplanche and Pontalis, 1967/1974):

> There is thus a *double inscription* of representations: in the unconscious, on the one hand, and in the preconscious-conscious system on the other. But Freud then notes that there are two coexistent hypotheses concerning the transposition from the unconscious system to the preconscious-conscious. From a topographical point of view, one would have to admit the existence of a second inscription or registration of the representation alongside which the unconscious

> inscription would persist. On the contrary, from a functional point of view, the transposition would consist in a change of state affecting the same material; in such a manner would there be a 'passage' between the unconscious and the conscious. The topographical hypothesis tends to keep the two instances radically separate, whereas the functional hypothesis tends to join them.

The perspective Lacan is defending in '*Science and Truth*' is clearly one that emphasizes the topographical perspective, and the separation between the unconscious and consciousness: although this separation should not be misunderstood, for as we know Lacan likes to configure it in terms of a Möbius strip. After mentioning his students, Lacan says he rejects a Gestaltist solution to the issue, which would presumably want to look at the psyche as a unified whole. Hence the reference, as Fink explains in his note, to the profile of Napoleon formed in the negative space between two trees on a plate. A solution like this would suggest that all one has to do is sort of shift perspectives to see the conscious or the unconscious (846, n864–4). The unconscious would not be "*ein anderer Schauplatz*," "an Other scene," as Lacan always liked to say it was (458, 5).

In order to account for how "inscriptions" in the two systems could still "commingle" Lacan again refers us to "topology, there being at hand's reach a surface in which front and back are situated so as to join up at all points" – the infamous Möbius strip (734, 4). He adds that such a topological figure is not just an "intuitive schema" or a way of thinking about things: psychoanalysis is practiced in a space like this (734, 5).

He uses his revision of Descartes from the previous year as another way of expressing the topological relationship he has just been discussing. What Lacan is doing with the Cartesian formula, by writing it as "*I am thinking: 'therefore I am'*" is supposed to show that "thought only grounds being by knotting itself in speech" – suggesting that the *cogito*'s connection to being is in fact more tenuous than Descartes wanted it to be, ensured only as it is through a linguistic act (734, 7). This idea of a knotted-up speech is an important one: Lacan refigures the expression of the Cartesian *cogito* into a speech act that is doubling back onto itself, like the Möbius strip or 'inner eight'. Against the manifest Cartesian conclusion, which posits, from the self-evidence of thinking, the equal self-evidence of being (with no loss in degree of certainty), the conclusion '*therefore I am*' is rendered by Lacan an embedded proposition articulated by a thinker. As Milner (2000: 38) wrote, with respect to Descartes's *cogito ergo sum*, what Lacan is trying to do is "suspend" the "passage from the first moment" (I think) "to the second" (I am). And to do so Lacan "confines the *cogito* to its strict enunciation; moreover, he buckles the enunciation back upon itself, making the conclusion ('therefore, I am') the pure *pronuntiatum* of the premise ('I think')" (Milner, 2000: 38).

Lacan observes that Heidegger presented the Cartesian formula several times in an abbreviated fashion, as *cogito sum*, leaving out the "ergo" (so it would read *I think, I am*) (the references in Fink's note are to the German page numbers of *Being and Time*, not the paragraph numbers (846, n865)). It nicely asserts the rapid equation of thinking and being that was important to Descartes; Heidegger, however, felt that the concept of being needed to be clarified before such a move could be made. Lacan refers to Heidegger's treatment of Descartes's phrase as an "algebrizing" and says that he wishes to highlight the remainder – the *ergo* that Heidegger leaves out – while linking it back to the *cogito* (734, 8). This would give us a "*cogito ergo*," an "I think therefore ...," in which "it is evident ... that nothing gets spoken without leaning on the cause" (734, 8). Or, to put it a bit differently, 'without being based on the cause' or 'without resting on the cause'. In this rendering, one can again see the emphasis on a thinking, a linguistic act, that is articulating a conclusion: ultimately about being, although the statement about being is entirely missing from this particular formulation (it is only *cogito ergo* ... no *sum*). We could say that Lacan is treating the 'therefore' here as something that establishes a causal link between two thoughts: the 'therefore' refers us back to the 'I think' and leads us forward to what can be drawn from the declaration that one is thinking. Without the 'therefore,' the cause of the subject's being remains obscure. One would get simply '*I think, I am*': which, without the '*ergo*' connector might read as two distinct claims without any logical connection.

It seems to me that Lacan has gone into this detail regarding Descartes in order to reconsider what Freud was doing with his '*Wo Es war, soll Ich werden*'. Returning to this, Lacan claims that Freud's "*soll Ich*" covers up the "cause" that Lacan himself wants to emphasize in the *cogito ergo* (734, 9). There is of course no 'therefore' in Freud's phrase, in other words. Notice that if one were to replace '*soll Ich*' with 'therefore,' one would get a phrase very close to Descartes's: '*Wo es war, therefore...werden*'. A grammatical and polyglot mess, perhaps, but it could be read as "*Where it was, therefore ... (I) am.*"

If we were to invert the '*soll Ich*' into '*Ich soll*' Freud's phrase would read "I must come to be where It was" and for Lacan this would be a "paradox of an imperative" since it "presses me to assume my own causality" – what caused me to come into being as a split subject, object *a*, would be where I would need to situate myself, as a subject; so it would sound like I am being called upon to become the cause of myself (734, 9). This leads Lacan to a series of associations, over the course of a page, ranging from Augustine, to Spinoza, back to Descartes, then to the mystic Angelus Silesius, and finally, to Schreber, culminating in Lacan's own effort to incarnate the truth as cause in his two presentations of his essay '*The Freudian Thing*' ten years earlier.

Before getting to this: given how important the idea of cause is going to be for what follows, why does the topic come up in the first place? This part of the essay started with an assertion regarding the object of psychoanalysis – it is object *a*, which is presented as the cause of the divided subject psychoanalysis treats. Science sutures this subject, yet this subject is the irrevocable other or after-effect of science's historical emergence. Lacan seems to be considering Freud's *Wo Es war* in two ways: on the one hand, it is about this subject's relationship to this object, and on the other it is a statement about the goal of psychoanalysis – to put the subject in the place of the object. Lacan seems to be saying instead that what occurs in psychoanalysis is that the object is put back in the place of the subject's division, and so he wants to highlight the importance of the cause, or the bringing forth of the cause, of the subject's divided state, which goes hand in hand with a further division, or maybe reduction, of the subject itself. Going back to his allusion to the talks his students Laplanche and Leclaire gave, and the controversy about the nature of double inscription, we can get a sense of what Lacan thought was at stake there. The error Lacan is concerned with, in Laplanche's treatment of language and the unconscious especially, is that it might be bringing thinking and being back together: this is precisely the sort of suturing of the subject's division that Lacan is accusing the sciences of engaging in.

So we can maybe appreciate now why Lacan wants to discuss various ways in which philosophy and religion have posited a self-causing being. For Lacan's view, the subject's division is going to be paramount. It is the inability to bring being and thinking, truth and knowledge, together, that is important, and is what will be essential about the subject of science. "I am not the cause of myself," he writes, and this is true, but not because "I am the creature" of myself – and we could take this to mean, a thing created by myself (734, 10). This echoes theological debates about the nature of God, especially in Augustine, who argues that it is an error to think of God as a creature able to generate itself. According to Augustine (*On the Trinity*, book 1: 1) "there is absolutely no thing whatever that brings itself into existence". Perhaps this is because if God were self-caused, this would leave open the possibility that God is not eternal: there may have been a void prior to God's self-creation, or, a time before God's existence ... which Augustine would reject.

This takes Lacan to Spinoza, who had notorious things to say about God and causality (and eternity). Lacan decides to call Spinoza's God "some-Thing else" – presumably with respect to created beings, and it is "some-Thing other" than "the Whole" as well (734, 11–735, 1). Lacan takes this to mean that Spinoza's philosophy is not pantheism. This is a rather unorthodox reading of Spinoza: at the end of his eleventh seminar Lacan claimed that this is the wrong interpretation because "what ... has been thought of in Spinoza as pantheism is simply the reduction of the field of God to the universality of the signifier" (S11: 275).

Continuing with the topic of the relationship of the *cogito* to God, Lacan goes back to Descartes and observes that the ego for Descartes, the first person Latin pronoun, is eliminated. In Latin it is not necessary to say '*ego cogito*' for example, just as the first person pronoun may be left out in Italian and Spanish. But the point Lacan seems to want to make in this paragraph is that the being of the Cartesian ego is "dependent on the god of religion" (735, 2). In a nice construction, he notes that the ego is a "curious scrap of ergo" and that Descartes is keen to protect it from "the deceitful God" (735, 2).

The Cartesian God is notoriously a voluntarist one: if God willed it, Descartes thought that mathematical truths such as 2 + 2 = 4 could be other than they currently are. This is why Lacan says that the ego's "partner" – God – is endowed "with the exorbitant privilege of guaranteeing the eternal truths only insofar as he is their creator" (735, 2). The same would hold true of the *cogito*'s very being, and so Lacan's take is that God is treated by Descartes as the cause of the *cogito*. That is, the being of the *cogito* is sustained by continuous acts of God's will (in what would come to be known as occasionalism).

Lacan then proceeds to compare Descartes's position on the relationship of the ego to God with that of the mystic Angelus Silesius (1624–1677), whose writings were overtly about attaining a mystical union with the divine. Silesius went much farther than Descartes did in this direction, but is perhaps, in Lacan's eyes, simply following through with what is already there in Descartes's work (again, following Descartes "according to the order of reasons"). As Fink observes in his note to the next paragraph, the discussion of Silesius occurs in Lacan's first seminar, not his third (in which Schreber is discussed) (846, n865). Schreber is relevant here since a significant part of his delusion was his becoming-woman in mystical union with God, with whom the world would be repopulated.

Lacan returns to what his perspective on all this is, which involves repeating that "the two sides do not fit together" – referring to the subject's division between truth and knowledge (or, in light of his recent points, between being and knowledge), and the cause of this (735, 6). And to do this he tells us that he is going to just "recall ... to mind" something he did already twice before – deliver, or perform, his essay '*The Freudian Thing*' in public (735, 7). Hence Lacan's reference to "repeating it twice": the second time he delivered it was a repetition, and if he actually were to deliver it again on this occasion this would make the performance into a *bis repetita*, a Latin phrase that is usually completed by either *placent* or *non placent*, meaning either that what is repeated twice is pleasing, or not (735, 7).

The talk was first delivered in November 1955 in Vienna, and Lacan also read the text out to his seminar on 21 December of the same year (seminar three, on the psychoses). Lacan discusses the context of the Vienna talk, his displeasure with the organizer (Hoff) and the audience there, and how what was important to him was to be present to render an "homage for the centennial of Freud's birth" in Vienna itself. The theme of the conference was "The meaning of a return to Freud in psychoanalysis" (S3, 71).

The audience in Vienna was unfamiliar with Lacan's claim that "the unconscious is language" (736, 1) (Lacan is usually careful to specify that his view is that it is 'structured like a language' and he will chastise people later on for misunderstanding him on this. Just a few paragraphs later, in this very essay in fact, he will present this idea in its more typical form). It occurred to him that if the unconscious is language, maybe he could, in his essay, present the truth (the unconscious being considered the truth of the subject) as speaking. So, in his paper, why not make truth into an "allegorical figure" who would give a speech (736, 1)? He says he was "playfully echoing" something Saint-Just (1767–1794) said in a speech during the French Revolution (736, 1). Saint-Just said:

> I detest the dust I am made of and which speaks to you. Let them persecute and kill that dust. But I defy them to wrest from me the independent life I gave myself before the centuries and the heavens.
> (Jaurès 1901: no page)

It is as if Saint-Just is letting the dust that he is speak for itself (as if dust is his cause!).

Such was the rationale, Lacan is saying here, behind his writing of the passage in '*The Freudian Thing*' that contains the phrase "I, truth, speak," which was a "prosopopoeia," a rhetorical figure in which an abstract thing is personified (736, 2). He adds that if there were an incarnation of truth, speaking, it would be the kind of thing that "would go right to the being of language" – and that we should be horrified by it (736, 2).

Lacan seems to understand why his Viennese audience would have reacted the way they did: they were not familiar with his thesis about the unconscious and language. But why did Lacan's second audience, at his seminar, also give it a "cool reception" (736, 4)? Lacan refers to the "oblative" value they acknowledged the text had, but that they were still deaf to its message (736, 4). If they weren't horrified by the presence of the truth speaking (being psychoanalysts they should not have been) it must have been something else that bothered at least one interlocuter (whom Fink identifies as the psychoanalyst Jean-Bertrand Pontalis (1924–2013)) – the reification of the unconscious and the analysand: consider Lacan's reference to "Jaspersian understanding and vacuous personalism" (736, 5). In all the dominant philosophical schools at the time, treating humans as things was regarded as the gravest of errors. And yet isn't this exactly what Lacan is doing? He turns truth into a thing that speaks. To tie this discussion back to what Lacan was saying about the human sciences, and the very concept of "man" used in them, this objection to Lacan could be taken as a humanist objection: Lacan is degrading the humanity of the analysand, and of what psychoanalysis does. Yet Lacan's view is that these concerns are vain, and get in the way of an appropriate understanding of psychoanalytic practice: "one does not see oneself as one is, and even less so when one approaches oneself wearing philosophical masks" (736, 6) – philosophical masks such as humanism, hiding the reality of what one is doing, and what one is working with.

But we finally get to the point Lacan really wanted to make here, the reason why he wanted to "recall to mind" what he was doing in the essay '*The Freudian Thing*'. It's the critique, uttered by Pontalis, that goes along these lines: Fine, psychoanalysis is about a speaking truth, and the view that the unconscious is structured like a language is thus very important … but still "why doesn't he say the truth about truth" (736, 7)?

That such a question emerged was evidence to Lacan that his rhetorical strategy was a failure. When Lacan "lent his voice" to the truth to say "I, truth, speak" the move should have been understood to be "beyond allegory" (736, 9). Does this mean it was literal? Not necessarily: it is beyond allegory because "there is no such thing as a metalanguage," and this is part of the point Lacan was making (737, 1). If there is no metalanguage, Lacan's statement cannot be allegorical: an allegory is, let's say, a use of language that involves a hidden meaning, such that an allegory is saying one thing but meaning something else, much like irony. We could think of an allegory as a coded speech, whose actual meaning would be deciphered, precisely, by a 'metalanguage,' a text or discourse that would deliver the true meaning of the allegorical text. So, generally speaking, a metalanguage is a discourse that is detached from a certain text, but in a privileged position to give a commentary on what that text might really be saying. In this way, a metalanguage could be taken to be saying 'the truth about truth' – whatever the truth is that is contained in an allegory is rendered more clear, and repeated, in the metalinguistic commentary. Lacan aligns such a project with logical positivism: in which an ordinary language proposition ('The tree is brown') would be rendered into a logical form ($\exists x \phi y$), reducing it to its logical meaning (737, 1). This is a similar sort of metalinguistic move.

Lacan is taking Pontalis's objection as the expression of a desire for a psychoanalytic metalanguage: such a theory should tell the truth about truth! But Lacan's view is that if the truth speaks (and recall, the idea here is that it does so in manifestations of the unconscious), it is impossible to say the truth about truth. From this perspective, the unconscious alone "tells the truth about truth" – it does not stop speaking, it does not stop producing (737, 2) (notice he does write here that the unconscious is "structured like a language" (737, 2)). There is no discourse, no speech, immune to the unconscious truth that may be speaking through it.

The absence of a metalanguage – the "lack of truth about truth" – is "the rightful place of *Urverdrängung*, that is, of primal repression" (737, 3). What makes metalanguages so appealing is precisely that they promise to overcome this lack (more like an inability) by replacing it with the truth about truth (in another language). Freud described primal repression as an act or event that forms the first cluster of unconscious representations, a repression that seems to be the very foundation of the unconscious. The rest of what is repressed in the unconscious might be taken as a sort of false knowledge, making up for the fundamentally repressed kernel. We can see here something like a suture again. Lacan's view, of course, is that psychoanalysis, not deploying a metalanguage, uses "other means to get to the bottom" of the repressed (737, 4).

We get a rather personal attack on Pontalis in what follows. Lacan says he is dubious that Pontalis was so naïve as to think it would be possible or easy to say the truth about truth. His "workaday role" in "a truth agency's offices" is probably referring to his membership in the Association Psychanalytique de France, which had ties to the IPA (737, 4). As an analysand and former student of his, Lacan felt quite betrayed by Pontalis not joining him in his own foundation of the École de la Cause Freudienne, and felt that Pontalis and others had conspired against him.

Lacan announces that he will be moving on to the topic of how "the subject of science" is the only thing we have left "to join knowledge and truth together" (737, 7). So he is "leaving my Thing to sort things out by itself with noumena" (737, 8). Noumena is, of course, in Kantian philosophy a word used for things-in-themselves, for what (depending on how Kant is read) perhaps causes the appearances of objects that we do experience. Noumena are inaccessible to experience but, Kant argued, things that we can be certain must exist (otherwise appearances would be appearances *of nothing* ...). Lacan's point then is that it is not difficult to see how his Truth-as-speaking-thing is different from the Kantian noumenon: the noumenon keeps "its mouth shut" while the Lacanian truth, of course, is far from silent (737, 8). (Also, we could add, the topology is different: in Kant the noumena seems like a radically inaccessible "other side" to phenomena, whereas Lacan would no doubt situate his Thing in a Möbius-like relationship to what it causes, the divided subject....)

Lacan wants to get back to the topic of cause, which, as he wants to consider it here is "not the cause as logical category, but as causing the whole effect" (738, 1). His discussion of the Cartesian '*ergo*' earlier might be an example of how cause functions as a logical category – how a thought, or claim, or belief, may entail and imply others, necessarily. Departing from this approach to cause, Lacan will use Aristotle's causes, which can be taken as reasons for why a thing is what it is, and the way that it is. This is an interesting move: Lacan is going back to Aristotle in an essay that is embracing the importance of the rise of the sciences for psychoanalysis! But at the same time, the move is understandable: if science gives rise to a mode of subjectivity that it at the same time sutures, in order to be effective, psychoanalysis, which deals with this subject, may have to take a different approach to the topic of cause. *Faute de mieux*, Lacan returns to Aristotle. And he exhorts psychoanalysts not to "refuse to take on the question of truth as cause when your very careers are built upon it" (738, 1), The truth, as cause, in the clinic "is supposed to act" (738, 1). And Lacan then gives us part of his rationale for returning to Aristotle: the notion of the truth as a cause that acts, and that especially speaks, "is veiled in science" (738, 2). So, psychoanalysis entails some departure from science.

Lacan then refers to Lenin's famous line that "'Marx's theory is omnipotent because it is true'" (from his 1913 '*The Three Sources and Three Component Parts of Marxism*') (738, 3). It is an interesting and relevant idea here, not because of what it is saying about Marx, but because of what it is saying about the connection between truth and causality, or better, efficacy. Marxism promotes a dialectical reading of history, of course, but if it took the truth it was articulating to be "mute" (as Lacan says science does) Lacan wonders how the efficacy of the theory could be asserted (738, 3). Or: if "the truth of materialism" were mute, then how could it be that just "theorizing" dialectical and historical materialism would be enough to "increase" the real world effectiveness of these theories (738, 3)? Lacan says that he would not be satisfied with an explanation that resorted to the capacities of a proletarian class consciousness, perhaps awakened by a group of informed Marxist militants.

Lacan finds in Marxism the same kind of distinction he is working with between truth and knowledge: a view in which truth is positively connected to causality. And the truth is not mute (but does it speak?). And what about the other side of the subject's division, knowledge? Truth as cause is distinguished from the "knowledge put into operation" in its wake – which Lacan characterizes here as a know-how, a practice (738, 4). For example, Lacan observes that an economic science based on Capital could be developed (a truth, say) that would be entirely disconnected from revolutionary politics (one variety of a knowledge-in-practice). Revolutions, as history shows us, "require help from something other" than a theory, however dialectical, and however true, it may be (738, 5). And so Marxism, like psychoanalysis, highlights the division between truth and knowledge (it would seem that Lacan is actually questioning Lenin's idea here: is the theory omnipotent just because it is true?).

Science is able to continue to develop its knowledge while forgetting "the circuitous path by which it came into being" (738, 5). Lacan takes this to mean that science can forget the dimension of truth as cause, and that this forgetting is positive for it, enabling, and connected to its efficacy. Yet this is exactly the dimension of truth "that psychoanalysis seriously puts to work": the efficacy of psychoanalysis relies on engaging with the truth as cause, and obviously, must involve something other than a forgetting of it (738, 5). We are getting a rather clear contrast here between science and psychoanalysis.

Lacan says that his point about the sciences is not some kind of critique according to which new theories in the sciences actually "maintain what they generalize" from a prior theory or "structure" – Lacan mentions theoretical physics and mathematics here specifically (738, 6). His points are not meant to be interventions into the history of science at all. What he is more interested in, regarding the sciences, is what he calls the "subjective toll" that crises in them have exerted on the individuals who work in their domains (738, 6). Lacan cites the cases of Mayer and Cantor as "tragedies, leading at times to the point of madness" (738, 6). Julius Von Mayer (1814–1878) was important in the field of thermodynamics, and his insights went unrecognized for much of his life; Georg Cantor (1845–1918) was a giant in mathematics and set theory, perhaps best known for his work on transfinite numbers. Both of them actually spent time in mental institutions.

Lacan thinks that at this point his "program" might be sufficiently clear, even if "it is not about to be realized" – the task of working on the links between the truth as cause, knowledge, and the subject of science (739, 1). He tells us he is "broaching" this topic "prudently," and that he is going to consider in what follows "other fields than psychoanalysis that lay claim to truth" (739, 2–3).

First up are disciplines that are "distinct from science" and generally considered inferior to it as far as their truth value goes (739, 4). Science and psychoanalysis, we already know, are on the agenda, and Lacan will consider them after considering "magic and religion" first (739, 4). Given the importance of Lévi-Strauss's work for Lacan throughout this entire essay, it is worth pointing out that part three of his *Structural Anthropology* is in fact entitled '*Magic and Religion*,' and starts with the essay '*The Sorcerer and his Magic*' (Lévi-Strauss, 1958/1963: 84–97). Magic in this context is referring to shamanism mainly, but something like alchemy would fall under its heading as well. Lacan observes that for the "subject of science" such disciplines are "will-o'-the-wisps," although "to the suffering subject with whom we deal" in psychoanalysis they are not; they still have an attraction, and even an efficacy (739, 4).

Having just mentioned suffering, Lacan imagines some hostile and critical reactions. Isn't Lacan's overly intellectual approach to things the least effective way to think about suffering? Do his "intellectualizations" give him any real "right" to address such a topic (739, 5)? Can this reduced, divided subject of science be said to suffer? Referring to the phenomenologist Michel Henry (1922–2002), who wrote in *The Essence of Manifestation* (1963) that "the truth of pain is pain itself," Lacan wants to say, in something he promises to work out later, that he could show how phenomenology offers a "counter-truth" (739, 6). The point Henry was making is worth going into, since it expresses a position on the relationship between truth and knowledge, and the body and language, that Lacan is criticizing. Henry is arguing against the philosopher Jules Lachelier's view (1832–1918) that the "knowledge of a pain is not painful, but true" (Henry 1963/1973: 676). Lachelier is defending a pretty straightforward distinction between intellect and affect, which Lacan is imagining himself being accused of upholding here. Henry (1963/1973: 678) wishes to say instead that "the truth of a pain is the pain itself … *the truth of pain is its affectivity*" – that is, as Heidegger had already argued, phenomenology advocates a notion of truth that is not propositional, or intellectual, but in and of things, perceptions, and experiences themselves. It promotes a truth that is an embedded, experiential, existential truth, we could say. This may seem like one way to get around the distinction between intellect and affect … but perhaps it assumes the distinction and simply locates truth on the other side of it – on the side of the experienced, the felt, or the perceived, rather than the known. Lacan does refer again to Henry's *The Essence of Manifestation* in his seminar on December 4th 1968 (S16: 69). There he names the book, but explicitly refuses to name its author. He seems to be taking Henry's point to be a banality – like saying that 'a toothache is a toothache' – and Lacan's rebuttal consists of saying: well, Henry, if you'd read Freud, you'd know better than that! Lacan of course would be more interested in seeing signifiers, so often (wrongly) associated with the intellect, at work in something like a pain. Thus Lacan's point seems to be that phenomenology actually keeps the intellect/affect divide intact, topologically speaking, whereas Lacan is interested in getting rid of it. In other words: from Lacan's perspective, the truth of pain is *not* pain itself … unless one adds that this pain is bound up with signifiers, or is not without them.

As we know, Lacan is working with the idea here of truth as a cause, moreover a linguistic, speaking cause, and when he gets to psychoanalysis and its relation to cause, we'll see that it involves material causes, which he will describe explicitly in terms of signifiers. Lacan asks the psychoanalysts in his audience whether the "truth of neurotic suffering lies in having the truth as cause" – and the implied answer is, of course, yes (739, 7).

Getting to the topics of magic and religion, he tells us that his approach to magic is going to be structuralist; it is going to be an interpretation of magical practices such that what is going on in them is that "signifiers answer as such to signifiers. Signifiers in nature are called up by incantatory signifiers. They are metaphorically mobilized" (739, 9). And so in magical practices "the Thing, insofar as it speaks, answers our insistent prayers" (739, 9). The idea that in magic the Thing is taken to be speaking is perhaps one of the reasons why Lacan wanted to tackle magic from this perspective first. For, unlike in religion and science, in psychoanalysis and magic the truth as cause speaks. The proximity of psychoanalysis to shamanism was one of the main points of Lévi-Strauss's essay on '*The Sorcerer and his Magic*' (1949) and his perspective in that essay was probably why Lacan is dealing with it here:

> the distressing trend which, for several years, has tended to transform the psychoanalytic system from a body of scientific hypotheses that are experimentally verifiable in certain specific and limited cases into a kind of diffuse mythology interpenetrating the consciousness of the group, could rapidly bring about a parallelism [between the analyst and the shaman – EP].
>
> (1958/1963: 183).

But a purely structuralist approach to magic – engaging in the type of "reduction" Lacan discussed earlier – "neglects the subject" of magic (739, 11). In magical practices Lacan points out that the "readying of the subject – the shamanizing subject – is essential" (739, 12). Perhaps Lacan's thoughts have turned to alchemy here. In the first session of *Seminar XI* he observed that what disqualified alchemy from being a science was "that the purity of the soul of the operator was, as such, and in a specific way, an essential element in the matter" (S11: 9). The subject of magic must be in a certain state for the efficacy of magic to happen. Lacan says the subject of science is "debarred" from doing this: the hewing, or placing in check, of his "corporeal medium", that seems to be what enables the subject of magic to approach the natural world, and himself, in terms of signifiers in the first place, is ruled out (739, 12–740, 1). In *Seminar XI* this consideration led him to contrast psychoanalysis and science, since for the former the role of the analyst's desire is rather important.

Lacan's remarks on magic are suggestive, and as I pointed out earlier he does not follow through with his discussion of magic elsewhere. He engages in a bit of speculation and offers some promissory notes in what follows. He wonders about the status of demand in magic, as well as desire, and wonders if his graph of desire would shed any light on the matter, or not. Such a consideration would, though, allow and qualify psychoanalysis to say something about magic and what is going on in it. Psychoanalysts have said "magic is always sexual" but Lacan thinks this observation, even if correct, lacks any real grounding (740, 6).

He concludes his discussion of magic with two points involving truth and knowledge: that magic "involves" the truth as "efficient cause", and that the knowledge involved in magic is not only obscure to the subject of science, but is essentially dissimulated, even to its practitioners (740, 7–8). Lévi-Strauss's essay deals with this issue quite a bit. He discusses the case of Quesalid, a member of the Kwakiutl people (in the Pacific Northwest) whose autobiography was discussed by Boaz (Lévi-Strauss, 1958/1963: 175). Quesalid was quite suspicious about shamanism, but became an apprentice and acquired a technique that was more effective than those of other shamans in other neighboring groups. He struggled with how to account for this, knowing that his technique consisted of a ruse – the extraction of a "bloody worm" that he would produce from his mouth and present to the patient and the community as the cause of the illness (Lévi-Strauss, 1958/19766: 175–6). Lacan is saying that the obscurity involved here, an obscurity about the very efficacy of magic, to all involved, is one of magic's "conditions": the knowledge in magic dissimulates itself "as such" (740, 8). As to why Aristotle's "efficient cause" is the "guise" under which truth works in magic, things are less clear (740, 7). Lacan says this without explaining it any further. In Aristotle, an efficient cause of a bronze statue would have been the artist. Should we take this to mean that the shaman is the efficient cause in magical practices? Dany Nobus (2002: 107) suggests the following: "The function of truth as an efficient cause in magic indicates that the truth of a magical phenomenon, whether a shamanistic healing practice or the cursing of natural forces, is always attributed to power, energy, or (super)natural abilities". In magic, agency is attributed to a sorcerer, a shaman, or natural forces, but the "how" of the efficacy remains a mystery to all.

Lacan then says that his discussion of religion will be informed by a similarly structuralist approach, and he clearly has much more to say about this topic. He wonders whether it is "possible to hope" that something about the status of religion might be clarified by science (740, 10). Lacan refers to some nameless "strange philosophers" who think that since science and religion are discourses about one and the "same world" religion should actually be considered the "more encompassing" discourse – presumably because it covers more ground than the natural sciences do, which limit themselves to the natural world and leave the supernatural out (740, 10).

Some might want Lacan to be neutral as an analyst and not chime in on debates about the relationship between religion and science, but Lacan observes that "befriending everyone" may make it difficult to keep "intact the position from which one must operate" (740, 11). We've seen that one of Lacan's main concerns in this entire essay has been to assert the importance of getting as clear as possible about the nature of psychoanalysis and what it works on (object *a*, and the subject of science). The reference to analytic neutrality is to Freud's idea that psychoanalysts must refrain from trying to impose their own beliefs and values, and especially their world-views, on their analysands. A critique of religion could be taken to be a violation of that.

Setting concerns about analytic neutrality aside, from the point of view of the subject of science, religion will appear to have traits similar to "obsessive neurosis" (740, 12). This is what Freud (1907) in fact claimed in '*Obsessive Actions and Religious Practices*.' Lacan describes Freud's take on religious belief and behavior as a "flash" that is more valuable than what "traditional criticism" was ever able to say about religion (740, 12). This perspective can see in religion a "negation of truth as cause," according to which a "revelation" negates "what grounds the subject" (for Lacan, the speaking truth) (741, 1). Unless such a perspective is adopted, Lacan does not think that a rigorous study of religion can take place. Moreover, the subject of religion "leaves responsibility for the cause to God" and "thereby bars his own access to truth" (741, 2). This could be taken as a challenge to analytic neutrality: is Lacan saying with this that the subject of religion is not analyzable? It could be the case that Lacan's remarks here are more about the limits of the discourse of religion itself (and similarly for magic, and science): within the limits of each discourse "access to truth" is barred: in magic knowledge is obscure, for example. But if these points about each discourse are coming from the point of view of a psychoanalytic discourse, does this then mean that psychoanalytic theory is the kind of metalanguage Lacan is saying does not exist? It does not seem to me that Lacan is saying enough about the relationships among these different discourses in this essay to decide the matter.

As he did in his discussion of magic, although obviously feeling that he can say more about it, he considers what status demand and desire have in religion, which will shed some light on his point about the status of the truth as cause in religion being negated – but what he describes sounds less like a negation and more like a transfer into the beyond. The subject of religion puts "the cause of his desire in God's hands": this is what sacrifices are about (741, 2). With the cause of his desire placed in the hands of an obscure God, the subject of religion's demands are "subordinated" to the task of trying to seduce this God (741, 2). "The game of love starts in this way," Lacan tells us (741, 2). Lacan's remarks here echo what he was saying at the end of his eleventh seminar, when he alluded to the temptation to make a sacrifice "to obscure gods" in order to "find evidence for the presence of" the Other's desire (S11: 275). He concludes there that in psychoanalysis the analyst's desire is not pure, but a desire to "obtain an absolute difference," one by means of which the analysand is able to "be confronted with the primary signifier" and "for the first time" is "in a position to subject himself to it. There only may the signification of a limitless love emerge, because it is outside the limits of the law, where alone it may live" (S11: 275–276). Here he is saying that the demands a religious person makes are "subordinated" to a "desire for a God who must then be seduced" (741, 2). Is Lacan associating the subject of religion with the structure of perversion, thereby calling into question Freud's claim about religion and obsessive neurosis?

For the subject of religion, the site of truth (the unconscious) instead becomes the locus of guilt (the subject of religion feels guilty for his or her unconscious desires). Lacan thinks this can explain the religious person's "distrust of knowledge," which he says is "most evident in the cases of those Church Fathers who proved to be the best reasoners" (741, 3). Lacan will return to the topic of knowledge in religion in a moment.

As far as causes go, truth appears in religion as a "final cause" – hence the importance of "eschatology" and "end-of-the-world judgment" for it (741, 4). This link between truth in the guise of final cause and religion is so strong Lacan thinks that even when the sciences take up the issue of final causes and purposes an "obscurantist stench" permeates their endeavors (741, 5).

Lacan then shifts from the topic of truth-as-cause in religion to the status knowledge has in it. He writes that we have much to learn "about the structure of the subject's relationship to truth as cause from the writing of the Church Fathers" and the resolutions to some of the most intense theological debates during the "first conciliar decisions" (741, 6). We subjects of science might think that these are among the most useless and academic of debates ('how many angels fit on the head of a pin?') but Lacan thinks there was more of importance in them than we might suspect. Fanciful as they may be, they can be understood as the putting into place of "a real that covers (over) the truth" (741, 7). It's very interesting that Lacan is associating the knowledge constructed in theological debates with "a real". From this point of view, one could shed some light on why "Christian Truth had to formulate the untenable notion of a Three and One God" (741, 8). The point of such a construct,

Lacan suggests, may have been precisely a "discouragement of thought" (741, 8). Tertullian's notorious *credo quia absurdum* could also be used as an excellent illustration of Lacan's point here: the intellectual absurdity and incomprehensibility of Christian doctrine were for him reasons to embrace it.

Rather than "accentuating the impasses of such a mystery" (as a classical philosophical critique might, as the sciences might) Lacan's orientation would emphasize "the necessity of this mystery's articulation" (741, 9). The slippage of dogma into heresy is particularly of interest, Lacan thinks: and something like the *Filioque* debate would even be susceptible of "explanation in topological terms" (741, 10). An interesting observation: the term means "and from the son" and is used in the Nicene creed to assert that the Holy Spirit proceeds not just from God the Father. The insertion of this term in the Creed was the cause of the schism between the Eastern and Western traditions: the Eastern Orthodox religions do not include it. A structural approach is important here because it would also help us to assess accurately "the function of images" in religion (741, 11). Augustine's *On the Trinity* is referred to as a model that would show us what Lacan wants us to see.

Lacan refers next to a tapestry that presents the trinity in the form of persons (there are several tapestries that can be found through an image search that do something like this, but I cannot figure out exactly which one Lacan might have been referring to). Evidently it also presented Adam and Eve "in the flower of their sin," and Lacan describes the overall effect of the personified trinity as "anxiety-provoking" (742, 1–2).

His comments on religion have focused, he admits, on what he calls "the Jewish tradition" and are "designed to show us" why that tradition is of interest (742, 4). He expresses regret, as he often does, at not being able to deliver the seminar he had planned on the Name-of-the-Father. Then he reiterates that the "key" to this tradition is the "relation of the subject to truth" (742, 5).

Lacan then takes up some remarks by Lévi-Struss on Buddhism, drawing I believe from the last chapter of *Tristes Tropiques*. In a passage that is interesting considering Lacan's discussion of knowledge and truth in this essay, Lévi-Strauss describes Buddhism as "this great religion of not-knowingness" that is not:

> based upon our incapacity to understand. It bears witness, rather, to our natural gifts, raising us to the point at which we discover truth in the guise of the mutual exclusiveness of being and knowing. And, by a further audacity, it has achieved something that, elsewhere, only Marxism has brought off: it has reconciled the problem of metaphysics with the problem of human behavior.
>
> (1955/2012: 395)

I cannot find any passage in *Tristes Tropiques* in which Lévi-Strauss broaches anything like the idea of "truth as cause," let alone what a "stopping down" of that would be, yet this is what Lacan says Lévi-Strauss's remarks on Buddhism amount to (742, 6). His remarks could indeed be taken to involve some view of a "generalized subject" – this is a big part of what structuralism does (742, 6). Lévi-Strauss (1955/2012: 395) does say the following about Marxism and Buddhism:

> Between Marxist criticism which sets Man free from his first chains, and Buddhist criticism, which completes that liberation, there is neither opposition nor contradiction. (The Marxist teaches that the apparent significance of Man's condition will vanish the moment he agrees to enlarge the object that he has under consideration.) Marxism and Buddhism are doing the same thing, but at different levels.

If Lévi-Strauss sees a sort of "universal reign of Marxism in society" foreshadowed by Buddhism, Lacan's rejoinder is that Lévi-Strauss actually misunderstands "the exigencies of the subject of science" – he is making "too little" of this subject's needs (742, 7). What does the "subject of science" require, in Lacan's opinion? A correctly conceived psychoanalytic practice, perhaps.

The rest of the seminar, Lacan suggests, is going to be dedicated to the question of how science relates to the truth as cause, but to open up the topic Lacan repeats his idea that part of science's success is due to its willful ignorance about the truth as cause: as he puts it, "science does-not-want-to-know-anything about the truth as cause" (742, 10). Lacan says that this recalls his discussion of foreclosure, which was one of a cluster of terms, along with repression and negation, that Lacan had dedicated much attention to in his earlier seminars and writings. His remarks about magic and religion earlier can be thought of in terms of repression and negation, respectively. While he was explicit about religion involving a negation of the truth as cause, the connection between magic and repression was never made clear. Perhaps his references to the status of knowledge in magic, as obscure, could be read as one of the consequences of this repression. Since the truth as cause is repressed in magic, knowledge about magic's efficacy – why it works – would remain a mystery to its practitioners and participants.

Lacan wonders now if what he is calling his "structural" take on magic, religion, and science is "at odds" with what he has said previously about foreclosure in psychosis, the foreclosure in question being that of the "Name-of-the-Father," since he is now claiming that science forecloses the truth as cause (742, 12). The structural resemblance of science to psychosis implied by his remarks is affirmed: science could be compared to "a successful paranoia" (742, 13). In a letter to Sándor Ferenczi discussing his relationship to Fliess and his self-analysis of that relationship, Freud (1996: xii) wrote that "a piece of homosexual development has been withdrawn and utilized for the enlargement of my own ego. I have succeeded where the paranoiac fails." The issue Lacan is concerned with here seems to be about a possible relationship between the foreclosure of the truth as cause in the sciences and the foreclosure of the Name-of-the-Father in psychosis. Can one be understood in terms of the other? The "closure" of science has a structure similar to psychosis: only, as is not the case in psychosis, it is a successful foreclosure, one in which what is foreclosed does not return to haunt it (742, 13). And the knowledge created by it turns out to be efficacious.

Shifting gears, Lacan notes that he will "have to indicate that the impact of truth as cause in science must be recognized in its guise as formal cause" (743, 3). Lacan does not say anything further about this in this essay. Dany Nobus (2002: 108) observes that "modern scientists are only willing to admit that they have discovered the true nature of a phenomenon if they have succeeded in formulating the laws governing its manifestations." We could add: the sciences develop mathemes or formulas for natural phenomena. The Aristotelian formal cause is perhaps the most obscure and abstract one. It is usually described as the shape of an object, or as what is responsible for the look of something, but Aristotle also argues that the ratio 2:1 is the formal cause of an octave in music (*Physics*, book II: 3).

Thinking about science's formal approach to truth would help make the distinction between science and psychoanalysis clear, and it would "clarify" that for psychoanalysis the truth is in the guise of a "material cause" – and this approach marks "psychoanalysis' originality in science" (743, 4). What Lacan has in mind with the material cause in psychoanalysis is the "impact of the signifier," in which the signifier acts "as if it were separate from its signification" (743, 5–6). As Nobus (2002: 108) points out, "for a psychoanalyst, the truth of a phenomenon, action, or process lies neither in the effort invested in it, nor in its goals or its logical plan, but only in its building-blocks, which are made up of speech and language." In this passage, Nobus is pointing out well how the material cause in psychoanalysis plays a role that would be different from how efficient, final, and formal causes might play a role in it, respectively. Just as the material cause of a brick house would be the pile of bricks that it constitutes (and one is reminded of the dust that makes up Saint-Just here), signifiers are the very stuff of psychoanalytic symptoms. The important aspect of a signifier in this respect is its materiality, or its thingliness, and not its signification.

Lacan declares that the phallus illustrates this idea. What Lacan calls the "copulatory signifier" is an example of the general autonomy of signifiers in that it represents something other than sex, and serves as something other than an individual's "biological sign" as well (743, 6). As a signifier, the phallus is detached from all that. Lacan reminds his audience of his views on the difference between the signifier and the sign. He defined the latter as something that represents something for someone, whereas a signifier represents a subject for another signifier (Cf. S20: 49). What is the upshot of this? Signs can be natural: they can also be more or less tied to their referent (as smoke is to fire, or a footstep is in some way to the foot that left it): signifiers for Lacan are autonomous from such links, and are characterized by their relation to a subject – which Lacan will even call in a moment not the subject of science but the subject of the signifier.

Lacan has already discussed how structuralism and psychoanalysis differ from psychology and other human sciences on issues like the development or progress of the intellect (childish vs. adult, 'primitive' vs. 'civilized'), and now he will consider the same issue regarding history. From the psychoanalytic point of view history is something that goes "against the rhythm of development" (743, 7). (So, the emergence of the subject of science should not be seen as progress?) Just as Lévi-Strauss's approach rids us of the idea that there is anything like intellectual progress in civilizations, the discipline of history too would benefit from a similar rejection. If history adopted this perspective it might be able to "escape the ever-present clutches of a providential conception of its course" (743, 7).

Psychoanalysis, with its attention to truth as material cause, in the guise of the signifier and its impact, is also best positioned to handle the topic of the subject of the signifier – another way of thinking about the subject of science. This subject is "conveyed by a signifier in its relation to another signifier" and "must be as rigorously distinguished from the biological individual as from any psychological evolution subsumable under the subject of understanding" (743, 8). These are points that should be clear enough by now. The subject of science, the subject psychoanalysis treats, is not the empirical or psychological individual.

Although it does not buy into a progressive view of history, Lacan thinks that his view of the function of "language in theory" would still be "compatible with historical materialism" – which, arguably, would have such a view (743, 9). This tradition has in fact left the topic of language "unaddressed," and Lacan speculates that along with language, maybe object *a* could find a place therein as well (743, 9). In fact he affirms that a linguistically informed historical materialism "is necessary to a correct integration of the function – from the standpoint of knowledge and the subject – of truth as cause" (743, 10).

And only now does Lacan explicitly point out the Aristotelian lineage of the four causes he's been discussing. He says this sampling of Aristotle makes sense because of Aristotle's "logicism," which was equally linked to a "grammaticism" (744, 2). The passage in Greek that Lacan gives is from Aristotle's *Physics*, in which the four causes are discussed (they are also discussed in *Metaphysics* book five). At the beginning of book two chapter seven Aristotle reiterates that he has got the number of causes right. The next line reads (depending on the translation): "the number is the same as that of the things comprehended under the question 'why'" (*Physics*, book II: 7) Aristotle seems to be arguing that in Greek the word or question 'why' can be said or asked in four different ways, or about four different aspects of things: and so it stands to reason that there are four 'causes' of objects (four reasons for the objects being as they are: 'why' with respect to what it is made of, what it looks like, how it was made, and for what purpose). Thus, the connection between grammar and logic Lacan is alluding to. Lacan's idea in the next paragraph, with its reference to a "polymerizing" of the cause, might be that with more complexity, or more ways of thinking about the word 'why,' perhaps we should wonder if there are only four causes (744, 4). Or perhaps that the link between our languages, and causes, may be ruptured. This perhaps would be another consequence of the sciences.

Not answering these questions, Lacan moves on. The point of this exercise is not just to give his audience "an elegant take" on other disciplines – those of magic, religion, and science (744, 5). The point is to express a warning. If one wants to remain within the framework provided by psychoanalysis (and Lacan continuously suggests in this essay how difficult that is, how fragile such a stance is) and to continue to think of things from the point of view of the subject of science, the "temptation of each of these relations to truth as cause" must be resisted (744, 6). And they are not tempting in the ways one might assume.

The temptation of magic within psychoanalysis or among psychoanalysts is to commit the error of psychologizing other subjects, positing their thinking as "'magical thinking'" (744, 9). If nobody is really free from engaging in such thinking, can it really be used as a "stigma" (744, 9)? We are all prone to it insofar as we are all involved in transferential relationships that make us susceptible to the effects of suggestion. So to be clear, the temptation here is not succumbing to magical thinking; the temptation is to use magical thinking as a label, maybe some sort of diagnostic tool. Moreover, such a labeling "explains nothing. What must be explained is its efficiency" (744, 10). And as we've seen, this is what part of Lacan's project is for this seminar.

The temptation regarding religion for psychoanalysis seems to involve something quite different – not a sort of bias or faulty assumption but an imitation, especially when it comes to organizational and institutional matters. Religious organizations create "a social hierarchy in which the tradition of a certain relation to truth as cause is preserved": psychoanalytic organizations do the same (744, 12). Lacan compares the IPA to the Catholic Church, claiming that both impose a "condition … upon communication," a sort of orthodoxy (744, 12). Lacan was personally familiar with this. But his idea seems to be that really nothing is communicated in such organizations (and this echoes his point about the status of knowledge in religion), for in the next sentence he asks: "need it be said that in science, as opposed to magic and religion, knowledge is communicated" (744, 13)? Of course it is, while it is not in magic and religion, although the communication of knowledge in science happens in a way that "sutures the subject it implies" (744, 14). This is ground Lacan has already covered: psychoanalysis, in contrast to science, would take on the divided subject implied, yet sutured, by science. The suturing of the subject is "the main problem raised by communication in psychoanalysis" in fact (744, 15). Evidently psychoanalysis should avoid doing this, but psychoanalysts themselves, having neglected "the relation to truth as cause, in its material guises," are partly to blame for the controversy surrounding the "scientific value" of their discipline (744, 16).

Returning to the topic of the subject and its division, and in closing, Lacan now describes the subject in terms of "a knot" of truth and knowledge (744, 17). Freud "unties" it when he discusses "the lack of the mother's penis," a discussion in which Lacan thinks "the nature of the phallus is revealed" (745, 1). I take Lacan to be giving us his interpretation here of how Freud accounts for the subject's division in '*The Splitting of the Ego*.' Part of it is worth quoting at length:

> Let us suppose … that a child's ego is under the sway of a powerful instinctual demand which it is accustomed to satisfy and that it is suddenly frightened by an experience which teaches it that the continuance of this satisfaction will result in an almost intolerable danger. It must now decide either to recognize the real danger, give way to it and do without the instinctual satisfaction, or to repudiate reality and persuade itself that there is no reason for fear, so that it may be able to retain the satisfaction. Thus there is a conflict between the demand of the instinct and the command of reality. But in fact the child takes neither course, or rather he takes both simultaneously, which comes to the same thing. He replies to the conflict with two contrary reactions both of which are valid and effective. On the one hand, with the help of certain mechanisms he rejects reality and refuses to accept any prohibition; on the other hand, in the same breath he recognizes the danger of reality, takes over the fear of that danger as a symptom and tries subsequently to divest himself of the fear. It must be confessed that this is a very ingenious solution of the difficulty. Both of the parties to the dispute obtain their share: the instinct is allowed to retain its satisfaction and proper respect is shown to reality. But everything has to be paid for in one way or another, and this success is achieved at the price of a rift in the ego which never heals but which increases as time goes on.
>
> (Freud, 1939/1964: 274–5)

Freud then discusses the case of a boy who developed a fetish in response to his perception of female genitals and his reaction to, and belief in, a castration threat from a nurse should he continue to masturbate. The creation of the fetish object allowed him to both deny and accept castration, and it enabled him to continue masturbation despite the threat. However, along with this fetish object, the boy developed a phobia of his father. Hence Lacan's discussion here of both phobic and fetish objects, and their differing roles. It would seem that the divided subject is accompanied by (even caused by?) a divided object. As Lacan describes it, the phobic object is a protection against the "abyss" of lack: it warns of an approaching encounter with it (745, 1). In Freud's study the phobic object, the father, is taken to be a castrating agent. The fetish object, however, covers lack up: as Lacan puts it, in language very close to Freud's, it maintains "the existence of the penis," "albeit displaced" (745, 1). The revelation of castration (the "(no-penis)") is suspended and is transformed instead into a positive lack of knowledge (the "no-knowledge") regarding the absence of the penis (745, 2).

But where there is a lack of knowledge Lacan also sees the construction of an alternative knowledge, a *gnomon* (which can mean "one who knows" but is also the word for the part of a sundial that casts a shadow) that "constantly indicates truth's site" to the subject in question (745, 3). And what it reveals about the "nature of the phallus" is that it is "nothing but the site of lack it indicates in the subject" (745, 4). This is a significant point, harking back to the discussion of suture earlier: we are dealing here with a lack and a supplement to the lack, a placeholder that also indicates lack's presence. Lacan says that psychoanalysts "shy away from" this revelation of lack even though they are "called forth as analysts" in it (745, 5).

Concluding remarks

As I said in my preamble, the status of '*Science and Truth*' is a bit strange: it is an official text in the *Écrits* that at the same time served as the opening to one of his seminars. There are many intriguing ideas and concepts discussed in it, with promises to develop them further that went unfulfilled. It does seem interesting to consider magic, religion, science, and psychoanalysis as precursors to the four discourses he would work out more systematically and in more detail later in his seventeenth seminar (the master's, hysteric's, university, and analyst's), with some significant modifications and eliminations.

Lacan does not broach this topic explicitly in this essay, but it is also interesting to ask: who is the subject of science? Not everyone, obviously – not historically speaking, since this subject emerged with the rise of the natural sciences, but even in the present not everyone in societies with advanced technologies, economies, etc., in which a scientific worldview is perhaps dominant is always, or ever, a subject of science, as Lacan himself suggests here. As one should expect with Lacan, there is an ambiguity in the phrase 'subject of science' that is being exploited, with both the subjective and objective genitive in play. The phrase refers both to the subject created by science, as an after-effect, but also to a subject who adheres to a scientific worldview. The two are not necessarily identical, and the latter is a worldview that Lacan seems to think is not fully worked out. I take his remark about the "exigencies of the subject of science," and Lévi-Strauss's misunderstanding of them, to suggest this (742, 7). One of Lacan's goals in this essay, and in the entire seminar, was to work out this position: he thinks we do not quite have that worldview yet, and that psychoanalysis is actually crucial to its development. Probably the later development of the "analyst's discourse" represents his more evolved position on this question (I'm using the term "worldview" consciously and guardedly, given Lacan's famous statement that "psycho-analysis is neither a *Weltanschauung*, nor a philosophy that claims to provide the key to the universe" (S11: 77). I think Lacan's position on this matter is far more ambiguous than this quote suggests.)

This brings me to my final point, about something like the subject of science as a subject-position, if not a worldview. Lévi-Strauss is obviously a very significant figure in this essay and I would argue that his work, or better the position from which he articulated some of his works, could well be a significant inspiration for the whole idea of a 'subject of science.' Lévi-Strauss was, after all, a structural anthropologist who reflected quite a bit about his own position as an anthropologist. His views at the end of a book like *Tristes tropiques* are what the subject of science might say if it spoke from a point of view that was specific to it: they are coming from the perspective of the subject of science that Lacan has in mind – perhaps crucial for the analyst to attain, even if Lacan will ultimately disagree with some of Lévi-Strauss's prognoses for this subject. This perspective entails an awareness of the determining influence of structures and signifiers, a possible detachment from them, and the attainment of a sort of general, depersonalized, object-like point of view, even (and maybe especially) regarding those structures and signifiers that are determinative for oneself. Lévi-Strauss (1958/1963: 117) at one point even refers to anthropology as a "*technique du dépaysement*," which could be translated as a disorientation-technique (as his translator notes, '*dépaysement*' suggests homelessness and uprooting, and might literally be rendered in English as a removal or alienation from one's home country). This might have served as a good phrase for what psychoanalysis does. One has not thought sufficiently perhaps about what the subject of structuralism is, and whether it is possible to take on a point of view that is appropriate to it. It seems to me that this is a topic Lacan is working on here and over the next several years of his seminar, when developing his notions of the psychoanalytic act and ultimately the analyst's discourse.

References

Aristotle. (1941) "The Physics". Trans. R. P. Hardie and R. K. Gaye. In Richard McKeon (Ed.), *The Basic Works of Aristotle*. New York: Random House.

Augustine. (1991) *The Trinity*. Intro and Trans. by Edmund Hill, O.P. Hyde Park: New City Press, 1991.

Canguilhem, Georges. (1958/2016) "What is Psychology". Trans. David M. Peña-Guzmán. *Foucault Studies*, 21, June, pp. 200–213.

de Saussure, Ferdinand. (1916/1986) *Course in General Linguistics*. Ed. Charles Bally and Albert Sechehaye. Trans. Roy Harris. La Salle, IL: Open Court Press.

Descartes, René. (1641/1979) *Meditations on First Philosophy*. Trans. Donald A. Cress. Indianapolis: Hackett.

Freud, Sigmund. (1907/1959) "Obsessive Actions and Religious Practices". In J. Strachey (Ed.), *The Standard Edition of the Complete Psychological Works of Sigmund Freud*, Vol. IX, London: The Hogarth Press and the Institute of Psycho-Analysis, pp. 115–128.

Freud, Sigmund. (1939/1964) "Splitting of the Ego in the Defensive Process". In J. Strachey (Ed.), *The Standard Edition of the Complete Psychological Works of Sigmund Freud*, Vol XXIII, London: The Hogarth Press and the Institute of Psycho-Analysis, pp. 271–278.

Freud, Sigmund and Sándor Ferenczi. (1996) *The Correspondence of Sigmund Freud and Sándor Ferenczi. Volume II. 1914–1919*. New York: Belknap.

Grigg, Russell. (2008) "Descartes and the Subject of Science". In *Lacan, Language, and Philosophy*. Albany, NY: State University of New York Press, pp. 133–149.

Henry, Michel. (1963/1973) *The Essence of Manifestation*. Trans. G. Etzkorn. The Hague: Nijhoff.

Hyppolite, Jean. (1946/1979) *Genesis and Structure of Hegel's "Phenomenology of Spirit"*. Trans. Samuel Cherniak and John Heckman. Chicago, IL: Northwestern University Press.

Jaurès, Jean. (1901) "Saint Just's Projects and Robespierre's Policies". Excerpt from *Histoire Socialiste de la Révolution Française*. Volume VI. Trans. Mitchell Abidor. Online. www.marxists.org/archive/jaures/1901/history/st-just.htm.

Kojève, Alexandre (1964) "L'origine chrétienne de la science moderne." In *Mélanges Alexandre Koyré*. Vol. II, pp. 295–306.

Koyré, Alexandre. (1959) *From the Closed World to the Infinite Universe*. Baltimore, MD: Johns Hopkins University Press.

Lamennais, Félicité Robert de. (1817/1895) *Essay on Indifference in Matters of Religion*. University of Michigan.

Laplanche, Jean and Jean-Bertrand Pontalis. (1967/1974) *The Language of Psychoanalysis*. Trans. Donald Nicholson-Smith. New York: W. W. Norton & Company.

Lévi-Strauss, Claude. (1949/1969) *The Elementary Structures of Kinship*. Trans. James Harle Bell and John Richard von Sturmer. Ed. Rodney Needham. Boston, MA: Beacon Press.

Lévi-Strauss, Claude. (1955/2012) *Tristes Tropiques*. Trans. John and Doreen Weightman. New York: Penguin.

Lévi-Strauss, Claude. (1958/1963) *Structural Anthropology*. Trans. Claire Jacobson and Brooke Grundfest Schoepf. New York: Basic Books.

Lévi-Strauss, Claude. (1962/1967) *The Savage Mind*. Chicago, IL: University of Chicago Press.

Lévi-Strauss, Claude. (1964/1983) *The Raw and the Cooked: Introduction to a Science of Mythology: Volume One*. Trans. John and Doreen Weightman. Chicago, IL: University of Chicago Press.

Lévy-Bruhl, Lucien. (1910/1966) *How Natives Think*. Trans. Lilian A. Clare. New York: Washington Square Press.

Miller, Jacques-Alain. (1966/2002) "Suture". *Un début dans la vie*. Paris: Gallimard, pp. 94–115.

Milner, Jean-Claude. (2000) "The Doctrine of Science". Trans. Oliver Feltham. *Umbr(a): A Journal of the Unconscious*. (No volume number), pp. 33–63.

Newman, John Henry. (1870/1947) *A Grammar of Assent*. New York: Longmans, Green and Co.

Nobus, Dany. (2002) "A Matter of Cause: Reflections on Lacan's 'Science and Truth'". In Jason Glynos and Stavrakakis Yannis (Eds.), *Lacan and Science*, pp. 89–118. London: Karnac.

Piaget, Jean. (1945/1962) *Plays, Dreams, and Imitation in Childhood*. New York: W. W. Norton & Company.

Ricoeur, Paul. (1965/1977) *Freud and Philosophy: An Essay on Interpretation*. Trans. Denis Savage. New Haven, CT: Yale University Press.

Roudinesco, Élisabeth. (1986/1990) *Jacques Lacan and Co.: A History of Psychoanalysis in France, 1925–1985*. Trans. Jeffrey Mehlman. Chicago, IL: University of Chicago Press.

Roudinesco, Élisabeth. (1993/1997) *Jacques Lacan: An Outline of a Life and a History of a System of Thought*. Trans. Barbara Bray. London: Polity.

11

METAPHOR OF THE SUBJECT

Stephanie Swales

Context

Lacan said that the text '*Metaphor of the Subject*,' which is included in the complete *Écrits* as an appendix (Appendix II), is related to '*The Instance of the Letter in the Unconscious, Or Reason Since Freud*' (hereafter referred to as *The Instance of the Letter*). Indeed, in both works he provides formulae for metaphor and is concerned with how the subject is structured by language. What is more, in the original French both of their titles allude to subjectivity; the French word '*Instance*' could also be translated as 'Agency,' just as it is used to refer to Freud's *Instanzen*, or agencies, of the id, ego, and superego. Bruce Fink, in his translator's notes to '*Metaphor of the Subject*', said '*La Métaphore du Sujet*' "could also be rendered, 'The Metaphor That Is the Subject,' 'The Subject's Metaphor,' or better still 'The Subject as Metaphor'" (848). And so the title promises to say something in the way of how the subject could be considered to be a metaphor. In Lacan's typical fashion, however, his allusive, dense text puts the reader to work.

'*Metaphor of the Subject*' was written in June of 1961, and is based on a presentation Lacan gave on June 23, 1960 to the French Philosophical Society. *The Instance of the Letter*, which Lacan links with '*Metaphor of the Subject*', was written in May 14–26 of 1957 and was based on a talk Lacan gave on May 9, 1957. In introducing *The Instance of the Letter*, Lacan said he situates "it between writing and speech—it will be halfway between the two" (493, 1). That being said, Lacan did not remark that '*Metaphor of the Subject*' was in between writing and speech just as he did not do so for other texts he rewrote after the original presentation, such as '*Position of the Unconscious*' (presented in the fall of 1960 and rewritten in 1964). It follows that in referring to *Instance of the Letter* as between writing and speech, Lacan was not simply referring to the fact that it had both written and spoken forms. Because '*Metaphor of the Subject*' was associated by Lacan with *Instance of the Letter*, however, we may be justified in wondering if any of the potential meanings of the latter being halfway between writing and speech are applicable to '*Metaphor of the Subject*.' Fink, in his chapter '*Reading "The Instance of the*

Letter in the Unconscious'" from *Lacan to the Letter: Reading Écrits Closely* (2004: 69), points out that the analysand's discourse can be understood as halfway between writing and speech. The analysand's discourse is spoken to the analyst, complete with intonations, hesitations, and so on, "and yet it is based on or dances around a kind of writing: the inscription of the subject's past and desire in the unconscious." Lacan might thus be characterizing what he says in *The Instance of the Letter* as the analysand's discourse just as he later does, for example, in *Seminar XVIII* (1971), *Seminar XIX* (1971–1972), and *Seminar XX* (1972–1973).

In '*Metaphor of the Subject*,' then, Lacan as analysand puts the listener/reader as analyst to work in trying to decipher it. What is more, since it was originally presented to the *French Philosophical Society* instead of an analytic audience he may be insisting that his audience try to listen on his terms—on psychoanalytic grounds rather than philosophical grounds—when he says "it is on the basis of the unconscious' manifestations, which I deal with as an analyst, that I have developed a theory of the effects of the signifier that intersects rhetoric" (755, 2). Lacan's '*Metaphor of the Subject*,' in fact, was developed in response to a talk given by philosopher and rhetorician Chaim Perelman. Perelman co-wrote, with Lucie Olbrechts-Tyteca, the book *The New Rhetoric: A Treatise on Argumentation* (1958/1969) with which Lacan was familiar. Just as the analysand's discourse necessitates that the analyst listen from the position of the analyst rather than with her own personal biases and modes of understanding, in '*Metaphor of the Subject*,' Lacan takes up what Perelman said about metaphor on his own terms—those of the unconscious—and asks philosophers and rhetoricians to suspend their frame of reference in favour of his. Because Lacan is the one who speaks, he is in the position of the analysand. Again, Lacan specifically speaks about "a theory of the effects of the signifier that intersects rhetoric" (755, 2). In a text in which the word 'subject' is only used on three occasions, it is words such as these that connect the dots between the title '*Metaphor of the Subject*' and the body of the text. Elsewhere in his work, for instance in *My Teaching* (1967/2008: 79), Lacan says, "The subject is what I define in the strict sense as an effect of the signifier" (a signifier being an element in language that might be a word or part of a word which refers to other signifiers within the structure of language rather than to something outside which would give a fixed meaning, or signified, to the signifier).

When Lacan tells us, at the start of '*Metaphor of the Subject*,' that he has "developed a theory of the effects of the signifier that intersects rhetoric" (755, 2), he is introducing the theme of this brief paper—a theme which emphasizes the inextricable link between the structure of language and the structure of the subject. Lacan was the first to argue this inextricable link and also to highlight the place of the subject in psychoanalysis. Lacan is careful to ground his theory in the work of Freud; for example, in paragraph 4 (755) Lacan alludes to Freud's discovery of condensation and displacement, "the two fundamental facets of the play of the unconscious" as discussed in *The Interpretation of Dreams* (1900/1953), and there Lacan links up metaphor with condensation and metonymy with displacement. Nevertheless, linking up the operation of language with the subject in psychoanalysis is, properly speaking, Lacan's innovation and part of what made him famous.

Out of all of the articles in the *Écrits*, Lacan wrote about metaphor most extensively in *The Instance of the Letter*, and so this, as Lacan tells us, is the text most crucial to consult in tandem with '*Metaphor of the Subject*' to learn about how the subject is a metaphor. In general, Lacan's early period (up through *Seminar XI*) makes substantial use of metaphor and metonymy toward the theory and practice of psychoanalysis. In addition to comparing '*Metaphor of the Subject*' with *The Instance of the Letter*, in this paper I will reference Lacan's usage of metaphor in *Desire and Its Interpretation: The Seminar of Jacques Lacan, Book VI* (1958–1959), *Transference: The Seminar of Jacques Lacan, Book VIII* (1960–1961), and '*The Signification of the Phallus*'. That being said, Lacan discusses metaphor in many of his texts in the 1950s and early 1960s, and so the references found in this paper are by no means an exhaustive list but rather function as closely connected texts which help elucidate '*Metaphor of the Subject*'. For example, in *Seminar VIII* (1960–1961), Lacan said that love is a metaphor, while at the end of *Instance of the Letter*, after having investigated the structure of metaphor in other ways, Lacan said, "For the symptom is a metaphor, whether one likes to admit it or not, just as desire is a metonymy, even if man scoffs at the idea" (439, 1). In '*Metaphor of the Subject*', Lacan alludes to both love as a metaphor and the symptom as a metaphor in unpacking how metaphor concerns the place of the subject.

'*Metaphor of the Subject*' is important to read in tandem with *The Instance of the Letter* because it gives a condensed version of the culmination of his 'early period' thought about the structure of metaphor and how the subject of the unconscious is an effect of metaphor. Although Lacan justifies highlighting the importance of metaphor in the creation and operation of the subject of the unconscious by referring to Freud's usage of condensation (along with displacement) in *The Interpretation of Dreams* (1900/1953), Lacan's concept of metaphor is not the same thing as Freud's concept of condensation. Lacan introduces two facets of metaphor that cannot be found in condensation. The first is the new meaning or creative spark that results from the operation of metaphor. The second is the elision or overwriting of something. This something, as negated and sometimes repressed, has significant effects. Lacan's '*Metaphor of the Subject*', then, is a text that provides psychoanalysts an orientation for clinical work and philosophers and linguists a ground for elucidating subjectivity. Through the process of analysis, the analysand comes into being where it was, recognizing himself as a metaphor and identifying with his symptom.

Commentaries on the text

For most of '*Metaphor of the Subject*', Lacan engages explicitly with Perelman's work on metaphor. Lacan begins (755, 1) by situating Perelman's project, that of "[p]rocedures of argumentation (755, 1)" within rhetoric as one which is wrongfully "scorned [*mépris*] by the scientific tradition" (755, 1). As such, we may note that Lacan's own project, that of psychoanalysis, has an analogous position. Since Freud's time, from the perspective of the natural sciences, psychoanalysis has been considered to be unscientific and dismissed on those grounds. Nevertheless, as Lacan points out near the end of his essay, "the discourse of science, insofar as it commends itself by its objectivity, neutrality, and dreariness, even of the Sulpician variety, is just as dishonest and ill-intentioned as any other rhetoric" (758, 4). Lacan's work within psychoanalysis is considered legitimate from other measures of truth, given that psychoanalysis follows the logic of the signifier and the operation of the unconscious (for more on this, see the commentary by Ed Pluth, Chapter 10 on '*Science and Truth*'; see also Eric Laurent's *Lost in Cognition: Psychoanalysis and the Cognitive Sciences*). As Lacan said in *Seminar XVII*, "the analytic discourse is specified, is distinguished by the fact that it raises the question of what the use is of this form of knowledge which rejects and excludes the dynamics of truth" (S17, 1969–1970: 91). In other words, analytic discourse is the only discourse that does not mistake itself for the truth.

Lacan criticizes Perelman for arguing "perhaps too cautiously" (755, 3) and not going "beyond defense" to "win us over to his side" (755, 2), perhaps meaning there is something lacking in Perelman's argumentation for the value of argumentation. Lacan goes on to introduce his own theory which "intersects rhetoric," seeming thus to make the case that with this theory he has been able to win people over to his side. Lacan here situates his work in psychoanalysis as being firmly rooted in Perelman's territory of rhetoric. What is more, as Lacan says his theory is one of the "effects of the signifier that intersects rhetoric" (755, 2), we recall that Lacan has defined the subject as an effect of the signifier; what is clearly at stake here is the subject in its relation to rhetoric.

Lacan continues on to engage with "the way Perelman deals with metaphor" (755, 5) after Lacan reminds us that he links up metaphor with condensation, one of Freud's "two fundamental facets of the play of the unconscious" (755, 4), the other facet being metonymy/displacement/desire. Specifically, Lacan takes issue with Perelman's reduction of metaphor "to the function of analogy" (755, 6).[1] In this vein, Perelman had said "we cannot better describe a metaphor than by conceiving it as a condensed analogy, resulting from the fusion of an element from the phoros with an element from the theme" (Perelman and Olbrechts-Tyteca, 1958/1969: 399).

According to Aristotle and Perelman, the structure of analogy can be represented by A/B and C/D or A:B::C:D. In an analogy, something is described by way of comparing it to something similar. For example, 'yellow'/'color' and 'orchid'/'flower.' The 'theme' is A/B or in this instance 'yellow'/'color,' while 'phoros,' which comes from *pherein* in Greek (translated as to carry or bear), refers to 'C/D' or 'orchid'/'flower.' 'Yellow's status as one of many colors is elucidated by way of comparison with 'orchid' in its relation to 'flower.' Lacan therefore says that "in the case of analogy, the specific effect of the relations A/B and D/C is sustained by the very heterogeneity by which they divide up into theme and phoros, this formalism is no longer valid for metaphor" (755, 7 and 756, 1). (It is notable that Lacan switches the given order of C and D in the phoros pair.) In other words, the two pairs which constitute the four terms are heterogeneous, each pair being neatly separated from the other. No new signification, no new meaning, no "poetic spark" associated with "metaphoric creation" (422, 2) results.

In contrast, although metaphor is also comprised of four terms, the terms are heterogeneous in a different way, "their heterogeneity involves a dividing line—three against one—and is tantamount to the dividing line between the signifier and the signified" (756, 2). Therefore, they have a different effect than that of "the relations A/B and D/C" (755, 7). Lacan tells us that in metaphor there is "nothing natural predestining the signifier for this function of phoros apart from the fact that two signifiers are involved, which can, as such be reduced to a phonemic opposition" (756, 4). The four terms of metaphor—S, S'_1, S'_2, and x—are heterogeneous insofar as there is "nothing natural" (756, 4) about their connection, there being no such thing, in Lacan's view, as a natural or fixed connection between signifiers. The structure of analogy as Perelman discussed it seems to operate with the erroneous idea that theme and phoros are neatly connected and differentiated from one another by way of a fixed meaning. Likewise, Lacan notes that Perelman himself gives us "the best proof" (756, 1) that analogy is different than metaphor by "the very illustrations" (756, 1) he provides. Before Lacan turns to consider one such illustration, he introduces a formula for metaphor, one which, in contrast to his formula in *The Instance of the Letter*, makes use of four terms.

Lacan tells us that he is going to "expand on a formula [he] gave for metaphor" (756, 3) in *The Instance of the Letter*. In *The Instance of the Letter*, Lacan's formula was [429, 1].

$$f\left(\frac{S'}{S}\right)\mathrm{S} \cong \mathrm{S}(+)s$$

This can be read as saying that metaphor is a function (*f*) of substituting one signifier (S) with another (S') in a way that S, the first signifier, remains present (hence the repetition of S before $\cong$), and this results in crossing the bar (+ being a cross) between signifier and signified and the creation of a new signification (+ also indicating something, *s*, which is added or new). The first signifier, S, remains alongside the new signification.

In '*Metaphor of the Subject*', Lacan's 'expansion' of his formula for metaphor is as follows: [756, 3].

$$\frac{S}{S_1'} \bullet \frac{S_2'}{x} \rightarrow S\left(\frac{1}{s''}\right)$$

Lacan posits, "[m]etaphor is, quite radically speaking, the effect of the substitution of one signifier for another in a chain" (756, 4). This is roughly the same definition he gave in *The Instance of the Letter*. Lacan tells us that the dividing line between the top and bottom terms (on the left side of the arrow) "is tantamount to the dividing line between the signifier and the signified" (756, 2). What is different or 'expanded' in the new formula? For starters, it is expanded in a quantitative sense since there are more signifiers involved in the example Lacan takes up from Perelman, who, in turn, borrowed it from George Berkeley. The example as initially provided by Lacan is "an ocean of false science." There are three signifiers here, 'ocean,' 'false,' and 'science.' When Lacan puts this metaphor into his formula, the fourth term becomes 'x,' which is below 'false.' The placement of this 'x' might function to signify that there is no term that opposes 'false' in the metaphor. 'Ocean' overwrites or is substituted for 'science,' but false is an adjective describing 'ocean' as well as 'science.'

$$\frac{\text{an ocean}}{\text{learning}} \text{ of } \frac{\text{false}}{x} \rightarrow \text{an ocean}\left(\frac{1}{?}\right)$$

We also notice in this formula that Lacan alters the signifier 'science' and changes it to 'learning.' Lacan tells us that he has done this intentionally when he says "it is better to restore what the French translation already tends to 'make dormant' [*endormir*], to do justice, along with Perelman, to a metaphor so felicitously found by rhetoricians" (756, 5). That is, in Berkeley's original work, *Three Dialogues between Hylas and Philonous in opposition to Sceptics and Atheists*, Hylas said, "What doubts, what hypotheses, what labyrinths of confusion, what fields of disputation, what *an ocean of false learning*, can be avoided by that single notion of immaterialism!" (my emphasis, 2016). Perelman, when translating this metaphor into French, used the word 'science' instead of 'learning,' referring to '*un océan de fausse science*[2]' (1958/1969). And so Lacan decided to restore 'learning' to the metaphor, saying that "[l]earning—*enseignement*[3]—indeed, is not science, and one senses even more clearly in the former that the term has no more to do with the ocean than a fish with a bicycle" (756, 6). One way we could read this is that Lacan is saying Perelman made his own metaphor when he substituted one signifier, 'science,' for another, 'learning.' These two terms having no more to do with one another "than a fish with a bicycle" (756, 6) is not problematic when making a metaphor, since in metaphor Lacan said there is "nothing natural predestining the signifier for this function of phoros apart from the fact that two signifiers are involved, which can, as such, be reduced to a phonemic opposition" (756, 4).

A key difference between Lacan's formula for metaphor in '*Metaphor of the Subject*' and *The Instance of the Letter* is that in the latter, S is the signifier that has been replaced by another signifier, S1, and yet it is S that remains present after the crossing of the bar and the creation of a new signification. In '*Metaphor of the Subject*,' S stands instead for the signifier that has replaced the original signifier (represented by S'_1) and it is the one that remains present after the crossing of the bar between signifier and signified and the creation of the new signification. Nevertheless, the overwritten signifier 'learning' is in both formulae positioned under the bar in the place of the signified. In the new formula, other than the addition of a third adjectival signifier, 'false,' the difference of interest to us is why 'learning,' the overwritten signifier, is no longer emphasized straightforwardly as remaining even after the crossing of the bar and the creation of the new signification. Why is it that 'ocean,' the signifier which is substituted for 'learning,' is what seems to be emphasized instead?

Perhaps the explanation lies in the '*s*"' or the '?' of Lacan's formula for metaphor, which, in addition to 'S' or 'ocean' is what results from the crossing of the bar. Although Lacan does not explicitly mention "the place of the question mark" (756, 9) until the end of the page, he leads up to it in the two preceding paragraphs. In the seventh paragraph of the page, Lacan says

> The sunken cathedral of what had been previously taught [*enseigné*] concerning this matter is still likely to ring fruitfully in our ears when it is reduced to the alteration of a muffled and sonorous bell by which the phrase penetrates us—lear-ning, lear-ning—not from the depths of a liquid layer, but due to the fallacy of its own arguments.
>
> (756, 7)

What does this paragraph have to do with the creation of a metaphor? One clue is provided by Fink's translator's endnotes (848), in which he informs us that "*La cathédrale engloutie* (The sunken cathedral) is the title of the Prelude for Piano, Book 1, Number 10 (1910) by Claude Debussy in which Debussy manages to make the piano sound very much like bells ringing. Lacan's use of 'the sunken cathedral' in paragraph 7 thus functions as a metaphor in which "what had previously been taught [*enseigné*] concerning this matter" (756, 7) is overwritten by the allusion to Debussy's prelude—a piece in which the piano notes are substituted for bells ringing, which is perhaps its own kind of metaphor. Fink, in his endnotes, also mentions that "Someone with a strong French accent in English is likely to emphasize the second syllable in 'learning,' making a ringing sort of sound ('ning, 'ning)" (848). Correspondingly, when Lacan mentions "the alternation of a muffled and sonorous bell by which the phrase penetrates us—lear-ning, lear-ning," (756, 7), he may be calling our attention to the materiality of the signifier (as he refers to it in *The Purloined Letter*). After all, it is through the voice that the subject first learns and internalizes language.

In contrast to this focus on the realm of the sonorous, Lacan goes on to introduce the metaphor as it relates to "a locus of deception" (756, 8), "nonmeaning" (756, 8), and something "unsoundable," (757, 1). Lacan says that what is produced "at the place of the question mark in the second part of my formula is a new species in signification: a falseness that disputation cannot fathom, for it is unsoundable" (756, 9 and 757, 1). 'S' or, to follow with our example, 'an ocean,' is what is produced via metaphor, but it is produced in tandem with the question mark, an 'unsoundable' 'new species in signification.' This unsoundable aspect of metaphor has to do with the real as an order; this unsoundable spark is something outside of the symbolic. In '*On a Question Prior to Any Possible Treatment of Psychosis*' (464–465), this unsoundable result of the metaphor is prefigured in Lacan's formula for the paternal metaphor, wherein the mother's desire is a signifier that is created reactively against the confrontation with the mother's *jouissance* (see also Vanheule, 2011).

What is crucial, then, in Lacan's definition of metaphor is its basis in nonmeaning. As Lacan put it in *Instance of the Letter*, "metaphor is situated at the precise point at which meaning is produced in nonmeaning" (423, 5). A signifier is only meaningful by virtue of its connection with, and difference from, other signifiers, and so we may understand nonmeaning as S1, a master signifier in its isolation from another signifier, S2, or as the absence of a pre-existing connection between two signifiers such as ocean and learning. Jacques-Alain Miller (2013) has formulated that the Lacanian subject is an empty set, a placeholder without any meaning of its own that yet grounds the subject in a kind of naming of the void.

The Lacanian subject, then, is born through making meaning out of nonmeaning, but the subject that results from this process (of substituting one signifier for another) is a subject that is paradoxically structured both by meaning (S) and by nonmeaning (*s*" or ?), or the unsoundable real. Indeed, the Lacanian subject is initially created during the process of primal repression, in which one signifier (e.g., 'big boy' as in 'be a big boy and let go of mommy') is substituted for another signifier ('momma's boy') in such a way that the original signifier is forced below the bar and becomes repressed. The repression of the original signifier is better demonstrated in Lacan's 'expanded' formula for metaphor in '*Metaphor of the Subject*' than the formula from *Instance of the Letter*, because in the former the new signifier is what persists after the crossing of the bar, not the original signifier. What results from the metaphorical process of primal repression is, of course, the subject, which is also known as the subject of the unconscious.

In describing the place of the question mark in the second part of Lacan's formula, Lacan said it is "a falseness that disputation cannot fathom, for it is unsoundable—the wave and depth of the imaginary's ἄπειρος[4] in which any vessel is swallowed up should it seek to draw forth something" (757, 1). Fink (848) says the "Greek Lacan provides here has many meanings, among which the Doric for ἤπειρος, meaning terra firma, continent, or land; infinite or immense; inextricable or without issue; and ignorance of or lacking in experience of." Notice that this Greek term has one of the meanings—'terra firma,' that Perelman, in his explication of his 'ocean of false science' metaphor, says could be gleaned from what he calls the "unexpressed inferior terms (B and D)" (1958/1969, 401). In terms of $\frac{A}{B}\frac{C}{D}$, Perelman says, 'ocean' stands in for 'A' and 'learning' for 'C,' and B and D can be implicitly assumed to be swim mer (B) and scholar (D), stream (B) and truth (D), or terra firma (B) and truth (D). Lacan's way of taking up a theory of the signifier that intersects rhetoric brings out the function and the importance of that unexpressed or hidden term. We can understand the terra firma of the imaginary in this sense to be the real as an order; Lacan likens efforts at taming the real with the symbolic to a vessel which "is swallowed up should it seek to draw forth something" (757, 1). Nevertheless, the real is the terra firma of the subject at the same time that the subject comes into being in the symbolic. Likewise, in '*The Subversion of the Subject and the Dialectic of Desire*,' presented between September 19 and 23 in 1960 (roughly contemporaneous with '*Metaphor of the Subject*'), Lacan says that the "cut made by the signifying chain is the only cut that verifies the structure of the subject as a discontinuity in the real" (678, 3).

In the third and fourth paragraphs on page 757 of '*Metaphor of the Subject*', Lacan refers to the use of metaphor in insults or swearing. Lacan refers to the Rat Man's temper tantrum as a child, in which the Rat Man angrily yelled at his father, "'*Du Lampe, du Handtuch, du Teller*' ("You lamp! You towel! You plate!" and so on), his father being unsure whether to consider this criminal or genius on his son's part [Freud, 1909/1957, 205]" (757, 3). Lacan then says that metaphor originates in "the dimension of insult" (757, 4). In other words, perhaps we can understand the process of metaphor, of substituting one signifier for another, whereby there is "nothing natural predestining" (756, 4) the relation between the two signifiers, as inherently insulting. Although this is easier to see when a human subject is being called something inanimate or lesser than in a case in which the two signifiers at stake are both in the realm of objects or ideas, the fact remains that calling one thing by what it is not can be a way of demeaning its nature. The possibility "of the dimension of insult [*injure*] in which metaphor originates" (757, 4) is owing to the fact that in language signifiers only have meaning by virtue of difference and deferral; there being no meta-language, no point outside of language which fixes signifiers to signifieds, a signifier lacks in any true essence which would protect it from the insult of being overwritten by another signifier. Bringing this point to the Lacanian subject, we may recall that the subject comes into being when it undergoes a first identification which forms the ego-ideal (see, for example, 684, 4), and that this identification, this overwriting of oneself with a signifier, is alienating. This first identification is a metaphor which is responsible for the creation of the subject, and since the unary trait is something that the subject initially was not, we can say that this crucial metaphor is one rooted in insult.

In the fourth paragraph of page 757, regarding metaphor's link to the dimension of insult, he said, "'The cat goes bow-wow, the dog goes meow, meow.' This is how the child spells out the powers of discourse and inaugurates thought" (757, 4). Lacan uses this same example in '*The Signification of the Phallus*' as well as commenting on it extensively in *Seminar VI* (S6, 1958–1959). In the 9th session of *Seminar VI*, given on January 21, 1959 (which is about a year and a half before the presentation version of '*Metaphor of the Subject*'), Lacan tells the story of a young child who learned from his father the signification of the word 'dog,' the family having a dog in their home, but who instead preferred to use the signifier 'bow-wow' to designate a dog. Lacan said that replacing 'dog' with 'bow-wow' is tantamount to creating the first metaphor. The child, who is learning language, has demonstrated a pragmatic understanding of "a structural necessity of language, a necessity which is such that in order for something to be generated in the realm of the signified, one signifier must be substituted for another" (S6, 1958–1959, session of January 21). Then, however, the child begins to call all kinds of things 'bow-wow,' and "the child declares with the greatest authority and insistence that 'the dog goes meow' and 'the cat goes bow-wow'" (S6, 1958–1959, session of January 21)—knowing full well that this is not true and that he is creating a metaphor. Lacan elaborates on this new development, saying,

> The enunciation 'the dog goes bowwow' is a simple imitative connection with respect to reality. From the moment the game begins, from the moment 'the dog goes meow' and the 'bowwow,' which is elided, sinks into what lies below the enunciation concerning the dog, the latter becomes a true signifying enunciation.
>
> (S6, 1958–1959, session of January 21)

To say a dog goes 'meow' and a cat goes 'bowwow' is to create a metaphor—an insulting one—and Lacan draws our attention to how common this phenomenon is in children who are learning to speak.

In '*Metaphor of the Subject*,' Lacan continues on to comment on an example from Aristotle's *Poetics* that Perelman uses. Perelman wrote, "Aristotle gives some examples of metaphors in which the analogical relation is made completely explicit. Thus, he writes: "As old age is to life, so is evening to day. One will accordingly describe evening as the 'old age of the day' and old age as the 'evening of life.' (Aristotle, *Poetics*, XXI, 1457b)" (Perelman and Olbrechts-Tyteca, 1958/1969: 399). In this example, we can see the logic of the metaphor 'the evening of life' spelled out, but Lacan says it "is quite telling in that it does not even point out the repression of the most unpleasant facet of the metaphorized term in order to bring out a sense of peacefulness that old age in no way implies in real life [*le réel*]" (757, 6). One reason, then, why metaphor cannot be reduced to the function of analogy is that metaphor involves hidden or repressed signifiers.

Lacan spoke at some length in *Seminar III* (S3, 1955–1956: 138–139) about the expression 'the peacefulness of the evening' which he brings up again here in relation to 'the evening of life.' The context in *Seminar III* is a question about the relationship between discourse and experience. Lacan says that the expression 'the peace of the evening' may come into our mind at a moment when "you are at the close of a stormy and tiring day" (S3, 1955–1956: 138) and anxiety or agitation are predominant in your experience. Language, then, as in the saying 'the peace of the evening,' has the power to substitute itself for something else in our experience, something that is not well-expressed by the words which overwrite it. The substitution of 'peace' for 'clamour' is a metaphor, and one which represses 'clamour.' The subject, then, being a metaphor, is founded by the process of repression.

In the last paragraph of page 757, Lacan references *The Instance of the Letter* in which he gave as an example of metaphor Victor Hugo's "His sheaf was neither miserly nor spiteful" from the poem 'Booz sleeping' or '*Booz endormi*.' Lacan says that this metaphor plays on the fact that "while language is essentially blah blah blah, it is nevertheless from language that having and being derive" (757, 8). We recall that for Lacan having the phallus versus being the phallus are two main positions which the subject can occupy, and so there is something important here in this metaphor about language and about the subject.

Hugo's poem tells the Biblical story of Booz and Ruth. Booz is an elderly (over eighty years old, we are told) farmer who worked hard caring for his barley and wheat fields. He is a moral man who is a 'good master,' a 'faithful friend,' 'frugal, yet generous' and would give from his crop to the poor. In the poem, Booz is sleeping by his harvested barley when he dreams that an enormously tall oak tree has sprouted from his loins and reaches all the way up to heaven. Booz marvels at the implied meaning of this since he is an old man who no longer has a wife and has no living son to carry on his name. God sends him Ruth, who steals away during the night to find Booz, and then the language of the poem makes it clear that their sexual union will result in a child. Although Booz does not have the vigor of youth to attract Ruth to him, he is depicted as having the phallus insofar as he is generous, good, and a hard worker.

The metaphor in question is "*Sa gerbe n'était point avare ni haineuse*[5]," or "His sheaf was neither miserly nor spiteful," in which 'sheaf' is substituted for 'Booz,' one signifier replacing another. When we read this line of the poem, the two words are condensed since we think of 'Booz' when we read 'sheaf.'

In *The Instance of the Letter*, Lacan highlights the negation in this line. Lacan suggests that the reader, rather than being skeptical of the negation, accepts his sheaf being *neither* miserly *nor* hateful because the sheaf, being an inanimate object "drawn from nature, knows neither our reserve nor our rejections, and even in its accumulation remains prodigal by our standards" (423, 1). If Booz's proper name were used instead of his 'sheaf' standing in for him, the reader would more readily associate Booz with miserliness and hatefulness. The fact remains, however, that as 'Booz' is the overwritten signifier in the metaphor, he is "ejected … into the outer darkness where miserliness and hatred harbor him in the hollow of their negation" (422, 7). That is, negating miserliness and hatred functions to solidify the connection between those negated terms and Booz himself, whereas we can think of his sheaf as being more generous and less hateful.

At the same time, since what interests Lacan in '*Metaphor of the Subject*' is what the sheaf/Booz metaphor reveals about being and having, his words at the top of 758 are a call for the reader to take a fresh look at the metaphor. Whereas typically, the negation of a signifier "would do no more here, as we know, than posit it" (758, 1) as I just delineated with the negation of miserliness and hatefulness, in this case the metaphor of sheaf/Booz brings "forth the only object the having of which necessitates the failure to be it—the phallus" (758, 1). Because the original French reads, "*nécessite le manqué à l'être*" (translated as "necessitates the failure to be it"), the lack-in-being or want-to-be is implied, so that having the phallus is only rendered possible on account of Booz's constitutive lack in being. In this special case of negation, instead of reading in negation an assertion, we are justified in reading the negation of having as asserting his lack of being. From this perspective, by virtue of not having it, Booz fantasized about being the phallus or the beloved for Ruth. (In this paragraph (758, 1), Lacan alludes to the roughly contemporaneous *Seminar VIII* (S6, 1960–1961): "The Psychology of the Rich: Pausanius," in which being rich and having it is portrayed as a surefire way to avoid being loved.)

Relevant to this discussion is Lacan's treatment of the metaphor of love in *Seminar VIII* (1960–1961). In this seminar, love begins with being loved, with the other reaching toward you as beloved object or *erómenos*, but it becomes a more elevated form of love when you become *erastés*, the lover or the one who desires. In other words, love, like a symptom (for the early Lacan) has the structure of a metaphor. Love is what occurs with the substitution of *erastés* for *erómenos*. Lacan's example for this is found in the actions of Achilles, who was said to have been in the position of *erómenos* because he was younger than Patroclus. In avenging the death of Patroclus, "he places himself not in the stead of, but rather in the wake of Patroclus. He makes of Patroclus' fate the debt he must pay, the debt with which he must come to terms" (Lacan, S8, 1960–1961: 70). In so doing, Achilles becomes *erastés*. The one who *has* it, much like Booz, renounces it, giving from his lack, since according to Lacan's formula, to love is to give what one does not have.

In '*Metaphor of the Subject*,' Lacan continues on in the second paragraph of page 758 to emphasize "that the most serious reality, and even the sole serious reality for man, if one considers its role in sustaining the metonymy of his desire, can only be retained in metaphor" (758, 2). This strong claim relates to Lacan's conception of the role of the ego versus that of the subject. Desire is associated with metonymy and with the ego, whereas the subject is associated with metaphor. Correspondingly, Lacan says that "enunciation can never be reduced to what is enunciated in any discourse" (758, 3). Enunciation, or the enunciating subject, is the subject of the unconscious, the metaphor that is the subject, and, through a slip of the tongue or an eruption of laughter, it will always say more than what is said. What is said or enunciated is uttered by the ego or the subject of the statement as indicated by a grammatical shifter such as 'I.' These are two very different types of subject. The analyst's job is not to prop up the deceptive ego by getting the analysand to perceive herself as desiring and encouraging the metonymy of its desire. Instead, the analyst should relate to the analysand in such a way that the analysand recognizes herself as a metaphor, or as a subject. In this, she recognizes herself as, or identifies with, her symptom. A symptom has the structure of a metaphor insofar as a compromise formation, such as obsessive handwashing (S), appears in the place of the subject of the unconscious ($\$$). The analysand, in order to gain some freedom from her symptom (S), must come into being where it was. This is what is meant by subjectifying her alienation; she assumes the position of the alienating signifier or symptom, thereby gaining some separation from it. It is through working in the realm of nonmeaning, on a discourse (like mathematical discourse) that "signifies nothing" (758, 6) that the analyst has effects on the subject as metaphor or as symptom.

Notes

1 At the time of Lacan's presentation of '*Metaphor of the Subject*' there was a large debate in the field of philosophy going on about the differences between analogical and metaphorical thought and which one was superior.

2 When spoken, the phrase '*un océan de fausse science*' sounds like a repetition of '*océan*,' since the 'ausse scien' in '*fausse science*' is pronounced the same way as '*océan*.' This near homonym is presumably an intentional play on words made by Lacan, such that his point that 'science' and 'ocean' have little to do with one another is underscored by a seemingly paradoxical linkage in spoken discourse. It is precisely such similarities, in sound but not in meaning, that can serve as part of the impetus for linking two signifiers in the creation of a metaphor.

3 Interestingly, *enseignement* means teaching, not learning; learning is, strangely enough, somewhat untranslatable into French! In certain contexts, one could use *connaissances* to refer to learning.

4 Lacan, following Heidegger, preferred to translate a word from its original language into French. Heidegger had pointed out that much work on philosophy had been done based on reading Latin translations of Greek texts, and that this had caused

significant distortions of interpretation. To take another pertinent example from this text, Lacan was aware that the Greek term for 'science' differed substantially from our contemporary definition of science. In ancient Greece, science was a much broader term, encompassing, to name a few, such things as logical thinking, mathematics, botany, and astronomy; consequently, in Greek, science was more akin to our contemporary notion of learning than our notion of science.

5 '*Point*,' in French, is an especially strong type of negation. In this metaphor, the subject is thus elided by the object, so that in a certain manner the phallus represents him.

Acknowledgments

I am thankful to Bruce Fink, Maria Cristina Aguirre, Francine Danniau, Charles Merward, and Renata Teixeira for their helpful comments on a draft version of this paper.

References

Berkeley, G. (2010) *Three dialogues between Hylas and Philonous in opposition to sceptics and Atheists*. Farmington Hills, MI: Gale ECCO.

Fink, B. (2004) *Lacan to the letter: Reading Écrits closely*. Minneapolis, MN: University of Minnesota Press.

Freud, S. (1900/1953) The interpretation of dreams, in J. Strachey (Ed.), *The Standard Edition of the Complete Psychological Works of Sigmund Freud*, Vols. 4/5. London: The Hogarth Press and the Institute of Psycho-Analysis.

Freud, S. (1909/1957) Two case histories ('Little Hans' and the 'Rat Man'), in J. Strachey (Ed.), *The Standard Edition of the Complete Psychological Works of Sigmund Freud*, Vol. 10. London: The Hogarth Press and the Institute of Psycho-Analysis.

Lacan, J. (1981/1997) *The seminar of Jacques Lacan. Book III: The Psychoses* (1955–1956), trans. R. Grigg. New York: W. W. Norton & Company.

Lacan, J. (1991/2007) *The seminar of Jacques Lacan. Book XVII: The Other Side of Psychoanalysis* (1969–1970), trans. R. Grigg. New York: W. W. Norton & Company.

Lacan, J. (2008) *My teaching*, trans. D. Macey. London/New York: Verso.

Lacan, J. (2015) The *seminar of Jacques Lacan. Book VIII: Transference (1960–1961)*, trans. B. Fink. Cambridge: Polity Press.

Lacan, J. (forthcoming) *The seminar of Jacques Lacan. Book VI: Desire and its interpretation (1958–1959)*, trans. B. Fink. Cambridge: Polity Press.

Laurent, E. (2014) *Lost in cognition: Psychoanalysis and the cognitive sciences*, trans. A.R. Price. London: Karnac.

Miller, J.-A. (2013) The experience of the real in psychoanalysis. In *The Symptom*, Volume 14, trans. J. Jauregui. Retrieved online from www.lacan.com/symptom14/the-experience.html.

Perelman, C.H. and Olbrechts-Tyteca, L. (1958/1969) *The new rhetoric: A treatise on argumentation*, trans. J. Wilkinson and P. Weaver. Notre Dame, IN: University of Notre Dame Press.

Vanheule, S. (2011) *The subject of psychosis: A Lacanian perspective*. New York: Palgrave Macmillan.

INDEX